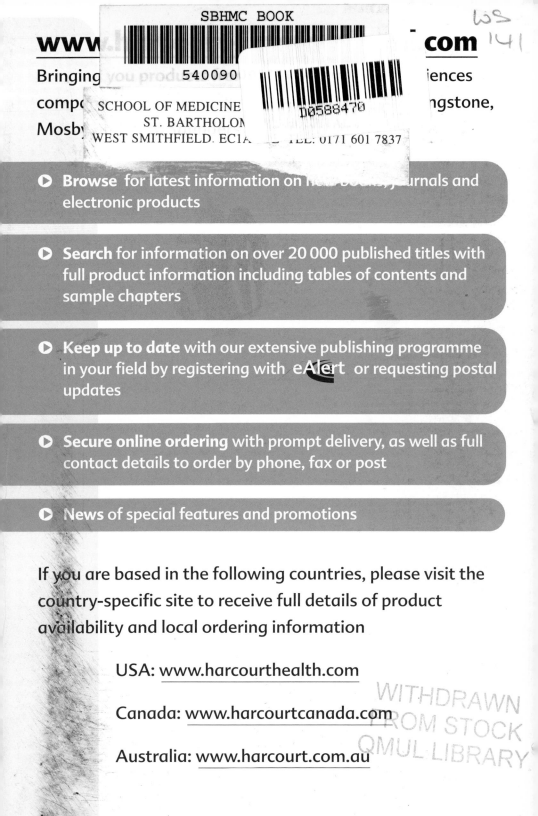

Handbook of
Paediatric
Investigations

Commissioning Editor: Deborah Russell
Project Development Manager: Tim Kimber
Project Manager: Kim Howell
Designer: Jayne Jones
Illustrator: Jenni Miller
Cover picture: Hatice Cinlar-Kaner, aged 10

Handbook of
Paediatric
Investigations

edited by

John Stroobant FRCP FRCPCH

Consultant Paediatrician and Honorary Senior Lecturer
University Hospital of Lewisham
London, UK

David J Field MBBS (Hons) DCH FRCPCH FRCP (Ed) DM

Professor of Neonatal Medicine
University of Leicester
Leicester Royal Infirmary
Leicester, UK

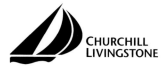

CHURCHILL
LIVINGSTONE

LONDON EDINBURGH NEW YORK PHILADELPHIA ST LOUIS SYDNEY TORONTO 2002

CHURCHILL LIVINGSTONE
An imprint of Harcourt Publishers Limited

© Harcourt Publishers Limited 2002

⬗ is a registered trademark of Harcourt Publishers Limited

The right of John Stroobant and David Field to be identified as editors of this work has been asserted by them in accordance with the Copyright, Designs and Patents Act 1988

First published 2002

ISBN 0 443 05143 7

British Library Cataloguing in Publication Data
A catalogue record for this book is available from the British Library

Library of Congress Cataloging in Publication Data
A catalog record for this book is available from the Library of Congress

Note
Medical knowledge is constantly changing. As new information becomes available, changes in treatment, procedures, equipment and the use of drugs become necessary. The editors/authors/ contributors and the publishers have taken care to ensure that the information given in this text is accurate and up to date. However, readers are strongly advised to confirm that the information, especially with regard to drug usage, complies with the latest legislation and standards of practice.

Existing UK nomenclature is changing to the system of Recommended International Nonproprietary Names (rINNs). Until the UK names are no longer in use, these more familiar names are used in this book in preference to rINNs, details of which may be obtained from the British National Formulary.

The
publisher's
policy is to use
**paper manufactured
from sustainable forests**

Printed in China by RDC Group Limited

Contents

Contributors

Huda Al-Ansari
Fellow in Paediatric Infectious Diseases
Great Ormond Street Hospital for
Children
London, UK

Eliza Alexander MB MRCPCH
Fellow
Department of Immunology and Infectious
Diseases
Royal Alexandra Hospital for Children
Westmead, Australia

Edward J Baker MA MD FRCP
Senior Lecturer and
Honorary Consultant Paediatric
Cardiologist
Department of Paediatric Cardiology
Guy's Hospital
London, UK

Colin S Ball BSc MBBS FRCP FRCPCH
Consultant Paediatrician and Paediatric
Hepatologist
Department of Child Health
King's College Hospital
London, UK

Philippe Bareille MD
Research Fellow
Great Ormond Street Hospital for Children
London, UK

Andrew Bush MBBS MA MD FRCP FRCPCH
Reader in Paediatric Respirology
Imperial College School of Medicine and
Honorary Consultant Paediatric Chest
Physician
Royal Brompton, National Heart and Lung
Hospital
London, UK

Antonia Calogeras MBBS BMedSci MRCP
(UK)
Consultant Rheumatologist
Southampton General Hospital
Southampton, UK

Jane Collins MSc MD FRCP FRCPCH
Director of Clinical Services and
Consultant in Metabolic Medicine
Great Ormond Street Hospital for Children
London, UK

Stefania Costa-Zaccarelli
Fellow in Paediatric Infectious Diseases
Great Ormond Street Hospital for Children
London, UK

Sean Devane MD FRCP (IRL) FRCPCH
Consultant Paediatrician
Department of Child Health
King's College Hospital
London, UK

Vijeya Ganesan
Institute of Child Health
The Wolfson Centre
London, UK

George Haycock MB BChir FRCP DCH
FRCPCH
Ferdinand James de Rothschild Professor of
Paediatrics and
Honorary Consultant
Guy's, King's and St Thomas'
Medical/Dental School
London, UK

David Isaacs MD FRCPCH
Associate Professor
Department of Immunology and Infectious
Diseases
Royal Alexandra Hospital for Children
Sydney, Australia

Gabrielle Kingsley MB CUB FRCP
Reader in Rheumatology and Consultant
Rheumatologist
Lewisham Hospital
Department of Rheumatology
Guy's, King's and St Thomas's School of
Medicine
Kings College London
London, UK

Fenella Kirkham MB BChir MRCP FRCP FRCPCH
Consultant Paediatric Neurologist
Great Ormond Street Hospital for Children
London, UK

Vas Novelli FRCP FRACP
Consultant in Paediatric Infectious
Disease
Great Ormond Street Hospital for Children
London, UK

Jon Skinner MD FRCPCH
Paediatric Cardiologist/Electrophysiologist
Green Lane Hospital
Auckland
New Zealand

Richard Stanhope BSc MD DCH FRCP FRCPCH
Consultant Paediatric Endocrinologist
Great Ormond Street Hospital for Children
London, UK

Richard F Stevens MB ChB FRCP FRCPCH FRCPath
Consultant Paediatric Haematologist
Royal Manchester Children's Hospital
Manchester, UK

Andrea Turner
Fellow
Department of Paediatrics
Guy's Hospital
London, UK

Preface

Performing tests is an integral component of the medical management of children. Investigations in any clinical situation should always be planned carefully, especially in children, who find many tests particularly unpleasant.

A decision to perform investigations should also be based on an understanding of the pathophysiology of the medical problem and the scientific basis of the test. Finally, it is crucial that once a decision has been made to carry out a test, it is done safely, accurately and with minimal distress.

This book, therefore, is designed to provide practical information relating to

- pathophysiology of medical conditions
- details of how to perform tests
- those investigations which should be performed in a wide range of clinical situations.

It is aimed largely at general paediatricians who need guidance on the investigation of both acute and chronic medical conditions and also an understanding of other investigations which might be carried out in tertiary paediatric units.

The authors are all practising clinicians who have particular expertise in the management of complex paediatric disorders.

We are most grateful to the authors for their contributions and to Deborah Russell, Tim Kimber, Maria Khan and many others at Harcourt Publishers Limited for their support and advice.

John Stroobant and David Field

1

Infectious Diseases

V Novelli, S Costa-Zaccarelli and H Al-Ansari

Introduction

Infectious diseases remain the leading cause of death worldwide, being responsible for some 17 million (32%) of the 52 million deaths each year. They account for around 25% of all visits to physicians. Whereas some 20–30 years ago it was thought that we had conquered all the major infectious diseases, the emergence of new infectious diseases and re-emergence of old ones, combined with increasing resistance to antibiotics, pose a significant threat to health. Fortunately most infections occurring in children, certainly in developed countries, are trivial, probably of viral origin, and do not require any investigations. However, in those children with serious or unusual infections who need admission to hospital, it is appropriate to obtain relevant investigations that will help in the diagnosis and management of that particular child, as well as addressing public health aspects. Major advances have occurred over the last few years in our ability to detect the presence of pathogens (e.g. polymerase chain reaction technology for the presence of viral DNA/RNA in clinical specimens). Other techniques to detect poorly-culturable or low-grade bacterial agents may also soon be available to clinicians.

In this chapter we describe:

1. A list of relevant tests
2. Details of tests and their use
3. Specific clinical problems and how to investigate them.

List of tests

BLOOD

Non-specific tests

1. Full blood count, including total white cell count, neutrophil, lymphocyte, monocyte and eosinophil counts, platelet count
2. Acute phase reactants
   a) Erythrocyte sedimentation rate (ESR)
   b) C-reactive protein (CRP)
3. Cytokines

Specific tests

1. Peripheral blood smear
2. Blood culture

3. Serology
   a) Tests to detect specific antibody titres (IgG, IgM, IgA)
   b) Rapid antigen detection tests such as:
      — Latex agglutination
      — Enzyme-linked immunosorbent assay (ELISA)
      — Radioimmunoassay (RIA)
4. Genome detection
   a) Polymerase chain reaction (PCR)
   b) Branched-DNA assay (b-DNA)

URINE

Bacterial infections (routine microscopy, Gram stain, rapid tests, culture)
Viruses (CNV Deaff test)
Fungi and parasites

STOOL

Routine microscopy (parasites, WBC)
Stool culture

Viral culture and electron microscopy
Toxin and antigen detection

CEREBROSPINAL FLUID

WBC, protein, glucose
Gram stain
Culture
Latex agglutination
Polymerase chain reaction

TISSUES

Immunofluorescence (IF)
Enzyme Immunoassay (EIA)
Solid-phase immunoelectron microscopy
Nucleic acid hybridization

IMAGING

Ultrasound
CT scan
MRI
Isotope studies

ABBREVIATIONS USED IN THIS CHAPTER

BAL — bronchoalveolar lavage
b-DNA — branched DNA
CFT — complement fixation test
CRP — C-reactive protein
EIA — enzyme immunoassay
ELISA — enzyme-linked immunosorbent assay
EM — electron microscopy
ESR — erythrocyte sedimentation rate
FNA — fine needle aspirate
FRA test — fluorescent rabies antibody test
FUO — fever of unknown origin

HAART — highly active anti-retroviral therapy
HAI — haemagglutin inhibition
IF — immunofluorescence
IFA — (indirect) immunofluorescent assay
LIP — lymphocytic interstitial pneumonitis
LPA — latex particle agglutination
NAH — nucleic acid hybridisation
NPCR — nested PCR
PCR — polymerase chain reaction
RIA — radioimmunoassay

Description and use of tests

BLOOD

Changes in the host inflammatory response to infection are usually monitored by a series of non-specific tests. Accordingly these should be interpreted in conjunction with the patient's history, physical examination and in the light of other investigations.

Full blood count

Infection usually leads to an increase in the white cell count with a resultant polymorphonuclear leukocytosis and often a 'shift to the left', indicating the presence of immature forms. This is mainly seen in bacterial infections. Neutrophils are mobile, short-lived cells (6–7 hours) that are responsible for phagocytosing pyogenic bacteria. They are present in the circulation and in the marginal pool, which are both supplied by the bone marrow. Bacterial infections result in the release of inflammatory mediators (TNF-alpha, IL-1, IL-8), which lead to margination and attachment of neutrophils to the endothelial lining of small blood vessels. They then migrate into the connective tissue spaces, through the blood vessel walls, via projecting pseudopodia. Occasionally, however, transient neutropenia may be seen in severe bacterial infections, due to increased margination and attachment of neutrophils to endothelial cells in capillary vessels of the pulmonary vasculature. Lymphocytosis is mainly seen in viral infections, with some notable exceptions, which include pertusis. Increased number of monocytes may be seen in tuberculosis, syphilis, brucellosis, protozoal and rickettsial diseases. Eosinophilia is usually suggestive of either tissue invasion by various helminths and worms or intestinal infestations (strongyloides, ascaris and hook worm). Red blood cells have a mean half-life of 120 days, so that it is only during a chronic and rarely during an acute infection (malaria), that there is an ensuing anaemia, the pathogenesis of which is either iron sequestration, haemorrhage or haemolysis. Iron sequestration, which is typical of a slow-onset anaemia, may be caused by some forms of tuberculosis, chronic pulmonary abscesses and parasitic infestations. In these conditions the anaemia is a hypochromic, microcytic picture. Haemorrhage on the other hand will lead to either a normochromic normocytic or hypochromic microcytic anaemia with reticulocytosis. This may occur in acute or chronic amoebiasis, leptospirosis and some intestinal infestations. Haemolysis may be seen in malaria or babesiosis due to intraerythrocytic parasitism; in mycoplasma pneumonia it may be due to the presence of cold agglutinins, whilst in infectious mononucleosis it may be associated with the production of auto-antibodies.

A reduction in the platelet count can occur in acute viral infections such as chicken pox, rubella, viral hepatitis, or infectious mononucleosis as well as in bacterial sepsis or in malaria. Chronic thrombocytopenia is seen in long-standing infections such as visceral leishmaniasis or brucellosis.

Acute phase reactants

a) Erythrocyte sedimentation rate   The ESR is a measure of the suspension stability of red blood cells in blood. It is a simple test to perform, highly sensitive but non-specific. It is elevated in many acute and chronic infections, and is a useful tool for measuring response to treatment. Other conditions in which it tends to be elevated include inflammatory/ collagen vascular disorders, neoplasms, renal diseases and anaemias. The units of measurement are mm/hr, and indeed anything which brings red cells together, such as rouleaux, will increase the ESR. High fibrinogen levels and immunoglobulin levels, as well as sickling, tend to result in a high ESR.

b) C-reactive protein (CRP) C-reactive protein is a molecule synthesised in the liver and released into the circulation within 6 hours of a stimulus, reaching peak levels within 2 days. It is found in both infectious and non-infectious inflammatory processes. It tends to be raised in most systemic microbial infections, especially in Gram-positive and Gram-negative bacteraemias. Levels in viral illnesses tend to be very low, whilst only moderate increases in CRP are seen in chronic infections such as tuberculosis. Deep-seated fungal infections in the immunocompromised host also induce high CRP values. There tends to be a good correlation between increased disease activity and high levels of CRP, whilst a response to treatment is usually followed by a rapid fall in the CRP. A persistently raised CRP suggests either uncontrolled infection or other pathology. Regular monitoring of infectious disease activity via CRP levels tends to be more sensitive than with the use of serial ESR.

c) Cytokines Cytokines are intracellular signalling polypeptides produced by activated monocytes and macrophages. Inflammation-associated cytokines include interleukin-1, interleukin-1b, tumour necrosis factor alpha, interferon gamma, transforming growth factor, and interleukin-8. Interleukin-6 is the chief stimulator of the production of most acute phase proteins. In clinical practice, measurements of cytokines and cytokine receptor levels are not usually carried out due to cost, limited availability and absence of standardisation.

Peripheral blood smear

Thick and thin blood films are the best method to diagnose a variety of parasitaemias, including malaria, filariasis (films need to be obtained at night), trypanosomiasis, and babesiosis. Specimens are obtained from a fresh fingerprick (two or three of each thick and thin film type for malaria diagnosis). One negative result does not rule out a parasitic infestation, and hence it is advisable that repeated samples are obtained for microscopic examination of thick and thin Giemsa-stained smears. In malaria, thick smears are examined to diagnose parasitaemia, whilst thin films are used to identify the type of malaria species.

Blood culture

Obtaining blood cultures (aerobic and anaerobic) is an important investigation in the work-up of a sick child, and forms part of the 'septic screen'. Following laboratory isolation and identification of the cause of the septicaemia or bacteraemia, antibiotic susceptibility testing is usually carried out on the isolate. The correct technique for obtaining blood culture is as follows. Blood has to be taken aseptically, so that the proposed site of the percutaneous needle aspiration should be cleansed first, using 70% isopropyl or ethyl alcohol, and then disinfected with 2%

tincture of iodine or an appropriate iodophor. The iodine should be allowed to dry prior to obtaining the cultures. Following aspiration, the blood should be inoculated into both aerobic and anaerobic bottles immediately. The major difficulty in the interpretation of blood cultures is contamination by skin flora. Careful attention to the technique described above should minimise the problem of contamination. Blood cultures should be taken prior to antibiotic administration; 1–5 ml are usually adequate in children.

Occasionally more than one sample is required:

- in suspected endocarditis, three sets of blood cultures are taken over several hours
- in immunocompromised patients with central lines (e.g. Hickman), often samples are obtained from the central line and peripherally.

It is better to avoid collecting blood cultures from femoral veins because disinfection of the skin over the groin is difficult, and there is no evidence that culturing arterial blood has any advantages over venous collection. Blood cultures from bacteraemic patients become positive within 24 hours in 65% of patients, and in 90% within 3 days. False positive blood cultures may occur, usually as a result of poor technique in collecting the blood. The organisms isolated in these circumstances are usually skin flora and consist of various Diphtheroids, *Bacillus* species or *Staphylococcus epidermidis*. In immunocompromised patients, and in those patients with central lines, these pathogens may be responsible for a true bacteraemia. Although yeasts can be isolated from routine blood cultures, often separate cultures are required. Special blood culture media are also ideally required for isolation of Mycobacteria. Certain laboratory methods (lysis centrifugation) have also been developed to increase the yield of more unusual organisms (fungi and mycobacteria) from blood cultures. Culturing for *Brucella* also requires special media for the blood culture bottle (Castanada bottle), as well as a special safety cabinet. An extended period of incubation (21 days) is required.

Serologic tests

a) Antibody tests Serologic methods are used to diagnose a current or recent infection (usually viruses) by quantifying specific antibodies in serum. They can also be used to assess susceptibility to an infectious agent. For a diagnosis of acute infection, the presence of an IgM response, or a four-fold or higher rise in specific IgG titres between acute and convalescent sera, is required. The most common method used for antibody detection is the ELISA (enzyme linked immunosorbent assay). Other methods used are the Complement fixation test (CFT), Haemagglutination inhibition (HAI), Indirect immunofluorescent assay (IFA). The CFT lacks sensitivity, and is not a very sensitive test for assaying susceptibility to an infectious agent (e.g. *Varicella*).

b) Rapid antigen detection tests

i) Latex particle agglutination assays (LPA)

This rapid method for detection of antigens in blood (and other body fluids) is applicable to bacterial, viral and fungal agents. It is a simple method and requires no special equipment. For the detection of bacterial antigens in blood, urine and CSF, it replaces other methods such as coagglutination and counter-immunoelectrophoresis. The clinical specimen containing antigen is added to a glass slide, which has latex particles with specific antibody bound to them. When antigen is present in the specimen, a visible, grainy, milky precipitate is formed. This test can be used for identification of *Streptococcus pneumoniae*, *Haemophilus influenzae* type b, *Neisseria meningitidis*, Group B streptococcus, and a number of viruses and fungi (e.g. *Cryptococcus neoformans*).

ii) Enzyme linked immunosorbent assay (ELISA)

The ELISA test can also be used as a quantitative test to detect the presence of specific antigen (e.g. Hepatitis B, Rotavirus). The test consists of an antigen capture system with the specific antibody bound to solid phase (wells of poly-styrene). Body fluid (usually serum) containing antigen is added and allowed to bind to antibody. A detector enzyme-labelled molecule is next added, followed by the addition of an appropriate substrate. A coloured reaction occurs when there is antigen present in the specimen. The amount of antigen can be measured by photometric methods, and compared to a standard curve.

ELISA for antigen detection can be used for the diagnosis of the following:

- Cytomegalovirus
- *Herpes simplex*
- Hepatitis B
- HIV
- Respiratory syncytial virus
- Rotavirus
- *Varicella Zoster*
- Chlamydia
- *Clostridium difficile* toxin
- *Giardia lamblia*
- Legionella
- Toxoplasmosis

iii) Radioimmunoassay (RIA)

RIA is a very sensitive assay for antigen quantitation; it is similar to ELISA except that the label used is a radioactive isotope such as radioactive iodine and the bound antibody is measured on a gamma counter. RIA has the advantage that it lends itself well to automation, but the disadvantages of high cost and potential health hazard.

c) Genome detection

i) Polymerase chain reaction (PCR)

PCR is a widely-used technique for amplifying microbial DNA or RNA in clinical specimens. It enables a single copy of any gene sequence to be amplified in vitro at least a million-fold, allowing the detection of small quantities of target DNA. PCR requires an enzyme, DNA polymerase (Taq polymerase), which is a heat-stable enzyme derived from a bacterium, *Thermus aquaticus*, that normally lives in hot springs. The amplified DNA can be detected as a fluorescent band in an electrophoretic gel or using labelled probes in a hybridisation assay. The technique can be used on blood, specifically for diagnosis of HIV, HCV and EBV, as well as other body fluids (CSF, sputum) and tissues (biopsy specimens). Virtually any micro-organism can be detected by the PCR technique if segments of its genome are known, and the relevant primers are constructed.

PCR TECHNIQUE

- The clinical specimen is treated to extract the microbial DNA.
- A mixture that contains oligonucleotide primers, nucleotide precursors, and a heat stable DNA polymerase is added.
- This mixture is heated to denature the microbial nucleic acid into single-stranded DNA, then cooled to allow the oligonucleotide primers to reanneal to the DNA area of interest.
- The mixture is reheated to eliminate non-specific primer binding and to allow the DNA polymerase to add complementary nucleotides.
- The reaction mixture is then heated to release new DNA chain from the original microbial DNA.
- This procedure is repeated in cycles to release millions of copies of the original DNA.
- The microbial DNA is now present in sufficient quantities for detection by hybridisation with oligonucleotide probes.

The PCR can be modified for the detection of viral RNA by incorporating a preliminary step in which reverse transcriptase is used to convert the RNA to DNA. Since PCR is a very sensitive test, slight contamination of the specimen with extraneous DNA may lead to amplification of DNA not in the original sample, and false positive result. It is possible to increase the sensitivity and specificity of the test by using a nested PCR (n PCR) which involves DNA amplification using complementary primers to internally amplified material. The quantitative PCR is a sophisticated technique that allows the detection of precise numbers of copies of DNA or RNA in the sample (copies per ml — in blood sample). This is now used routinely in the assessment and treatment of patients with HIV/AIDS. It is also being used to assess disease burden in immunocompromised patients with CMV and EBV infection, as well as in patients with Hepatitis C.

ii) Branched DNA assay (b-DNA)

b-DNA is a new sandwich hybridisation assay, used for the detection of HIV, HCV, and CMV. In this technique, instead of amplification of target taking place(as occurs in the PCR), there is amplification of the hybridisation signal. The extracted viral RNA is linked to synthetic b-DNA molecules and amplified using an alkaline-phosphatase-linked synthetic probe. After incubation with a chemiluminescent substrate (dioxetane), light emission is measured and is proportional to the concentration of the target nucleic acid in the specimen. It is a very rapid and highly sensitive test, with a good linear relationship between levels of amplified product and target.

URINE

Bacterial infections

Urine analysis, microscopy and culture are the mainstays in the diagnosis of a urinary tract infection. Rapid screening methods to diagnose urinary tract infection (UTI) are available — see also chapter 5 — and depend on the presence of bacteria or leukocytes or both in the urine.

These simple tests can be used in the doctor's office:

- Gram stain of uncentrifuged urine sample examined under oil immersion
- Biochemical screening dipstick methods which detect the presence of either bacteria (nitrite test) or white cells (leukocyte esterase test). These are not recommended in children under 2 years of age.

Children less than 2 years of age should have a urine culture performed. Urine can be collected by either midstream clean catch, catheterisation or suprapubic puncture. Specimens should be despatched to the laboratory within an hour, otherwise they should be refrigerated at 4°C. Cultures are usually available within 48 hours, and most children with UTI have bacterial counts of > 100,000 cfu/ml of a pure culture of bacteria. Cultures obtained by suprapubic aspiration and catheterisation will be significant if bacterial growths are more than 1000 cfu/ml and 10,000 cfu/ml, respectively, with several logs less bacterial growth. The only useful information gleaned from a 'bag' specimen is if it is negative, which would rule out the presence of a UTI. The presence of a pyuria (WBC) also supports the diagnosis of a UTI: >10 WBC/hpf on examination of uncentrifuged urinary sediment is suggestive of a UTI, but its absence does not rule out the diagnosis. Organisms most frequently causing UTI are usually spread via the ascending route:

E. coli, *Proteus* spp, *Klebsiella*, *Enterobacter*, *Citrobacter*, *Providencia*, *Pseudomonas* spp, *Staphylococcus aureus*, *S. saprophyticus*, *S. epidermidis*, *Streptococcus faecalis*, *S. agalactiae*.

Other bacterial infections that can be diagnosed via the urine include *Legionella pneumophila*, which can be diagnosed by a rapid urinary antigen screen using RIA. An early-morning urine examination for acid-fast staining (Auramine–Rhodamine stain, Fluorochrome stain) will be positive in 80% of cases of renal tuberculosis. *Mycoplasma urealyticum* can also be cultured from the urine.

Viruses

Cytomegalovirus can be cultured from the urine as well as identified via rapid antigen and shell vial culture methods (DEAFF test). Other viruses that can also be cultured from the urine include Adenovirus, Enteroviruses, Mumps and Rubella.

Fungi and parasites

Candida albicans, other Candida spp as well as *Aspergillus* and *Cryptococcus*, can be cultured from urine. They are usually grown from immunosuppressed individuals or those with obstruction to the urinary tract. Freshly voided urine specimens may also be examined for ova of *Schistosoma haematobium* (Bilharzia) in patients with haematuria and exposure to the parasite.

STOOLS

Stools should be collected, free of urine, in a plastic container and sent to the laboratory immediately. If this is not possible then the specimen should be refrigerated.

Routine microscopy

i) Faecal stains

The detection of faecal leucocytes in a stool smear (Gram stain) is suggestive of a bacterial pathogen (e.g. *Shigella, Campylobacter*) as a cause of the diarrhoea. A modified acid-fast stain (Kinyoun) is used for examination of cysts of *Cryptosporidium* (a monoclonal fluorescein-conjugated stain, and ELISA is also available) and *Isospora belli*.

ii) Ova and parasites detection

Examination of a fresh stool specimen. Wet mounts, concentration techniques and H+E stains will detect ova and parasites such as amoebae (e.g. *E. histolytica*), coccidia (e.g. *Balantidium coli*), and the flagellates (e.g. *G. lamblia*). If threadworms are suspected, then a scotch tape preparation (from the perianal area) is submitted to the laboratory for identification of *Enterobius vermicularis*. Characteristic eggs of *Schistosomiasis mansoni* can also be identified in concentrated stool specimens.

Stool culture

Apart from routine stool cultures which will detect enteric pathogens including *Salmonella, Shigella*, and *Campylobacter*, some laboratories are equipped to characterise the different diarrhoeagenic *E. coli* into their various categories, i.e. enterotoxigenic, enteropathogenic, enterohaemorrhagic and enteroinvasive. This is done through sub-culture techniques, serotyping and *Shiga* toxin detection.

Viral culture

Stool or rectal swabs can be cultured for a number of viruses such as Adenoviruses, Enteroviruses, and Polioviruses. Specimens are inoculated into cell cultures and are then observed for typical cytopathic effects. The virus is then identified through the use of monoclonal antibody fluorescence.

Electron microscopy (EM)

Many enteric viruses can also be detected in the stools through the use of Electron Microscopy. Characteristic viral particles can be directly visualised in the stools of children with diarrhoeal symptoms: Rotavirus, Astrovirus, Calicivirus, Norwalk virus, Adenovirus. This technique is not as sensitive as viral culture, as more than 10 to 6 virions/ml are required for detection via EM. The specimens are first clarified by low-speed centrifugation, then the supernatant is subjected to ultracentrifugation to deposit the virion. The specimen is then negatively stained with phosphotungstate or uranyl acetate and scanned by EM. The sensitivity of the technique can be greatly enhanced by the addition of antibody to the clinical specimen (immunoelectron microscopy). EM can also routinely be performed on vesicle fluid for detection of Herpesviruses, on urine for detection of Adenovirus and Papova, and on blood for detection of Parvovirus.

Toxin and antigen detection

Detection of *Shiga* toxin in the stools via enzyme immunoassay indicates the presence of enterohaemorrhagic *E. coli*, often the 0157:H7 serotype, responsible for haemolytic uraemic syndrome. In antibiotic-associated colitis, *C. difficile* toxin can be demonstrated in the stools via a latex agglutination test. The diagnosis is questionable if *C. difficile* is present in stools, without toxin production. Rotavirus, the most common infective cause of infantile diarrhoea, is detected in stool specimens via rapid antigen rest (enzyme immunoassay). It is also identified via electron microscopy.

CEREBROSPINAL FLUID

Examination and culture of CSF is essential for the management of children with signs and symptoms of CNS infections. CSF specimens should be collected aseptically and transported promptly to the laboratory. At least 2 ml of CSF need to be obtained for protein and glucose analysis (a plasma glucose should be obtained simultaneously) and cell count, as well as for microbiological studies. For virological studies, CSF specimens need to be frozen ($-25°C$ to $-70°C$).

Cerebrospinal fluid analysis/microscopy

In general, CSF appears turbid in bacterial meningitis (>500 cells/mm^3), clear in viral meningitis and clear or viscous (with fibrin strands) in TB meningitis. Xanthochromia (yellowish colour of CSF) is due to either the presence of bilirubin or haemolysed red cells following recent bleeding.

i) Cells

The number of white cells in a normal CSF is usually <5 cells/mm^3 (all lymphocytes); in neonates up to 30 cells/mm^3 are considered normal. Any number of neutrophils in the CSF is abnormal. The predominant cell in bacterial meningitis is the neutrophil ($>50\%$ of total); usually 500–1000 cells/mm^3. TB and fungal meningitis have a predominance of lymphocytes. In viral meningitis, there may be an initial neutrophil preponderance, which is followed by a lymphocyte preponderance.

ii) Proteins

Protein levels above 50 mg/dl, outside the neonatal period, are indicative of increased permeability of the blood–brain barrier, suggestive of an infection. CSF protein levels are increased in bacterial meningitis, marginally elevated in viral meningitis and extremely high in TB meningitis.

iii) Glucose

Normal ranges are 50–80 mg/dl. In patients with bacterial meningitis and TBM, levels tend to be less than 40 mg/dl; CSF/blood glucose ratios are $<50\%$. Some patients with viral meningitis caused by the following may have low CSF glucose levels: HSV, VZV, enteroviruses.

iv) Bacteria/fungi

A Gram stain is used to detect bacteria in a spun deposit of CSF. Each of the major pathogens causing meningitis has differing characteristics. An acid-fast stain (Ziehl–Neelsen) of the CSF is carried out to detect any Mycobacteria. These organisms are resistant to destaining by acid-alcohol. Culture is more sensitive than smears for diagnosis of TB; positive smears have been reported in 60%–70% of culture-proven TBM. An India ink preparation is used to detect the presence of *Cryptococcus* spp in CSF. Unfortunately this test is not very sensitive (30–50%); latex antigen testing and culture are much more sensitive.

Culture

i) Bacterial/fungal culture

The gold standard for a diagnosis of bacterial meningitis is isolation of bacteria from the CSF. Success in the isolation of fungi (Cryptococcus) and mycobacteria is dependent on the amount of CSF submitted for culture. At least 10 ml should be obtained. Mycobacterial culture may take up to 6 weeks to be reported as negative.

ii) Viral culture

Specimens are inoculated into tissue culture, incubated and examined periodically for the appearance of typical cytopathic changes. Identification of the isolate is then carried out with the use of monoclonal antibodies or haemadsorption techniques. The most likely causes of viral meningitis include the Enteroviruses (Coxsackieviruses, Echoviruses), Adenoviruses and occasionally the group of Herpesviruses (HSV, VZV, CMV). Additional specimens that may be helpful in making a diagnosis include viral cultures of throat, stool, urine and fluid from vesicles (if present).

Antigen detection

i) Bacteria

The CSF latex agglutination test for bacterial antigens is not meant to supplant the 'gold standard' of Gram stain and CSF bacterial culture. The test detects the presence of bacterial antigens in the CSF, for the rapid diagnosis of meningitis. Available assays can detect antigens of *Haemophilus influenzae* type b, *Streptococcus pneumoniae*, *Neisseria meningitidis*, Group B Streptococcus, and *E. coli* K1. The latter two assays are particularly relevant for the neonatal population. Sensitivity of the tests varies from 60% to100% (Hib test most sensitive). Cross reactions occur between *E. coli* K1 and *Neisseria meningitidis*, group B. The latex agglutination test is particularly useful in those situations where patients have already received some antibiotics prior to admission (partially-treated meningitis) and the CSF culture is negative. Other body fluids (blood, urine) can also be tested for the presence of bacterial antigens.

ii) Cryptococcal latex agglutination

This test is positive in cases of Cryptococcal meningitis, which is caused by *Cryptococcus neoformans*, an encapsulated yeast, and is usually seen in immunosuppressed patients (e.g. AIDS). The assay has a sensitivity of around 90%, and is suitable for detection of antigen in both CSF and serum.

Polymerase chain reaction

This technique detects the presence of nucleic acid of a microorganism present in CSF. The DNA, which is amplified via the use of specially-constructed primers and a heat-stable enzyme (Taq polymerase), is detected using radiolabelled probes in a hybridisation assay. The list of infectious neurotropic agents which can be diagnosed via PCR technology continues to grow and includes the following:

- *Neisseria meningitidis*
- Borrelia (Lyme disease)
- *Mycobacterium tuberculosis*
- Toxoplasma
- Viruses — HSV, CMV, EBV, VZV, HIV, enteroviruses

TISSUE

Gross and histological examination of various tissue specimens and biopsies may lead to a diagnosis of a specific infection (e.g. caseating granulomas and Mycobacterial infection); however, the assays and techniques described below have been found to be very useful for the direct detection of particular micro-organisms or specific antigens in tissue specimens. The relevant specimens are as follows:

- Nasopharyngeal aspirates
- Gastric aspirates
- Bronchoalveolar lavage
- Fine needle aspirate (FNA)
- Bone marrow aspiration
- Tissue biopsy (lymph node, liver, brain).

Methenamine silver stain

This test is used for the rapid diagnosis of *Pneumocystis carinii* pneumonia. Organisms present in a smear (touch preparations) or histologic sections of lung, or in BAL fluid, are stained with a silver precipitate. Pneumocystis organisms stain black and appear as rounded objects of about 5–8 µm diameter. Other methods used for identification of *Pneumocystis carinii* include Toluidine Blue stain, Giemsa stain, and monoclonal antibodies to *Pneumocystis carinii*.

Immunofluorescence (IF)

If is used for the early identification of viral antigens (or protozoal antigens) in infected cells and tissues. Infected cells for examination (e.g. nasopharyngeal aspi-rate) can be obtained simply by swabbing or scraping the infected mucous membranes at different sites:

- Upper respiratory tract
- Genital tract
- Conjunctivae

- Skin
- Mucus aspirated from nasopharynx.

IF is used for the rapid identification of the following:

- RSV
- Parainfluenzae
- Mumps
- Measles
- Paramyxoviruses
- Influenzae
- Herpesviruses
- *Legionella pneumophila*
- *Pneumocystis carinii.*

Brain biopsy specimens from patients with encephalitis can also be tested via direct immunofluorescence for the presence of *Herpes simplex* virus. Brain specimens of potentially rabid animals who may have bitten humans can be tested for the presence of rabies virus via the Fluorescent Rabies Antibody Test (FRA Test). In humans a rabies diagnosis can be confirmed by FRA staining of skin biopsy tissue taken from the back of the neck.

There are two main variants of the IF technique: direct and indirect methods, as described in the information box.

DIRECT IF

1. A frozen tissue section or an acetone fixed cell smear is exposed to antibody labelled with fluorochrome (fluorescein-tagged antiviral antibody).
2. Unbound antibody is washed away.
3. The cells are inspected by light microscopy using a powerful ultraviolet/blue light source; the antigen–antibody complex is revealed as an apple-green coloured light against a black background.

INDIRECT IF

The indirect IF differs in that the antiviral antibody is untagged. The antibody binds to the antigen in the tissue and is recognised by the addition of a fluorescein-conjugated anti-immunoglobulin.

Enzyme-immunoassay (EIA)

This technique detects relevant antigens in various tissues. It can be performed instead of the IFA for a number of microorganisms. It is particularly useful for a number of viruses, bacteria and fungi including Adenovirus, RSV, Group A Streptococcus (throat), Histoplasma. The technique involves:

- The addition of specimen (e.g. naso-pharyngeal aspirate, BAL fluid, throat washing) to a solid phase which has capture antibody attached to it.
- Unattached antigen is washed out.

- An enzyme-labelled indicator antibody is added.
- An appropriate substrate is added which gives a colour signal if antigen is present.

Solid-phase immunoelectron microscopy

This is a technique that is being developed in which virus-specific antibody is fixed to the plastic supporting film on the copper grid of the electron microscope. This enables the technique of immunoelectron microscopy to be used to examine specimens and tissues, other than faeces, urine, serum and vesicle fluid, for the presence of microorganisms.

Nucleic acid hybridisation

Nucleic acid hybridisation tests are based on the ability of complementary nucleic acid strands to align specifically and associate to form stable double-stranded complexes. The clinical specimen is tested for the presence of nucleic acid of the pathogen by specific microbial RNA or DNA radiolabelled probes. The probes hybridise to specific complementary sequences on the sample nucleic acid bound to the filter. Hybridisation is detected by autoradiography, or colour development on the membrane. Probes may also be used to hybridise nucleic acids within cells or histologic sections. DNA probes are available for the detection of a number of viruses and bacteria including HSV, EBV, CMV, human papillomavirus, *Legionella* species, *Mycoplasma pneumoniae*, *Neisseria gonorrhoeae*, *Mycobacterium tuberculosis* and MAI. A major disadvantage of this method is the short half-life of radio-labelled probes, difficulties in handling and disposing of radioactive substances, and the requirement for a scintillation counter or darkroom facility. New probes, incorporating biotinylated nucleotides into DNA, or biotin labelling of RNA, have been developed for easy use and rapid diagnosis.

DIAGNOSTIC IMAGING

In the assessment of a child with a probable serious infection, a thorough history and physical examination is usually followed by requests for a number of laboratory investigations. Additional investigations, often requested, are for diagnostic imaging. There have been great strides in this field over the last 20 years. The introduction of CT and MRI scanning, as well as the numerous isotopic studies available today, have created a revolution in our ability to detect occult disease or visualise diseased tissues or organs.

Ultrasound (abdomen)

One of the commonest requests for imaging in the field of paediatric infectious diseases is for an ultrasound of the abdomen. Organs such as the liver, spleen and kidneys are imaged via the use of sound waves. The test is particularly useful for detecting the presence of intra-abdominal lymphadenopathy (suggestive of either TB or a lymphoma), abnormalities of the liver and spleen (hepatosplenomegaly, miliary disease, candidiasis), fluid collections, abscess or malignancy. The use of a doppler to assess flow in vessels, e.g. portal vein, may also be helpful. Imaging of the kidneys is carried out to exclude the presence of scarred, shrunken kidneys, hydronephrosis and hydroureter in patients with a history of urinary tract infections.

CT scan/MRI scan

i) Neuroimaging

CT and MRI are the investigations of choice for neuroimaging, and are particularly useful in assessing patients with CNS infections. Both modalities are able to show up fluid collections, brain oedema, abscess formation with ring enhancement, and diffuse meningeal enhancement suggestive of meningitis. The administration of intravenous contrast, during the CT scan, is an essential part of the investigation of CNS infections. This is also applicable to Gadolinium administration during an MRI scan. MRI scanning is especially helpful in the early detection of diffuse viral encephalitis. Intracranial calcification suggestive of intrauterine infections is readily detectable by CT. MRI scanning has become the imaging modality of choice for the spinal cord; patients with myelitis/myelopathy are readily diagnosed.

ii) Respiratory tract imaging

The plain chest X-ray is obviously the most widely used diagnostic imaging technique for assessment of the respiratory tract. A CT of the chest is often used to determine the presence or absence of bronchiectasis, especially in immunocompromised patients. It is also helpful in the management of patients with empyema.

Indium-labelled white cell scan

This technique is used for determining the site of an occult infection or in confirming the presence of an infection at a suspected site. Blood is initially drawn from the patient; the white cells are separated and then labelled with ^{111}I. These are then injected into the patient and images are obtained over the next 24 hours. Focal accumulations of leucocytes will occur at inflamed sites, as well as in the tissues of the reticuloendothelial system. If there is extensive uptake in the colon, a diagnosis of ulcerative colitis is likely. This test has replaced the Gallium-67 scan. The presence of a leucocytosis is necessary for the test to be done.

Bone scan

A bone scan is obtained to confirm a diagnosis of acute or chronic osteomyelitis. The patient receives an intravenous injection of a ^{99m}-Tc-labelled compound. This localises in bone, in proportion to the degree of bone turnover. Early blood pool images may be taken, followed by definitive bony images after 3–4 hours. Bone scan abnormalities seen in osteomyelitis (increased uptake) are obvious long before changes are seen on the plain X-rays of the bone.

Gallium scan

This consists of an intravenous injection of Gallium-67 citrate, with images taken over the next 2–3 days. Gallium localises to sites of inflammation, infection and neoplasm as well as to sites in RES. It is a non-specific test but is often carried out in the investigation of the child with a fever of unknown origin (FUO). It can be performed, in lieu of a white cell scan, when the neutrophil count is not raised. After a Gallium scan, other isotope studies need to be postponed for at least 7 days.

Clinical problems and how to investigate them

- Kawasaki disease
- Encephalitis
- Fever of unknown origin
- Fever in the returning traveller
- Child with recurrent infections
- HIV/AIDS.

KAWASAKI DISEASE

Kawasaki disease is an acute febrile illness of unknown aetiology affecting predominantly infants and young children. Its clinical manifestations are of a vasculitis affecting medium-sized vessels but with a predilection for the coronary arteries. It is the leading cause of acquired heart disease in children from the developed countries. The disease is most prevalent in Japan where epidemics occur every 3 years. In the UK around 100–200 cases are reported on a yearly basis. The clinical diagnosis is based on the presence of 5 of 6 principal criteria (Table 1.1), one of which should include fever, without other explanation for the illness. Cardiac involvement, with coronary arteritis and aneurysm formation, may occur with fatal consequences.

Laboratory investigations

There is no diagnostic test for Kawasaki Disease; laboratory tests are non-specific, but indicative of an acute inflammatory response. There is usually a normocytic, normochromic anaemia, leucocytosis, thrombocytosis (usually in the second week), raised ESR and CRP, and hypoalbuminaemia. The main differential diagnosis consists of infection with Group A beta-haemolytic Streptococcus (Scarlet fever), Staphylococcal scalded skin syndrome, toxic shock syndrome, other viral

Table 1.1   **Diagnostic criteria for Kawasaki disease**
Fever (lasting for more than 5 days)
Conjunctivitis (without exudate)
Cervical lymphadenopathy (unilateral, > 1.5 cm)
Mucositis (red cracked lips, strawberry tongue)
Swelling of hands and feet (desquamation follows)
Polymorphous rash

infections, rickettsial disease, leptospirosis, Still's disease and drug reaction (e.g. Steven–Johnson syndrome). Further tests that may be obtained include the following: ASOT + throat swab (most relevant), nasal swab, viral titres, ANA and rheumatoid factor. An echocardiogram is obtained at baseline, and then repeated in 1–2 weeks, 4 weeks and at 6–8 weeks. An ECG, chest X-ray and cardiac enzymes are also obtained at baseline and repeated if necessary.

Monitoring

The disease is thought to be due to a circulating toxin (? staphylococcal, ? streptococcal) which acts as a superantigen, causing generalised immune activation and cytokine release. This results in the initiation of generalised inflammatory changes and vasculitis. Although treatment with immunoglobulin and aspirin may produce an improvement in the clinical status, the ESR tends to remain elevated for some time, often up to 4–6 weeks. If the echocardiogram is normal at 4 weeks, it is very unlikely that any cardiac abnormalities will develop after this. Atypical cases of Kawasaki disease can occur, with fewer than the required number of diagnostic features.

ENCEPHALITIS

Acute encephalitis is an inflammation of the brain induced directly or indirectly by microbial agents. Clinical symptoms and signs in children include headache, fever, photophobia, vomiting, focal seizures, alterations in conscious level and personality changes. Other manifestations which may also occur include hemiplegia, ataxia, cranial nerve palsies, and bowel and bladder dysfunction. The incidence in developed countries is around 1 per 10,000 children. Although most cases of encephalitis are caused by direct invasion of a microorganism (usually viruses) into the CNS, a proportion are the result of an inflammatory reaction, leading to areas of demyelination (post-infectious encephalomyelitis). Table 1.2 shows the most common causes of encephalitis. In developed countries, an aetiology for the encephalitis is not identified in up to 60% of cases.

Table 1.2 **Common infective causes of acute encephalitis**	
Viruses	HSV, CMV, EBV, VZV, enteroviruses, mumps, measles, rubella, HIV, arboviruses, rabies
Bacteria/parasites	*Mycoplasma pneumoniae*, Borrelia (Lyme disease), *Toxoplasma gondii*, leptospirosis, brucella, typhus, trypanosomiasis, Rocky Mountain spotted fever, TB
Post-infectious causes	Measles, mumps, rubella, influenza, VZV, enteroviruses

Laboratory investigations

- MRI scan or CT scan of head (with contrast)
- EEG
- Chest X-ray
- Throat swab + stool for viral culture
- Serum — acute and convalescent samples for
  - ▲ Neurotropic viruses: HSV, CMV, EBV, VZV, influenza, measles, mumps, rubella, enteroviruses, arboviruses (if appropriate)
  - ▲ Lyme disease
  - ▲ *Mycoplasma pneumoniae*
- CSF — (if not contraindicated) — cell counts, bacterial culture, TB culture, viral culture, PCR (HSV, CMV, EBV, toxoplasma, enteroviruses).

FEVER OF UNKNOWN ORIGIN

Fever of unknown origin (FUO) is a fever of more than 38.5°C, present for more than 2 weeks in a child in whom a thorough history, physical examination and preliminary laboratory tests have failed to reveal an aetiology. A number of studies have shown that an infective aetiology is responsible for around 40% of these cases, a collagen-vascular disorder 16%, a neoplastic disorder 9%, miscellaneous causes 15%, and undiagnosed 20%. Although in younger children (<6 years) infection tends to be the most common cause of an FUO, in the older age group (6–14 years) collagen–vascular and inflammatory bowel disease are more common. A good history is essential in the initial evaluation of the patient. Particular emphasis should be given to questions about any foreign travel, contact with animals (including pets), and family history of TB or fevers. A history of swimming in a river or lake, or a visit to an area of Lyme disease, is obviously relevant information in assessing the possibility of acute leptospirosis or Lyme disease being the cause of the FUO. During the physical examination, it is important to look for evidence of hepatosplenomegaly, generalised or localised lymphadenopathy, and signs of cutaneous disease or joint swellings.

Laboratory investigations

Investigations are chosen initially to evaluate those systems that are found to be abnormal. In general, one should proceed with a multiple-tiered approach to the investigations required, with latter tiers involving the more invasive procedures (e.g. bone marrow). Some very basic information can be obtained immediately to distinguish between the presence of an infection and an inflammatory disorder: a very high ESR with a normal or low CRP is very suggestive of an inflammatory disorder.

First tier

FBC + film, ESR, CRP
Blood cultures, urine microscopy and culture, throat swab, stool microscopy and culture
Liver function tests
Mononucleosis screen (EBV, CMV, toxoplasmosis)

Viral serology (including HIV, enteroviruses, HHV-6, parvovirus B19)
Other serology (brucella, rickettsiae, borrelia, and mycoplasma)
Auto-immune screen (including DNA antibodies, ANCA)
Chest X-ray
Mantoux test (1:1000)
Ultrasound of the abdomen (? lymphadenopathy)
Urine for VMAs.

Second tier

Echocardiography
Bone or gallium scan
White-cell labelled scan
CT/MRI scans.

Third tier

Colonoscopy/endoscopy
Biopsies (e.g. lymph node)
Bone marrow examination/trephine
Visceral angiography (for vasculitis).

Additional investigations

a) It may be appropriate to consider a number of basic immunology tests as a part of the first tier investigations, in certain patients. These would include the following: immunoglobulins, immunoglobulin G subclasses, IgE, NBT, vaccine responses, T-cell subsets.
b) There are also a number of conditions which fall into the miscellaneous category that need to be considered and screened for, for example:
   Cyclic neutropenia (twice weekly FBC for 6 weeks)
   Familial Mediterranean fever (genetic screening test)
   Hyper IgE syndrome (IgE levels).

FEVER IN THE RETURNING TRAVELLER

There has been a very large increase in international travel and thus in the prevalence of travel-related diseases seen in the UK. Generally, the risk of developing a travel-related illness increases the further south and east the destination. It is estimated that travel-related infections cause up to 50 deaths per year in the UK. Fevers of acute onset may be the most difficult to diagnose as these may be due to many conditions ranging from self-limiting viral infections to more serious, life-threatening conditions that have not yet manifested themselves. Fevers that have been present for more than a few days will be associated with other symptoms, that may be helpful in identifying a focus. Conditions such as TB, salmonellosis, rickettsial infections and hepatitis may be associated with a fever of unknown origin (FUO), i.e. fever without localising signs present for longer than 2 weeks. The pattern of fever is often not very helpful, although a fever of a relapsing or intermittent nature is present in the conditions shown in Table 1.3.

Table 1.3   Relapsing/intermittent fever: possible conditions
Malaria
Visceral Leishmaniasis
Trypanosomiasis
Relapsing fever
Brucellosis
Filariasis
Acute bacterial endocarditis
Pyogenic infections
Typhoid

A biphasic fever is very suggestive of dengue fever. The presence of associated symptoms such as a rash may be due to the viral haemorrhagic fevers, rickettsial or meningococcal disease. Protracted diarrhoea is suggestive of a parasitic infection (amoebic dysentery, giardiasis), whilst bloody diarrhoea is also suggestive of either amoebic or bacillary dysentery. Contact with water may cause schistosomiasis (especially holidays in Lake Malawi), or leptospirosis. Arthropod-borne infections may occur following visits to game parks. Disease transmitted by the various vectors are shown in Table 1.4.

In the examination, a relative bradycardia in response to fever is noted in typhoid. Generalised lymphadenopathy is not a usual finding in malaria and an

Table 1.4 Arthropod-borne diseases	
Vector	**Disease transmitted**
Ticks (hard)	Spotted fever, Q fever, Lyme disease, viral encephalitis
Tick (soft)	Relapsing fever
Mites	Scrub typhus
Lice	Epidemic typhus, relapsing fever
Mosquito	Malaria, filariasis, arboviruses
Fleas	Plague
Sandfly	Visceral leishmaniasis

Table 1.5 Splenomegaly	
Bacterial	Septicaemia, typhoid, SBE
Viral	EBV, CMV, toxoplasmosis
Protozoa	Malaria, visceral Leishmaniasis
Other	Schistosomiasis

alternative explanation should be sought (concurrent EBV, CMV, HIV, typhoid or TB). Splenomegaly may occur in a number of infections, as listed in Table 1.5.

Laboratory investigations

If diagnosis is not clear after a thorough history and physical examination, the following **first-line investigations** should be obtained:

FBC, differential, ESR
CRP
Thick and thin blood smear (repeated)
Urine microscopy and culture
CXR
Blood cultures (repeated)
Stool for ova, cysts and parasites + culture
Echocardiogram

Table 1.6   Causes of peripheral eosinophilia

- **Parasitic infections**
  Ascariasis
  Strongyloides
  Toxocariasis
  Trichinellosis
  Schistosomiasis
  Filariasis
  Cutaneous larva migrans

- **Allergy**
- **Polyarteritis nodosa**
- **Malignancy (Hodgkin's disease)**

Table 1.7   Second-line investigations of fever in the returning traveller

Investigation	Diagnostic possibilities
Bone marrow + culture	TB, typhoid, visceral Leishmaniasis
Lymph node biopsy	TB, atypical TB, cat-scratch disease
Liver biopsy	Brucella, TB, visceral Leishmaniasis, chronic viral hepatitis
Imaging (CT, MRI)	Thoracic/abdominal lymphadenopathy, Deep seated infections (abdo, head)
Bone scan	Osteomyelitis
White cell scan	Deep-seated pyogenic infections

Ultrasound (abdomen)
Mantoux test
Lumbar puncture (if indicated) + rapid antigen screen.

Table 1.8 **Investigations for specific diseases**

Disease	Investigation
Amoebiasis	Stool for trophozoites/cysts (intestinal)
	Serology/ultrasound or CT scan (extra-intestinal)
Arbovirus (dengue, yellow fever)	Serology/viral isolation
Borreliosis	Thick/thin blood smear, blood culture
Brucellosis	Serology, blood/bone marrow/tissue culture
Cholera	Stool culture
Diphtheria	Nose/throat swab
Filariasis	Blood smear for microfilaria (night)
	Serology
Hepatitis	Antigen/antibody test, PCR
HIV	Antibody test, Western blot, PCR
Infectious mononucleosis	EBV-specific antibody tests, monospot
Leishmaniasis	Splenic/bone marrow aspirate/liver biopsy
	Skin biopsy
Lyme disease	Serology/Western blot
Malaria	Thick and thin blood smears
Meningococcal disease	Blood/CSF microscopy + culture
	Antigen test (blood/CSF), PCR
Rickettsial diseases (Q fever, typhus, RMSF)	Serology
Salmonella (typhoid)	Stool, blood, urine + bone marrow culture
Schistosomiasis	Urine/stool for ova, rectal/bladder biopsy
	Serology
Shigellosis	Stool culture
Trypanosomiasis	Blood/CSF/lymph node microscopy
Tuberculosis	Sputum/gastric aspirates/urine/CSF
	Microscopy/culture, PCR
	Mantoux skin test (5 TU or 10 TU)

A peripheral eosinophilia is often found in numerous parasitic infections but other conditions can also lead to this picture, as listed in Table 1.6.

In cases where first-line investigations have not revealed an aetiology for the fever and the patient remains febrile and unwell, **second-line investigations** should be considered, as in Table 1.7.

Table 1.8 gives a list of **investigations for specific diseases**, if these are suspected from the location of travel or the presence of clinical findings.

The major infections prevalent in those areas more commonly visited by UK residents are set out in Table 1.9.

THE CHILD WITH RECURRENT INFECTIONS

Children are often referred to paediatricians with a history of recurrent infections. It is important to determine if the number of severity of infections is

Table 1.9 **Major infections prevalent in areas commonly visited from the UK**	
Country	**Major infections**
Europe (including Cyprus + former Soviet Union)	Dysentery, typhoid, hepatitis A, tick typhus, Lyme, Leishmaniasis*, tick-borne encephalitis, polio, diphtheria, brucella
North Africa/Middle East	Diarrhoeal diseases, dysentery, hepatitis A, intestinal parasites, typhoid, malaria (v, f), TB, Leishmaniasis*, tick typhus, relapsing Fever, brucella, schistosomiasis
Sub-Saharan Africa	Diarrhoeal diseases, dysentery, typhoid, hepatitis A, amoebiasis, cholera, malaria (f), Leishmaniasis*, yellow fever, typhus, TB, HIV, trypanosomiasis, meningococcaemia, schistosomiasis
South Asia (Indian subcontinent + Nepal, Sri Lanka)	Diarrhoeal diseases, dysentery, typhoid, intestinal parasites, hepatitis A, cholera, malaria (v, f), filariasis, Leishmaniasis*, TB, dengue, Japanese encephalitis
South-east Asia/Far East	Diarrhoeal diseases, cholera, dysentery, typhoid, amoebiasis, intestinal parasites, malaria (f), filariasis, Japanese encephalitis, dengue, Leishmaniasis*, TB, schistosomiasis
North America	Viral encephalitis, Lyme, Rocky Mountain spotted fever
*Visceral Leishmaniasis; (f) *Falciparum*; (v) *vivax*	

greater than expected. In young infants and children, up to 7–8 infections per year (mainly upper respiratory tract) are considered normal. Older children often experience 4–5 minor infections per year. The child with an unusual frequency, character, or severity of infection should be suspected of having an underlying problem. A complete history and physical examination will be required to ascertain whether there is any abnormality of host defence. A localised anatomical, physiological or immunological defect may be present. The majority of children with recurrent infections do not have an immune defect.

Normal host defences

The immune system can be divided into specific and non-specific components. Non-specific immunity refers to the first line of defence against pathogens, such as skin, mucus, tears and acidity of gastric fluid. If these anatomic barriers are breached, then specific immune responses are activated. Second-line non-specific components include serum complement, neutrophils and cytokines. Specific immunity is divided into humoral and cellular arms. Cellular immunity is mediated by the cells of the immune system, while humoral immunity refers to the production of antibody specific for a particular invading pathogen. This adaptive immune response leads to recruitment of inflammatory cells at sites of infection, as well as the development of immunological memory.

Clinical assessment

1. Determine whether the number and type of infections are significant (see Table 1.10), for example the identification of *Pneumocystis carinii* in a broncho-alveolar lavage specimen in a child with interstitial pneumonia. This would be suggestive of immunodeficiency (T-cell disorder).
2. Check for anatomical or physiological abnormalities of the skin, respiratory system, gastrointestinal or genitourinary tract that may result in recurrent infections. Such abnormalities may involve lack of adequate drainage, stasis

Table 1.10   **Microorganisms commonly causing infection in specific immunodeficiencies**

Cell-mediated immunity	Viruses (CMV, HSV, RSV, enteroviruses, rotavirus). Fungi (candida, aspergillus, nocardia, cryptococcus). Bacteria (mycobacteria, listeria). Protozoa (pneumocystis, cryptosporidium).
Humoral immunity (antibody deficiency)	Bacteria (staphylococci, streptococcus, Hib). Viruses (ECHO, polio). Protozoa (giardia, cryptosporidium).
Phagocytes	Bacteria (staphylococci, Gram–ve bacteria) Fungi (candida, aspergillus)
Complement	Bacteria (Neisseria, pneumococcus)

in ducts and passages, abnormal communications or disruption of normally impermeable barriers.
3. General examination, including assessment of growth and development.
4. Specific history and examination looking for evidence of an immunodeficiency disorder. Particular attention is given to the presence or absence of lymphoid tissue, such as tonsils and lymph nodes (SCID, X-linked agammaglobulinaemia), any nail and skin changes (mucocutaneous candidiasis), abnormal facial features (DiGeorge syndrome, Hyper IgE syndrome), CNS (Ataxiatelangiectasia) or cardiac abnormalities (DiGeorge syndrome). A history of consanguineous marriage or a family history of deaths in infancy may be relevant.

Laboratory investigations

Investigations of the immune system can be organised into several tiers of increasing complexity (Table 1.11), with the most sophisticated tests only being available at tertiary referral centres. The latter tend to be confirmatory tests (Table 1.12).

First-tier investigations are available in most laboratories. These will detect neutropenia (will need several counts to exclude cyclic neutropenia), lymphopenia (SCID), thrombocytopenia and small-sized platelets in a child with eczema (Wiskott–Aldrich syndrome), giant neutrophil granules (Chediak–Higashi syndrome); low or absent immunoglobulins in X-linked agammaglobulinaemia, hypogammaglobulinaemia, common variable immunodeficiency, and IgG subclass deficiency. Measuring IgG levels and IgG subclasses is not very helpful in patients under 6 months of age, as these are mainly of maternal origin. Isohaemagglutinins are a measure of natural IgM antibodies; patients with blood group AB will obviously not produce any isohaemagglutinins. Some patients with normal immunoglobulin levels and recurrent infections have an inability to mount antibody responses to particular antigens. In these patients, it is important to evaluate antigen-specific responses.

Complement deficiencies are seen in recurrent Neisserial infections (C5, C6, C7); low C3, C4 may be seen in lupus-like syndromes. The NBT test (nitroblue

Table 1.11 **Investigations of the immune system**
First-tier investigations
• Full blood count and film
• Immunoglobulins (IgG, IgA, IgM), IgE
• IgG subclasses
• Isohaemagglutinins
• Vaccine responses (diphtheria, tetanus, Hib)
• Immune response panel to common antigens (HSV, VZV, other viruses)
• Total haemolytic complement
• NBT test
• HIV antibody test/HIV PCR (if appropriate)
• Basic T-cell subset panel

tetrazolium) is used to screen patients with phagocytic abnormalities due to chronic granulomatous disease (CGD). An HIV antibody test is the appropriate screening test, for patients over 18 months of age, suspected of HIV infection. HIV PCR is used to diagnose HIV infection in patients <18 months. A basic T-cell panel will give some information in those patients suspected of a T-cell immuno-deficiency, including SCID, CID and HIV.

The above tests are usually available in those centres with specialised immunology laboratories. They should be done in consultation with a paediatric immunologist. Treatment of immunodeficiencies consists of either regular replacement therapy (IVIG), antibiotic prophylaxis, bone marrow transplantation, or for the future, gene therapy.

HIV/AIDS

One to two million children worldwide have been infected with HIV, and most (80%) have acquired the disease through mother-to-child transmission.

Table 1.12 **Second-tier (confirmatory immunological tests)**	
Antibody deficiencies (humoral immunity)	• B-cell numbers and phenotype (CD19, CD20) • Pneumococcal antibody response to administration of Pneumovax
Phagocytic abnormalities	• Adhesion molecules expression • CD11/CD18 (e.g. LFA-1) • Functional assays (mobility, chemotaxis) • Phagocytosis (NBT, luminescence) • Phagocyte enzyme analysis
Cell-mediated immunity	• T-cell numbers and phenotype (CD3, CD4, CD8) Natural killer cells (CD16) Monocyte (CD14) • T-cell function PHA test (non-specific) In-vitro proliferative responses (Candida, PPD) Mixed lymphocyte reaction IL-2 stimulation test Markers of activation (CD25, IL-2 receptor) DR expression (MHC class II) • Enzyme and surface molecule expression (ADA, PNP, CD40 ligand expression, CD3 intensity)

Clinical manifestations

The majority of infected children are asymptomatic for the first few years of life. Generalised lymphadenopathy, hepatosplenomegaly, failure to thrive, parotitis and lymphocytic interstitial pneumonitis are often seen in combination, when children become symptomatic. Paediatricians thus need to consider HIV infection, amongst the differential diagnoses, when infants and children present with these clinical signs. This is especially the case if families are from those areas of the world with high HIV prevalence. Around 25% of children present in the first year of life with an AIDS-defining illness (PCP, CMV disease, including CMV retinitis, HIV encephalopathy, etc.) A particularly common presentation is of an infant, usually under the age of 6 months, who is admitted to a PICU with increasing respiratory distress, and a chest X-ray suggestive of interstitial pneumonitis. Subsequent investigations (e.g. BAL) confirm the pneumonitis as being due to *Pneumocystis carinii*, and it usually emerges that this is the first presentation of HIV infection in that particular family. With the advent of widespread HIV screening being available to pregnant women in the UK, it is hoped that the above clinical scenario will become increasingly rare. The introduction of HAART (highly active anti-retroviral therapy) will also, no doubt, lead to a changing natural history of HIV infection in children.

Laboratory investigations

1) Diagnosis in infants born to HIV positive mothers

HIV antibodies (IgG) are passively transferred across the placenta to the fetus and may persist for up to 18 months, in infants born to HIV positive mothers. Thus, it is not possible to diagnose HIV infection, in infants under 18 months, via an HIV antibody (ELISA) test. What is required is a test to show the presence of virus in the blood. This is possible via an HIV viral culture, p24 antigen testing and HIV PCR. The detection of HIV proviral DNA (HIV DNA integrated into the host genome), through PCR techniques, is now the diagnostic test of choice to diagnose HIV infection in infants <18 months. What is required, for a 'safe diagnosis', are the results of 2 HIV PCR tests, done at least 1 month apart, with at least one set being performed at or after 3 months of age. It is therefore possible

Table 1.13 **Establishing diagnosis of HIV in children born to HIV positive mothers**

Age	Test
Birth (1–2 days)	HIV PCR test
4 weeks	HIV PCR test
2–3 months	HIV PCR test
6–18 months	HIV antibody (ELISA) test*

*This is obtained on a 3–6 monthly basis in those infants who are PCR negative, i.e. uninfected, to follow-up for loss of HIV antibody

to be fairly certain of a child's HIV status, by around 3 months of age. In children over 18 months, a positive HIV antibody test (ELISA) is diagnostic of HIV infection. Confirmatory tests are often carried out to make the diagnosis secure (e.g. Western blot, IFA). A suggested regimen for follow-up/establishing diagnosis of HIV in children born to HIV positive mothers is given in Table 1.13.

Investigations in HIV-infected children are set out in Table 1.14.

Table 1.14 **Investigations in HIV-infected children**	
Initial visit	FBC, urea + electrolytes, liver function tests, amylase, T-cell subsets (CD4% of total lymphocytes, total CD4 count), HIV viral load, hepatitis B, C screen, CMV antibodies, *Toxoplasma* antibodies, baseline Chest X-ray
At each visit	FBC, urea + electrolytes, liver function tests, amylase T-cell subsets (CD4% of total lymphocytes, total CD4 count), HIV viral load
Prior to changing anti-retroviral Rx (failing regimen)	HIV resistance testing (usually Genotypic testing)

Table 1.15 **Respiratory problems in HIV: tests and diagnoses**	
Test	**Diagnosis**
Chest X-ray	Reticulonodular infiltrates suggest LIP, but miliary TB/PCP needs to be ruled out. Interstitial pneumonitis suggests PCP, CMV or LIP. Lobar or bronchopneumonia suggests bacterial infection. Hilar adenopathy suggests TB.
Nasopharyngeal aspirate (viral immunofluorescence)	RSV, CMV, other viruses, PCP
Bronchoalveolar lavage (viral immunofluorescence, PCP stain/fluorescence, bacterial + fungal culture)	PCP, CMV, Candida, Aspergillus, other viruses
Gastric aspirates/sputum: (bacterial + fungal culture)	TB, atypical TB, *S. pneumoniae*
Blood (culture, serology antigen testing)	*S. pneumoniae*, other bacteria, adenovirus, CMV
Mantoux test (10 TU)	TB (patient may be anergic if CD4 counts low)

Table 1.16 **Neurological tests in HIV**	
CT scan/MRI scan	There may be evidence of a space-occupying lesion (lymphoma, toxoplasmosis, tuberculoma), or white matter changes (progressive multifocal leuco-encephalopathy), cerebral atrophy or basal ganglia enhancement/calcification (HIV encephalopathy). MRI scan of spinal cord may show evidence of myelitis (CMV)
Brain biopsy	Histological examination for lymphoma, PML, toxoplasmosis
CSF	Bacterial/TB/Fungal culture; *Cryptococcus* latex antigen levels; PCR for CMV, EBV, papovavirus (JC strain); CSF HIV viral load
Blood	Serology for toxoplasmosis, CMV, EBV, antigen for *Cryptococcus*

2) Specific clinical syndromes

a) Respiratory infections/distress

The most likely respiratory problems in HIV-infected patients are recurrent bacterial infections, lymphocytic interstitial pneumonitis (LIP), *Pneumocystis carinii* pneumonia and CMV pneumonitis. Tuberculosis and atypical TB are also possible agents. Tests and diagnoses are listed in Table 1.15.

b) Chronic diarrhoea

The most likely agents causing chronic diarrhoea in the HIV-infected child are *Cryptosporidium, Isospora, Microsporidia, Salmonella, Shigella, Campylobacter, Clostridium difficile* and atypical TB. HIV itself is also a cause of chronic diarrhoea.

The following investigations may be helpful:

- Stool cultures and examination for ova and parasites; *C. difficile* toxin
- Acid-fast stain of stool for *Cryptosporidium/Isospora*/atypical TB
- Colonoscopy (biopsy + culture) for CMV, Cryptosporidia and atypical TB
- Jejunal biopsy — histology for Criptosporidia; subtotal villous atrophy (HIV).

c) Neurological syndromes

Table 1.16 sets out neurological tests in HIV. Spastic diplegia, delayed developmental milestones, ataxia and focal seizures are not uncommon symptoms and signs in HIV-infected patients. The most common agents causing neurological problems are HIV itself, toxoplasmosis, CMV, *Cryptococcus neoformans*, papovavirus (PML) lymphoma (often EBV-associated).

FURTHER READING

Davies, E.G., Elliman, D.A.C., Hart, C.A., Nicoll, A., Rudd, P.T. (1996) *Manual of Childhood Infections*. London: W.B. Saunders.

Gaspar, H.B., Goldblatt, D. (1997) Investigation of the immune system in recurrent infection. *British Journal of Hospital Medicine* 58: 517–520.

Isada, C.M., Kasten, B.L., Goldman, M.P., Gray, L.D., Aberg, J.A. (1999) *Infectious Diseases Handbook*, 3rd edn. Hudson, Ohio: Lexi-Comp.

Novelli, V., Peters, M.J., Dobson, S. (1999) Infectious diseases. In: Macnab, A.J., Macrae, D.J., Henning, R. (eds) *Care of the Critically Ill Child*, pp 281–298. London: Churchill Livingstone.

Rudd, P. (1996) Pyrexia of unknown origin (PUO). *Current Paediatrics* 6: 105–107.

Shingadia, D., Al-Ansari, H., Novelli, V. (1996) Investigation and diagnosis of fever in the returning traveller. *Current Paediatrics* 6: 108–113.

2

Immunology

E Alexander and D Isaacs

Introduction and basic physiology

The immune system provides complex defence against foreign antigens and hence microorganisms. The normal immune response incorporates the activities of antigen recognition, signal transduction, cell adhesion, cell proliferation and maturation, cytokine production, controlled inflammation, complement activation and secretion of effector molecules. Different mechanisms have evolved for dealing with extracellular organisms such as streptococci, intracellular organisms such as viruses, and parasites. It is important to look at the clinical picture before deciding which immunological tests are necessary, as the clinical pattern of infection is often a strong pointer to the nature of the underlying immune deficiency.

INVESTIGATING THE CHILD WITH SUSPECTED IMMUNE DEFICIENCY

It is important to know when to investigate and which specific investigations are indicated. Normal children have up to 12 respiratory infections each year in the first five years of life. Factors affecting the frequency of infections include presence of older siblings, attendance at childcare, and environmental exposure to tobacco smoke. It may be difficult to define a normal frequency of infection, especially when different parental expectations result in pressure on GPs to prescribe multiple courses of antibiotics and to explain why the child always has an infection. Clues that the child is infection-prone but otherwise normal are:

1. Infections are mild, acute and probably viral
2. Child usually recovers without sequelae
3. Growth pattern is normal
4. Infections restricted to a single site suggest local obstruction, i.e. an anatomical problem.

There is a percentage of children with unusually frequent, severe, chronic or recurrent infections (usually of the sino-pulmonary system, skin or intestinal tract), which are resistant to therapy, or opportunistic infections, in which an underlying immunodeficiency must be suspected. The ten warning signs of primary immune deficiency are given in the information box.

PRIMARY IMMUNE DEFICIENCY: WARNING SIGNS

1. Multiple ear infections (perhaps 6 to 8 in one year)
2. Several proven serious sinus infections (2 to 4 in one year)
3. Need for prolonged oral antibiotics to clear infections (for longer than 2 months)
4. More than 2 episodes of proven pneumonia
5. Failure of an infant to gain weight or grow normally
6. Recurrent, deep skin or organ abscesses
7. Persistent thrush in mouth or elsewhere on skin after the age of one year
8. Need for prolonged intravenous antibiotics to clear infections
9. Two or more deep-seated infections such as meningitis, osteomyelitis, cellulitis or sepsis
10. Family history of primary immune deficiency.

The presence of two or more of the above demands further investigation, and even one is a strong indication.

PHYSIOLOGY OF THE IMMUNE SYSTEM

Mature host defence mechanisms to overcome infections can be divided into immune and non-immune, and invading organisms into intracellular and extracellular. The extracellular organisms are mainly bacteria, both Gram-negative and Gram-positive, and are predominantly cleared by phagocytosis ± opsonisation with antibody and complement. Intracellular organisms such as *Listeria*, *Salmonella*, *Mycobacterium tuberculosis* and viruses are protected from these mechanisms once inside the cell, and the body relies on other defence mechanisms which depend on recognition of infected cells. This consists of immune and non-immune recognition of the infected cells and a subsequent amplification of the immune response.

Immunological response to infection

Pyogenic bacteria are extracellular organisms. Once they are established, the most important defence mechanism is phagocytosis and killing by neutrophils, enhanced by specific antibody and complement. Viruses are intracellular organisms. Apart from antibody, important early mechanisms in limiting viral replication are interferons, natural killer (NK) cells and antibody-dependent cellular cytotoxicity. Immunological response to intracellular pathogens is predominantly mediated by cellular immunity. Monocytes and macrophages produce interleukins, which activate T cells, while T cells produce lymphokines, which activate macrophages and T cells, thus producing an amplification of the cellular response to infections (see Fig. 2.1).

Defects in the immune system which result in recurrent infections can be in one or more of:

▲ T cells (T lymphocytes) which deal with intracellular pathogens. Defective T cell immunity, as in AIDS, results in infections with fungi like *Candida* and

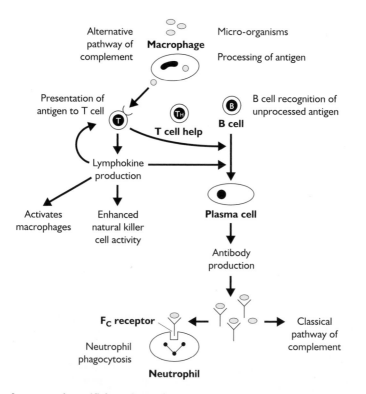

Fig. 2.1   **Immune (specific) and non-immune mechanisms interacting in response to infection. (Reproduced with permission from Isaacs, D., Moxon, E.R. (1999)** *Handbook of Neonatal Infections.* **London: W.B. Saunders.)**

Pneumocystis carinii, parasites like *Toxoplasma gondii*, and viruses like cytomegalovirus and *herpes simplex* virus. T cells also help B cells produce antibody, so defective T cell function may also result in defective humoral immunity, as in HIV/AIDS and severe combined immune deficiency (SCID).

▲ B cells which produce antibodies. Pure B cell deficiency occurs in X-linked agammaglobulinaemia, and results in sino-pulmonary infections (otitis media, sinusitis, pneumonia) but normal recovery from viral infections including measles and chickenpox.

▲ The complement system. Defects in terminal components of the complement cascade are rare and result in recurrent neisserial infections, meningococcal or gonococcal. Defects in early complement factors result in recurrent bacterial infections and/or systemic lupus erythematosus.

▲ The phagocytic system. Neutropenic patients are at risk of severe Gram-negative bacillary infections and fungal infections as well as staphylococcal infections. Susceptibility to a similar spectrum of organisms is seen in chronic granulomatous disease, although the two above conditions present with somewhat different clinical manifestations, particularly in terms of severity.

Early evaluation will allow early identification of affected children and subsequently lead to proper treatment before devastating infections cause irreversible organ damage. In general, infants with humoral deficiencies such as X-linked agammaglobulinaemia do not become unwell until maternal antibody begins to decline at 3 months. Combined immunodeficiencies, T cell defects, defects of adhesion molecules or phagocytic cells usually become evident in the first few months of life.

List of tests

IMMUNE FUNCTION TESTS

Cellular immunity
Lymphocyte count
Platelet count
Serum immunoglobulins G, A, M
HIV serology
T and B cell subsets
T cell proliferation
CD40-ligand

Humoral immunity
IgG, A, M
IgG subclasses
B & T cell numbers
Functional antibodies
Response to immunisation
HIV antibodies

Complement system
CH_{50}/CH_{100}
C_3 or C_4
Complement components (rare)
Properdin, Factors B, D

Phagocytic system
Neutrophil count
Serum IgE
NBT
Neutrophil function tests
Weekly neutrophil counts
CD11, CD18

Natural killer cell function
T and B cell subsets, CD 16/56
NK cell function

ABBREVIATIONS USED IN THIS CHAPTER

CGD — chronic granulomatous disease
FACS — fluorescent-activated cell sorter

SCID — severe combined immunodeficiency
URTI — upper respiratory tract infection

Tests

IMMUNE FUNCTION TESTS

There are a very large number of immune function tests available. It is important not simply to request a battery of immune tests without thought. The tests requested should reflect the clinical scenario. For example, recurrent boils suggest a phagocyte defect and tests of humoral and cellular immunity are not indicated.

Defects of antibody production are the commonest defects (about 50% of all cases): therefore, tests to evaluate humoral immunity take precedence over those used to test cell-mediated immunity, especially as they are simpler and cheaper.

All immune function tests must be reported in context of appropriate normal range, as this varies with age and sex.

Initial evaluation

▲ History and physical examination including weight and height
▲ Family history
▲ Chest X-ray looking for presence or absence of thymus.

Which form of immunity seems to be involved?

A. Cellular immunity

▲ Cells involved: T lymphocytes 'educated in thymus', CD4 and CD8 cells. T cell help required for B cells to function normally, so B cell problems often occur concurrently (SCID, HIV)
▲ Clinical picture: *Pneumocystis carinii* pneumonia, persistent oral candidiasis, persistent diarrhoea (rotavirus or other viruses), failure to thrive, e.g. SCID, HIV.

Tests to distinguish the form of immunity are listed in Tables 2.1 and 2.2.

Table 2.1 First-line screening tests	
Test	**Interpretation**
Differential white blood cell count	Lymphopenia ($< 1 \times 10^9$/L) common in SCID
Platelet count	Thrombocytopenia common in HIV, SCID, other congenital immunodeficiencies
Serum immunoglobulins G,A,M	Absent or very low in SCID, high in HIV infection. IgM normal or high in hyper IgM syndrome (with absent G or A)
HIV serology	

Table 2.2 Second-line immunological tests (specialist advice strongly advised)		
Test	**How performed**	**Interpretation**
T and B cell subsets	Fluorescent-activated cell sorter (FACS)	CD4 low in SCID, HIV
T cell proliferation	^{3}H-thymidine incorporation into mitogen-stimulated (PHA, ConA) lymphocytes	Low in T cell defects
CD40-ligand		Absent in X-linked hyper-IgM syndrome

B. Humoral immunity

▲ Cells involved: B cells from bone marrow, produce antibodies but need T cell help
▲ Clinical picture: sino-pulmonary infections (otitis media, sinusitis, pneumonia), especially with encapsulated pyogenic bacteria, seronegative sterile arthritis, recurrent bacterial conjunctivitis and sometimes other serious infections such as osteomyelitis, septic arthritis or meningitis.

Tests for humoral immunity are given in Tables 2.3 and 2.4.

Table 2.3 **First-line investigations**		
Test	**How performed**	**Interpretation**
IgG, IgA, IgM	Nephelometry, ELISA	In X-linked hypogammaglobulinaemia, maternal IgG may persist for up to 9 months.
IgG subclasses	Nephelometry, ELISA	Very important to compare to paediatric reference range. Low IgG$_4$ is normal.

Table 2.4 **Second-line investigations**		
Test	**How performed**	**Interpretation**
B&T cell numbers	FACS	In X-linked hypogammaglobulinaemia no B cells present.
Functional antibodies, i.e. antibodies to previous vaccines, haemolysins	Usually ELISA	Absent in X-linked hypogammaglobulinaemia and Nezelof's
Response to immunisation, e.g. Pneumovax, boosters of tetanus, diphtheria, Hib.	ELISA	If absent indicates impaired functional antibody production
HIV antibodies	ELISA, Western blot (pre-test counselling essential)	If present requires confirmation

If a child has proven sub-class deficiency, they should be referred for follow-up.
NB If all humoral immunity studies are normal, consider sweat test and ciliary studies. (See Chapter 10.)

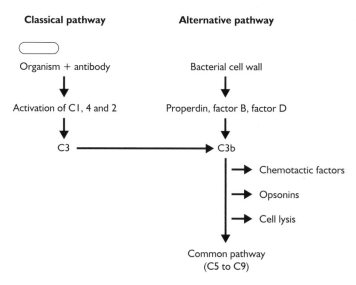

Fig. 2.2 Simplified representation of the complement cascade. (Reproduced with permission from Isaacs, D., Moxon, E.R. (1999) *Handbook of Neonatal Infections*. London: W.B. Saunders.)

C. Complement system

▲ Consists of a series of proteins which interact sequentially on the cell surface in a cascade starting with either classical or alternative pathways and leading to a common pathway, which generates chemotactic factors, opsonins and causes cell lysis (see Fig. 2.2).

▲ Clinical picture: recurrent bacteraemia and meningitis, especially neisserial infections, recurrent infections, systemic lupus erythematosus.

Tables 2.5 and 2.6 set out investigations in the complement system.

Table 2.5 **First-line investigations**		
Test	**How performed**	**Interpretation**
CH_{50} or CH_{100} C_3 or C_4	Blood sample	Easily artificially low if serum left sitting without separation of blood

Table 2.6 **Second-line investigations**		
Test	**How performed**	**Interpretation**
Individual complement components (very rarely needed)	Blood sample	If any component of complement missing then CH_{50} and CH_{100} are usually zero

D. Phagocytic system

▲ Cells involved: neutrophils (see Fig. 2.3)
▲ Clinical picture: boils, furunculosis, mouth ulcers, gingivitis and sometimes deep-seated abscesses. Increased susceptibility to *Staphylococcus aureus*, Gram-negative bacilli, (e.g. *Pseudomonas*) and fungi (e.g. *Aspergillus*).

Tables 2.7 and 2.8 set out investigations in the phagocytic system.

E. Natural killer cell function (always needs specialist advice)

▲ Cells involved: natural killer cells kill virus-infected cells, some micro-organisms and tumour cells spontaneously, with stimulation by interferon
▲ Clinical picture: important in recovery from herpes infection (HSV, CMV, and VZV) especially when haemophagocytosis is suspected.

Natural killer cell function tests appear in Table 2.9.

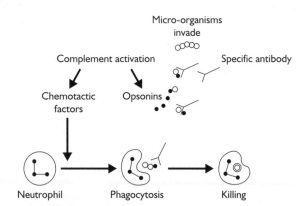

Fig. 2.3 Host defences against infection with pyogenic bacteria. (Reproduced with permission from Isaacs, D., Moxon, E.R. (1999) *Handbook of Neonatal Infections*. London: W.B. Saunders.)

Table 2.7	First-line investigations	
Test	**How performed**	**Interpretation**
Neutrophil count	Blood film	Congenital and acquired neutropenia
Serum IgE	Nephelometry or ELISA	Very high in hyper-IgE syndrome

Table 2.8 Second-line investigations

Test	How performed	Interpretation
Nitroblue tetrazolium (NBT) test	Specialised laboratory	Chronic granulomatous disease
Neutrophil function tests e.g. chemotaxis, chemiluminescence	Specialised laboratory	If NBT negative and suspected neutrophil defect
Weekly neutrophil counts × 6 weeks	Blood film	Suspected cyclical neutropenia (fever ± infection ± mouth ulcers every 3 weeks)
CD11, CD18	FACS	Suspected leucocyte adhesion defect (delayed separation of umbilical cord, severe early infections)

Table 2.9   NK cell function tests

Test	How performed	Interpretation
T&B cell sub-sets with CD16/56	FACS	NK cell deficiency
NK cell function	Cr^{51} release assay using target cells	Very low or absent when functional NK cell defect

Clinical problems

Recurrent infections 6–10 per year are usually due to viral URTIs, but they may be diagnosed as acute otitis media and treated with antibiotics (child may have a history of attendance at day care, or older siblings, therefore increased exposure, parental smoking); no failure to thrive; normal examination. *Conclusion*: normal child, no investigations required, parental reassurance only.

Recurrent ear infections (4 per year): ± purulent discharge — may be bacterial or viral. Check immunoglobulins and IgG sub-classes only.

Sino-pulmonary disease (ears, sinuses, chest) — may be associated with joint disease, bacterial conjunctivitis. On examination look for tonsillar tissue. *Investigations*: serum immunoglobulins and IgG subclasses, complement, also sweat test, CXR. Ciliary studies if other tests are normal, but as the first-line investigation if dextrocardia is present.

Opportunistic infections: thrush, failure to thrive, rash and chronic diarrhoea strongly suggest a T cell problem but usually there are associated B cell problems. In the history ask specifically about consanguinity, family history of similar disorders or unexplained infant death, risk factors for HIV. On examination look for purpura and eczema (Wiskott–Aldrich).

Investigations:

B&T cell subsets

HIV serology

IgG, A, M, E, and IgG sub-classes

CXR

Consider bronchoscopy with bronco-alveolar lavage for *Pneumocystis carinii* (Fig. 2.4) (infection often indolent initially).

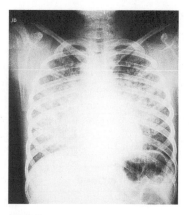

Fig. 2.4 **Pneumocystis carinii.**

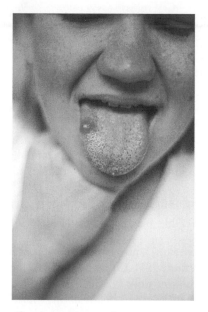

Fig. 2.5 **Tongue ulceration in neutropenia.**

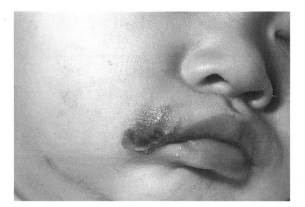

Fig. 2.6 **Ecthyma gangrenosum in neutropenia.**

Boils and fevers: suggests a possible neutrophil problem (Figs 2.5, 2.6). Can be suspected from history of gingivitis, mouth ulcers. Cyclical neutropenia presents with ulcers and boils every 4–6 weeks. Chronic granulomatous disease (CGD) can present with peri-anal abscesses, sometimes with unusual organisms, e.g. *Pseudomonas* and *Serratia* in boils, abdominal pain, deep abscesses, etc.

Investigations: FBC — 1–2 per week for 4–6 weeks if looking for cyclical neutropenia. NBT and other neutrophil function tests if available for CGD and other rare neutrophil defects.

FURTHER READING

Stiehm, E.R. (1995) *Immunologic Disorders in Infants and Children*, 4th edn. Philadelphia: W.B. Saunders.

Stiehm, E.R. (1995) *Immunologic Disorders in Infants and Children*, 4th edn. Philadelphia: W.B. Saunders.

3

Haematology and Oncology

R F Stevens

Introduction

The investigation of children with haematological and oncological disorders is not always the same as in adults. Sampling methods may be different, normal values are not always comparable and disease entities may be unfamiliar.

In this chapter haematological and oncological investigations will be considered, and how they relate to the appropriate diagnosis of childhood conditions.

Physiology/anatomy/principles of tests

THE BONE MARROW

The bone marrow is the factory for blood cell production, although in situations of marrow replacement the child may revert to more embryonic haematopoiesis with blood cell formation in extra-medullary sites such as the spleen and liver.

The concept of bone marrow stem cells has developed over the past 50 years, although these vital precursors are still not morphologically identifiable in the blood or bone marrow. Pluripotential stem cells have the capacity to divide so as to maintain the stem cell population, and also produce daughter cells which can differentiate into a variety of cell lines: a) erythroid, b) granulocytic and monocytic, and c) megakaryocytic, as well as to a common stem cell. Committed stem cells can only develop along specific maturation lines whilst maintaining a population of progenitors. The precursor cells are capable of responding to haemopoietic growth factors with increased production of one or other cell line when the need arises. A variety of stem cell assays have been developed which are useful in detecting qualitative and quantitative marrow defects. These assays are usually based on liquid marrow techniques but must still be considered as specialised rather than routine investigations.

Defects of pluripotential stem cells may present as aplastic anaemia (reduced numbers) or chronic myeloid leukaemia (abnormal maturation). Defects of committed stem cells may present as red cell aplasia (Diamond–Blackfan anaemia) or acute lymphoblastic leukaemia, for example.

THE PERIPHERAL BLOOD

Red cells

Mature red cells are anucleate and do not have the capacity of protein synthesis. They can however change their shape under certain circumstances (e.g. fragmentation). In terms of cellular differentiation, once a red cell has reached maturation (e.g. become a macrocyte) it will remain in this state and cannot return to normality.

The mature red cells can provide vital information in the diagnosis of haematological disorders. Their colour, size and shape can go a long way in defining haematological abnormalities and hence clinical disease. Normocytic, microcytic and macrocytic red cells each suggest pointers towards underlying pathology. Likewise normochromic, hypochromic and hyperchromic red cells are indicative of other diseases. It is important to remember that once a red cell has achieved its final configuration then it must remain in this form until it is removed from the circulation. The presence of more than one population of cells (diamorphic blood picture) is also indicative of some abnormality.

White blood cells

The total white cell count can vary considerably in childhood disease. Similarly variations in the individual cellular components may indicate certain pathological processes. Whereas normal red cells have a circulating survival time of 3 months, white cell survival varies remarkably depending on subtype. Neutrophils survive in the circulation for only 6 to 10 hours before moving into the tissues, where they perform their phagocytic function. They then spend about 5 days in the tissues before death. Monocytes circulate for up to 40 hours before entering the tissues. They can perform a variety of functions depending on their final resting place. The majority of lymphocytes in the peripheral blood are T cells which recirculate through the lymphatic system. The majority of B lymphocytes are more sedentary and spend longer periods in the spleen and lymph nodes.

Platelets

Platelets are cytoplasmic fragments which are produced as a result of 'budding' from their multinucleate bone marrow giant cells known as megakaryocytes. Under normal circumstances they have a circulating life span of up to 10 days, although this may be shortened considerably in disease. Although anucleate they have active metabolic enzyme systems. The normal platelet has a volume of approximately 6 fl, which compares with a red cell volume of between 75 and 95 fl. Some modern FBC machines are able to estimate the size of platelets and this is sometimes useful in disease diagnosis (e.g. small platelets in the Wiskott–Aldrich syndrome).

Increased peripheral destruction of platelets may be associated with a compensatory increase in bone marrow megakaryocytes, assuming the marrow has the capacity to increase production.

Platelets have a vital role in primary haemostasis and the formation of the platelet thrombus. As a result of blood vessel damage, platelets adhere to subendothelial tissues. Through a series of reactions involving platelet membrane glycoproteins and both circulating plasma and endothelial von Willebrand factor (VWF), platelet adhesion to subendothelial tissues is facilitated. Exposed tissue collagen or the action of thrombin results in the release of platelet granule contents including ADP, serotonin, fibrinogen, thromboglobulin and platelet factor 4. Collagen and thrombin stimulate platelet prostaglandin synthesis. Platelet arachidonic acid is also converted into thromboxane A2 in the platelet, and this, together with released ADP, results in further platelet aggregation at the site of injury. This in turn stimulates further platelet release and hence a positive feedback system culminating in a platelet plug at the site of vessel injury.

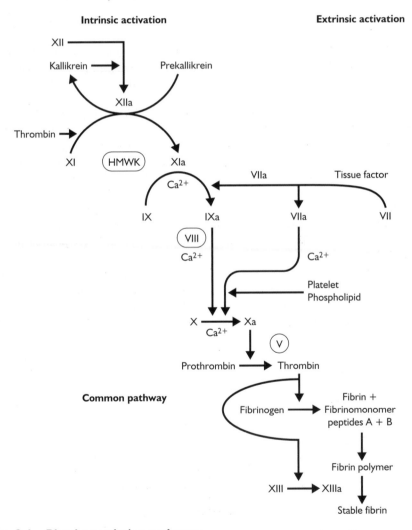

Fig. 3.1   **Blood coagulation pathways.**

Blood coagulation tests

Blood coagulation involves a biological amplification system in which activation of a cascade of coagulation enzymes is stimulated, culminating in the formation of thrombin which then converts soluble plasma fibrinogen into insoluble fibrin. This enmeshes with platelets to convert the primary haemostatic platelet plug into a stable haemostatic thrombus. For many years it was thought that in the intrinsic system, collagen and other negatively-charged tissue components activated factor XII, which then in turn activated factor XI and subsequently factor IX and factor X (in the presence of calcium and factor VIII). It is now thought that this reaction is only relevant in vitro, and that in vivo activation of factor XI occurs via factor VII activated by tissue factor. This is probably the major pathway for blood coagulation, and in vivo activation of factor XI by thrombin only becomes important in situations of major haemorrhage (Fig. 3.1).

Factor VIII coagulant protein (Factor VIII:c) is made up of 2332 amino acids and is coded by a 186-kb gene on the long arm of the X chromosome. It is synthesised in the liver, and in the plasma is bound to von Willebrand factor.

As part of the extrinsic pathway, tissue factor on the surface of vascular cells binds to factor VII, which then activates factor X and also results in activated factor VIIa. The main role of in vivo factor VII is to activate factor IX rather than activate factor X directly.

In the final common pathway, the complex of factor Xa and factor V on the phospholipid surface (together with calcium) converts prothrombin to thrombin, which in turn hydrolyses the arginine–glycine bonds of fibrinogen, releasing fibrinopeptides A and B to form fibrin monomers. These form cross linkages to form a loose, insoluble fibrin polymer which is then stabilised by the action of factor XIII (Fig. 3.2).

Fibrinogen is made up of two similar sub-units, each consisting of the polypeptide chains linked by disulphide bonds. After cleavage by thrombin of fibrinopeptides A and B, fibrin monomer consists of three paired alpha, beta, and gamma chains.

In summary, the intrinsic and extrinsic coagulation systems complement each other. Also factor VIIa generated in the extrinsic system activates factor IX in the intrinsic system. The thrombin then generated also positively feeds back to activate factors V and VIII, and also activates factor XI. It is therefore apparent that

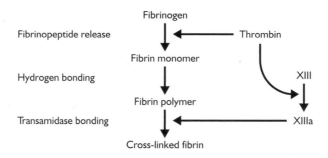

Fig. 3.2   **The formation of stable fibrin.**

an intact intrinsic and extrinsic system are both necessary for normal haemostasis.

Factors II, VII, IX and X are known as the vitamin K-dependent coagulation factors. Vitamin K is responsible for the carboxylation of these factors. In the absence of vitamin K no carboxylation of glutamic acid residues takes place, calcium is not bound and the coagulation factors are not linked to platelet phospholipid. Normal conversion of thrombin to prothrombin is restricted.

ONCOLOGY PATHOLOGICAL INVESTIGATIONS

The basic approach to tumour diagnosis is illustrated in Table 3.1. Although most tumours will require only a few of the investigations listed, certain cases may require a more extensive range of tests.

Table 3.1   **Methods in the diagnosis of small round-cell tumours**
Light microscopy
Electron microscopy
Immunochemistry (paraffin sections)
Immunophenotyping (monoclonal antibodies; frozen sections)
Tumour imprints (special stains; immunophenotyping; in situ hybridisation)
Viable tumour (cytogenetics; molecular genetic analysis; tissue culture)
Biochemical analysis (neurotransmitters; protein synthesis)

Light microscopy

There is a truism in tumour diagnosis: the most profitable route to diagnosis is a multidisciplinary approach, beginning with conventional light microscopy in the context of the clinical history. The newer technological methods should complement and not compromise the standard techniques. This being said, the desired aim is for the newer techniques to aid confirmation and not increase diagnostic uncertainty.

Electron microscopy

The main value of electron microscopy is not in answering the question of benign versus malignant, rather that it is a more accurate determinant of histogenesis. For example, neuroblastoma is more easily diagnosed when dense core granules are seen on EM, myofilaments in rhabdomyosarcoma, or platelet granules in acute megakaryocytic leukaemia.

Immunochemistry

The introduction of immunochemistry in light microscopy has been a major development. It is a non-morphological method intended to detect the tumour cell content of a marker substance (usually an antigen) that will react with an antibody presumed specific for that substance. The antigen must be stable and resist fixation and tissue preparation. Many substances detectable by radioim-

Table 3.2 Some antibodies used in the diagnosis of small round cell tumours	
Antibody	**Specificity**
Neurone-specific enolase	Found in nearly all neuroepithelial tumours
Leu 7 (human natural killer cell)	Found on T killer lymphoid cells, in nerve and neural tumours
Desmin	Found in myogenous tissues but not specific for skeletal muscle
Vimentin	Found in mesenchymal tissue, sarcomas and lymphoid malignancies
Keratin	Found in epithelial tissues, benign and malignant

munoassay or enzyme-linked immunosorbent assay (ELISA) are not detectable in fixed tissue.

The list of antibodies is ever-increasing. Table 3.2 lists just some of the more commonly used ones.

Biological markers in paediatric oncology
Biological markers may be present in the cell, on the cell surface or secreted into body fluids. They have not been identified in all malignancies and are of variable usefulness in diagnosis. They can be divided into tissue and serum proteins, hormones, enzymes and oncogenes.

Proteins
Several proteins have been identified as important markers.

Alpha-fetoprotein (AFP)
AFP is a serum protein synthesised by fetal liver cells and yolk sac tissues. AFP appears to behave as a fetal albumin and is found in high concentration in hepatoblastoma, hepatocellular carcinoma, and teratocarcinoma. The half-life of the protein is between 4 and 9 days, and levels usually fall to normal in 4 to 6 weeks following surgery. Normal physiological levels of AFP fall progressively after birth. Normal decay curves are available.

Ferritin
Raised ferritin levels may be found in malignancy, particularly those associated with necrosis or increased iron storage. This is particularly true of neuroblastoma.

Hormones
Catecholamines and human chorionic gonadotrophin are the most important hormones used in the identification of paediatric malignancy.

Catecholamines

Malignant cells derived from neural crest tissue are able to take up, synthesise and also break down catecholamines. Paediatric neuroblastoma is of neural crest origin and is often active in producing catecholamines and their metabolites. Raised levels are also seen in phaeochromocytoma, although this is a rare paediatric tumour. The most commonly measured metabolites are dopamine, vanillylmandelic acid (VMA) and homovanillic acid (HVA). They have a short half-life, and 24-hour urine collection is probably the most accurate, although shorter-term or even spot collections are helpful.

Human chorionic gonadotrophin (HCG)

HCG is usually produced by human placental trophoblast. Characteristically, tumours arising from trophoblastic tissues are associated with elevated HCG. High levels are also seen in embryonal carcinoma.

Enzymes

Neuron-specific enolase (NSE)

NSE represents a marker for both neurons and neuroendocrine cells. Various endocrine tissues including the adrenal, pituitary, pineal and thyroid glands may have significant levels of NSE but the levels may not be particularly high.

Lactic dehydrogenase (LDH)

A raised LDH is of limited value in tumour diagnosis but raised levels may be seen in leukaemias, lymphomas, Ewing's sarcoma, rhabdomyosarcoma and neuroblastoma. Changes in concentration are sometimes helpful in monitoring therapy.

Oncogenes

It is postulated that tumour formation is associated with activation of cellular genes called oncogenes. Activation can occur at the original chromosomal site or after translocation to other parts of the genome. Increasing use is being made of the new, sophisticated molecular techniques using copy DNA probes, etc.

Two oncogenes have been associated with paediatric tumours, namely N-ras and N-myc in neuroblastoma. The latter is associated with an inferior prognosis.

List of tests

HAEMATOLOGICAL TESTS

Full blood count
Blood film
Differential count
Bone marrow examination
Coagulation tests

Screening tests for haemostasis
  Bleeding time
  Prothrombin time
  Partial thromboplastin time
  Thrombin time
  Fibrinogen level
  Platelet count and blood film examination

Specific coagulation tests
Specialist haematological
tests

ONCOLOGICAL TESTS

Imaging
Specialist imaging
Tumour biopsy

ABBREVIATIONS USED IN THIS CHAPTER

AIHA — autoimmune haemolytic anaemia

EDTA — ethylenediaminetetraacetic acid

FDPs — fibrin degradation products

HbAS — sickle-cell trait

HbSS — sickle-cell disease

HCG — human chorionic gonadotrophin

HS — hereditary spherocytosis

HVA — homovanillic acid

ITP — idiopathic immune thrombo-cytopenia

LDH — lactic dehydrogenase

MAHA — microangiopathic haemolytic anaemia

NSE — neuron-specific enolase

PT — prothrombin time

PTT/APTT — partial thromboplastin time

TIBC — total iron-binding capacity

TT — thrombin time

VMA — vanillylmandelic acid

VWF — von Willebrand factor

Tests

HAEMATOLOGICAL TESTS

Full blood count (FBC)

The full blood count is often treated almost with contempt, particularly as it is one of the most frequently requested laboratory investigations. In paediatric prac-

Table 3.3 **Full blood count: age-related normal values**

Age	Hb (g/dl) Mean (range)	Haematocrit Mean (range)	MCV (fl) Mean (range)
Birth (cord)	16.5 (13.5–19.5)	0.51 (0.42–0.62)	108 (98–135)
I day	18.5 (14.5–21.5)	0.56 (0.45–0.66)	108 (95–135)
I week	17.5 (13.5–20.5)	0.54 (0.42–0.62)	107 (88–115)
I month	14.0 (10.0–16.5)	0.43 (0.31–0.51)	104 (85–108)
6 months	11.5 (9.5–13.5)	0.35 (0.29–0.45)	91 (74–96)
I year	12.0 (10.5–13.5)	0.36 (0.33–0.42)	78 (70–86)
5 years	12.5 (11.5–14.0)	0.37 (0.34–0.41)	81 (75–88)
10 years	13.5 (11.5–14.5)	0.40 (0.35–0.45)	86 (77–94)
15 years:			
female	14.0 (12.0–15.5)	0.41 (0.36–0.46)	88 (78–96)
male	14.5 (13.0–16.0)	0.43 (0.37–0.50)	90 (78–96)

tice it is important to have at least a basic perception of age-related normal values (Table 3.3).

The full blood count can be estimated from capillary or venous blood samples. The former has obvious practical advantages but is subject to greater technical errors. Poor peripheral circulation and excessive squeezing may cause haemo-concentration. Slow sample-bottle filling or inadequate mixing may result in fibrin clots and therefore reduced haemoglobin and platelet counts.

EDTA samples are 'stable' for several hours. After this period morphological changes occur (e.g. red cell crenation) which might be confused with pathological processes.

The blood film

If the sample is large enough to perform an FBC then there is usually sufficient to make a film which can then be stained to allow microscopic examination of the cellular morphology.

There are certain things which can and cannot be seen on a blood film (Table 3.4). For example, reticulocytes can only be visualised after staining with a special (supravital) stain.

Examination of the blood film requires skill and experience. Many of the newer blood count machines are able to give a good estimate of red cell and white cell morphology. This is often necessary because of the ever-increasing workloads on laboratories. Nevertheless there is no substitute for direct micro-scope morphological identification, particularly when other haematological parameters are abnormal.

Reticulocytes are red cell precursors which are present in the peripheral blood and which can be visualised with supravital stains. The normal count is 0.5–2.0%, and the absolute count $25–75 \times 10^9/l$. The reticulocyte count should rise in anaemia and bone marrow erythroid hyperplasia. If there is not a reticulo-cyte response, this suggests impaired marrow function or a lack of erythropoietin stimulus.

Differential count

The differential white blood cell count is an expression of the ratio of white blood cells in the peripheral blood. A total of 100 cells are usually counted (although a more accurate differential can be obtained by counting a larger number) and the various types (neutrophils, lymphocytes, monocytes, etc.) expressed as a per-centage or as an absolute figure. Modern blood count machines may be able to

Table 3.4 **Present on a blood film or bone marrow (routine haematological stain)**

Visible	Not visible
Howell–Jolly bodies	Reticulocytes
Malarial parasites	Heinz bodies
Marrow storage cells	Ring sideroblasts

Table 3.5 Normal leukocyte counts ($\times 10^9/l$)

Age	Total Leukocytes		Neutrophils			Lymphocytes		
	Mean	Range	Mean	Range	(%)	Mean	Range	(%)
Birth	15.0	10–26	8.0	2.5–15	(60)	5.5	2.0–7.5	(30)
1 month	11.0	5–20	4.0	1.0–9.0	(35)	6.0	2.5–16.5	(56)
6 months	12.0	6–18	4.0	1.0–8.5	(32)	7.3	4.0–14.0	(61)
1 year	11.5	6–18	3.5	1.5–8.5	(31)	7.0	4.0–11.0	(61)
5 years	9.0	5–15	4.0	1.5–8.0	(50)	4.0	2.0–8.0	(50)
10 years	8.0	4.5–14	4.5	2.0–8.0	(55)	3.1	1.5–6.5	(38)
15 years	7.5	4.5–13	4.5	2.0–8.0	(58)	2.8	1.2–5.3	(35)

perform simple or more comprehensive differential counts based on counting sometimes many thousands of cells. However, they cannot identify all morphological types and routine microscopy is often then necessary.

Like haemoglobin levels there are important age-dependent variations in the differential count (Table 3.5). In general there is an increase in the percentage of lymphocytes during the first year of life which reflects the child's early antigenic exposure. The association of a mild anaemia (when compared to adults), relative lymphocytosis, and cervical lymphadenopathy can lead to clinical anxiety when in fact it may be entirely normal.

Bone marrow examination

Bone marrow aspiration is usually not a difficult procedure but does require a little familiarity both in aspiration and spreading the slides. Trephine biopsy is more tricky but is particularly useful in assessing marrow cellularity and detecting infiltration. Without a general anaesthetic or suitable sedation a bone marrow test is a traumatic experience for a child, particularly if it needs to be repeated in the future as in children with leukaemia. The subsequent staining, examination and interpretation of the bone marrow is best left to the haematologist. Bone marrow samples are important for other reasons, including:

◆ Iron stain (a crude quantitation of iron stores)
◆ Leukaemia special stains
◆ Leukaemia cell markers (immunophenotype)
◆ Cytogenetics (important in leukaemia diagnosis)
◆ Marrow culture
◆ Marrow genetics (e.g. detection of minimal residual disease in leukaemia).

Coagulation tests

Care has to be taken to ensure that samples are taken into the correct specimen bottles (usually sodium citrate), with the correct volumes (avoiding over- or under-filling), and transported to the laboratory without undue delay. Heparin contamination must also be avoided as this will produce erroneous results.

Screening tests for haemostasis

These include:

◆ Bleeding time
◆ Prothrombin time (PT)
◆ Partial thromboplastin time (PTT, APTT)
◆ Thrombin time (TT)
◆ Fibrinogen level
◆ Platelet count and blood film examination.

Values for screening coagulation tests in children are set out in Table 3.6.

Prothrombin Time (PT)

The prothrombin time is a measurement of the plasma clotting time after the addition of thromboplastin (a tissue–brain extract). It is a non-specific indicator of the extrinsic blood coagulation mechanism.

Partial thromboplastin time (PTT or APTT)

The partial thromboplastin time is a quick, non-specific indicator of defects in the intrinsic coagulation pathway.

Thrombin time

In this test, exogenous thrombin is added to the patient's plasma and the clotting time measured. The thrombin time is affected by the concentration and functional activity of fibrinogen, and by the presence of circulating inhibitor substances.

Specific coagulation tests

Specific assay of the concentration of a particular clotting factor in plasma may be necessary:

1) To confirm the diagnosis of a bleeding disorder
2) To assess the laboratory severity of the disorder
3) To monitor replacement therapy for the disorder.

Table 3.6 **Values for screening coagulation tests in children (all values in seconds)**

Age	PT		PTT		TT		Fibrinogen	
	Mean	Range	Mean	Range	Mean	Range	Mean	Range
30 weeks	13	10–17	54	27–80	25	19–30	2.4	1.5–3.8
Birth	13	11–15	43	37–49	24	21–27	2.8	2.2–3.6
3 months	12	11–13	37	32–43	25	22–28	2.4	1.7–3.1
1–5 years	11	10–12	30	24–36	25	20–28	2.7	1.7–4.0
6–10 years	11	10–12	31	26–36	25	21–28	2.8	1.6–4.0
Adult	12	11–14	33	27–40	25	22–27	2.8	1.7–4.0

The results of assays may be informative in isolation (e.g. Factor VIII:c assay in diagnosing haemophilia), or may be used in combination (e.g. Factor VIII:c, VW:Ag, and Ristocetin co-factor (VW:Activity) assay in the diagnosis of von Willebrand's disease).

Platelet function tests including the bleeding time may be important investigations in the child with bruising and purpura. Abnormal bleeding associated with a prolonged bleeding time may result from thrombocytopenia or platelet dysfunction. In the latter the platelets are often present in normal numbers but fail to aggregate or adhere to the blood vessel walls.

Specialist haematological tests

There are many specialist haematological investigations which may be helpful or even essential in the diagnosis of haematological disorders. Some of these tests are not specific to blood disorders, whereas others are truly diagnostic. In the main they will be considered later under specific disease headings, e.g. Leukaemia, Hypoplastic anaemia, Immune defects (both cellular and humoral) and Anaemias.

ONCOLOGICAL TESTS

Oncology is the study of cancer and is therefore more often involved in the diagnosis of 'solid' tumours as compared with the haematological 'liquid' malignancies. In the same way that many haematological diagnoses depend on examination of the blood and possibly the bone marrow, tumour biopsy and histology are the mainstay of paediatric oncological diagnosis. Routine oncological investigations also include several imaging techniques.

Imaging

Routine X-rays are necessary in virtually every child with cancer, either in defining primary disease or estimating the degree of metastatic spread. This being said, many of the previously routine X-rays (e.g. IVUs, barium studies) have been replaced by newer imaging techniques such as ultrasound, CT scan and MRI scan.

Specialist imaging

Ultrasound is non-invasive, quick and rarely intimidating to children. However, it is usually necessary to follow ultrasound with more detailed imaging if a lesion is suspected. CT and MRI scanning usually require intravenous contrast and take longer to perform. The machinery itself may be frightening to children, and in some cases general anaesthesia may be necessary. Nevertheless expert imaging and reporting have revolutionised the diagnosis, localisation and follow-up of paediatric solid tumours.

Tumour biopsy

With very few exceptions, tumour histology is vital in the management of paediatric malignancies. In some cases total tumour resection may be possible and beneficial. More often a biopsy is appropriate. This can be performed by needle

Table 3.7 Small round-cell tumours of childhood: classifications	
Traditional	**Revised**
Ewing's sarcoma	Ewing's sarcoma
Neuroblastoma	Metastatic neuroblastoma
Lymphoma	Extranodal lymphoma
Rhabdomyosarcoma	Metastatic alveolar rhabdomyosarcoma
	Small-cell osteosarcoma
	Primitive neuroectodermal tumour of bone
	'Askin' tumour of bone
	Peripheral neuroepithelioma

(e.g. 'Tru-cut') or open biopsy. The latter means that more tissue is available for histological diagnosis and subsequent biological studies and an open biopsy often means that the risk of complications such as bleeding is lower. In many instances complete surgical removal offers no survival advantage over subsequent chemotherapy, and may carry a greater risk of complications.

Over the last 30 years there have been major advances from the pathological background of gross specimen examination and light microscopy. Histochemistry, electron microscopy, immunochemistry, cytogenetics, and molecular genetics are all now part of the diagnostic armamentarium. An example of one of the diagnostic problems in paediatric pathology is the 'small round-cell tumour' which in itself is misleading as the cells are often neither small nor round. Nonetheless they are primitive or embryonal in appearance and lack any specific morphological features to make a diagnosis. As such, they provide a model system to demonstrate the benefits of a multi-disciplinary approach to tumour diagnosis. Some of the methods now used in the diagnosis of small round-cell tumours were listed above (Table 3.1); Table 3.7 gives the revised classifications which resulted.

Clinical problems and how to investigate them

ANAEMIA

With the advent of modern-generation automated haematological analysers, more screening tests for anaemia and other haematological abnormalities are becoming available. Values obtainable for the red cell count, mean corpuscular volume (MCV) and mean corpuscular haemoglobin (MCH) are far more reliable than those by visual estimation. However, it is still important to examine the blood film as certain conditions may otherwise be missed.

Hypochromic anaemia

Hypochromasia is present when red cells stain palely. It is due either (and more commonly) to a low haemoglobin concentration (low MCH) or to abnormal thinness of the red cells. Hypochromia is frequently associated with microcytosis, and iron deficiency is the most common, but not the only, cause of this red cell appearance. In hypochromic microcytic anaemias all three red cell indices (the MCV, MCH and MCHC) are reduced and the blood film shows small pale red cells.

It is important to remember that the MCV in healthy children is very much age-dependent. In the context of diagnosing a hypochromic microcytic anaemia the following values are useful.

Hypochromic microcytic anaemia:

6 months to 2 years	MCV<70fl
2–5 years	MCV<73fl
5–12 years	MCV<75fl

Table 3.8 Differential diagnosis of hypochromic anaemia

Condition	MCV	Serum iron	TIBC	Ferritin	Iron stores
Iron deficiency	↓	↓	↑	↓	Absent
Anaemia of chronic disorders	↓ or N	↓	↓	↑ or N	↑ or N
β thalassaemia	↓	↑	N	↑	↑ or N
Sideroblastic anaemia	↓ or ↑	↑	N	↑	↑

Table 3.8 gives the differential diagnosis of hypochromic anaemia.

Iron deficiency

Iron deficiency is the commonest cause of anaemia in the world. As already mentioned, hypochromic microcytic anaemia is not synonymous with iron deficiency. In particular, thalassaemia may be confused with iron deficiency. The red cell

Table 3.9 Disorders which may be confused with iron deficiency

	Iron deficiency	Thalassaemia minor	Anaemia of chronic disorders
MCV	↓	↓	N or ↓
Serum iron	↓	N	↓
TIBC	↑	N	↓
TS[†]	↓	N	N or ↓
FEP[*]	↑	N	↓
Serum ferritin	↓	N	N or ↑

*FEP = Free erythrocyte protoporphyrin
†TS = Transferin saturation

indices start to fall before anaemia develops, and then fall progressively. The reticulocyte count is low in relation to the anaemia. The blood film shows hypochromic, microcytic cells and occasional target cells and pencil-shaped poikilocytes (although never more than 25% of total red cells as seen in elliptocytosis). It is important to remember that a) up to 20% of cases of iron deficiency may be associated with a normal blood film, b) blood films of normal children may sometimes show some morphological features of iron deficiency, and c) thrombocytosis (platelet count $>350 \times 10^9/l$) in association with iron deficiency may be indicative of gastrointestinal blood loss.

Table 3.9 sets out disorders which may be confused with iron deficiency.

Serum iron and iron-binding capacity (TIBC)

In children with true iron deficiency the serum iron is reduced (<13 µmol/l) and the iron binding capacity is raised (>70 µmol/l). However, these values are influenced by physiological factors such as age, sex, and time of day, as well as laboratory methodology and disease processes. Calculation of the transferrin saturation increases the usefulness of the serum iron and TIBC.

$$\text{Transferrin saturation (TS)} = \frac{\text{Serum iron} \times 100}{\text{TIBC}}$$

The TIBC is inversely related to the amount of storage iron. Typical iron deficiency is marked by a low serum iron, raised TIBC and consequently a low TS. A low serum iron and a low TS cannot be taken in isolation to diagnose iron deficiency, unless associated with a raised TIBC.

Table 3.10 Serum iron	
Reduced serum iron	**Raised serum iron**
Iron deficiency	Acute leukaemia
Chronic infection and inflammation	Hypoplastic anaemia
Debilitating conditions, e.g. malignancy, uraemia	Haemolytic anaemia
	Megaloblastic anaemia
	Iron overload
	Hepatitis (acute)
	Cirrhosis

Table 3.11 Iron binding capacity	
Reduced iron binding capacity	**Raised iron binding capacity**
Infection	Iron deficiency
Haemolysis	Pregnancy
Cirrhosis	
Debilitating conditions	
Iron overload	

There are two main drawbacks with the serum iron and TIBC. Firstly the day-to-day fluctuations in serum iron and wide range in transferrin concentration, and secondly many coincidental illnesses, may make interpretation difficult (see Tables 3.10, 3.11).

Serum ferritin Only a small fraction of the total body ferritin circulates in the serum but nevertheless is related to total iron stores, particularly storage iron. In the majority of situations the serum ferritin is a sensitive, reproducible, quantitative assay of body iron stores which requires only small blood samples. The normal values in children are similar to those in adult females (15–140 μg/l), with higher levels in infants between the ages of 1 and 3 months (up to 350 μg/l) but falling again to adult levels by 6 months.

The differentiation between iron deficiency and the anaemia of chronic disorders may be difficult on the basis of the serum iron, iron binding capacity and percentage saturation. The serum ferritin is most helpful as it is normal or raised in the anaemia of chronic disorders. It is also very useful in assessing iron overload in thalassaemia and other haemolytic anaemias. In a few situations the serum ferritin may not be a true reflection of body iron stores. These include acute and chronic leukaemia, some malignancies (e.g. neuroblastoma) and acute hepatic failure.

Erythrocyte protoporphyrin The incorporation of iron into protoporphyrin is the final step in the formation of the haemoglobin molecule. With reduced supplies of iron, red cells accentuate free protoporphyrin and zinc protoporphyrin. Free and zinc erythrocyte protoporphyrin increases early in iron deficiency before the anaemia develops, and is therefore a sensitive measure. Raised levels are however seen in lead poisoning, erythropoietic porphyria and some rare forms of sideroblastic anaemia. Measurement of the erythrocyte protoporphyrin level can be made from small capillary EDTA samples without the need for venous blood and is a very useful and relatively reliable screening test for iron deficiency.

Macrocytic anaemia

It is important to remember that macrocytosis (MCV >96fl) is not synonymous with vitamin B12 or folic acid deficiency (Table 3.12).

Table 3.12 **Commoner causes of macrocytosis**	
Causes of macrocytosis	**Associated blood features**
Vit B12 deficiency Folate deficiency	Hypersegmented neutrophils, leukopenia and thrombocytopenia
Liver disease	Target cells
Hypothyroidism	Target cells, occasional acanthocytes
Hypoplastic anaemia	Leukopenia and thrombocytopenia
Reticulocytosis (haemolysis)	Polychromasia

In megaloblastic anaemia the red cells are abnormally large and may be oval in shape. Red cell precursors (erythroblasts) in the bone marrow show the characteristic abnormality of delayed nuclear maturation as compared to that of the cytoplasm.

The bone marrow is often hypercellular, and characteristic changes are seen in the erythroblasts with a primitive, open nuclear chromatin pattern but relatively normal haemoglobinisation. Changes are also seen in other cell lines with hyper-

---

Table 3.13   Diagnostic approach to megaloblastic anaemia

Tests to establish diagnosis	FBC (MCV) including platelets
	Reticulocyte count
	Examination of blood film
	Bone marrow examination
	Serum ferritin
	Bilirubin (and possibly LDH)
Tests to differentiate B12 from folate deficiency	Serum B12 level
	Serum and red cell folate levels
	Vit B12 binding proteins (transcobalamins)
Tests to establish cause of deficiency	Barium meal and small bowel radiology
	Chest X-ray and urine analysis
	Autoantibodies (intrinsic factor, parietal, thyroid)
	Tests of malabsorption (e.g. immune reactive trypsin)
	Vit B12 absorption test with and without intrinsic factor (Schilling test).

It is important to remember that true megaloblastic anaemia in children is rare and therefore a selective approach to investigation should be adopted.

Table 3.14   Megaloblastic anaemia with normal vitamin B12 and folate levels

Congenital
Defective Vit B12 transport (transcobalamin II deficiency)
Orotic aciduria
Congenital dyserythropoietic anaemia
Rare metabolic disorders of B12 or folate metabolism (e.g. Lesch–Nyhan syndrome)

Acquired
Associated with blood dyscrasias (e.g. leukaemia, sideroblastic anaemia, aplastic anaemia)
Drugs (cytotoxics in particular)

Table 3.15 Vitamin B12 malabsorption in childhood			
	Age of onset (years)	**Intrinsic factor**	**Intrinsic factor antibodies**	**Associated features**
Congenital pernicious anaemia	3	Absent	Absent	Immunodeficiency
Immerslund–Gräsbeck syndrome	2	Present	Absent	Proteinuria
Juvenile pernicious anaemia	10+	Absent	Present	Polyendocrine failure, immunodeficiency
Defects of the terminal ileum		Absent	Absent	Inflammatory bowel disease
Inadequate dietary intake		Absent	Absent	Ethnic or cultural associations

segmented neutrophils (with 6 or more lobes), and sometimes dysplastic megakaryocytes. Giant and abnormal metamyelocytes are also seen and are a strong pointer to Vit B12 or folate deficiency as opposed to other causes of 'megaloblastoid' marrow changes, such as dyserythropoietic anaemias or drug effects (e.g. cytotoxics) (see Tables 3.13, 3.14, 3.15).

Haemolytic anaemia

The basic definition of haemolytic anaemias are those that result from an increase in the rate of red cell destruction. Under normal circumstances the bone marrow has a great capacity for increasing red cell production and therefore avoiding anaemia. In children the diagnosis of haemolytic anaemia is influenced by several factors. For example, in the newborn an obstetric history may be of particular importance, and in the older child the ethnic origin may provide an important clue.

The investigation of haemolytic anaemia is a good example of a coordinated logical approach where investigations should be performed in a logical sequence.

Evidence of haemolysis

Reduced haemoglobin level
Abnormal red cell morphology (e.g. spherocytes, elliptocytes, sickle cells, fragmented cells, red cell agglutination)
Raised serum bilirubin.

Evidence of increased bone marrow activity

Reticulocytosis and polychromasia
Bone marrow erythroid hyperplasia.

Specific diagnosis of haemolytic anaemia

The subsequent investigations necessary for the precise diagnosis of haemolytic anaemia will be largely dependent on the results of initial tests, and it is important to remember that not all investigations are indicated in every case.

1) Where a hereditary haaemolytic anaemia is suspected

a) *Osmotic fragility*. This investigation has been largely superseded by the confirmation of spherocytes on the blood film and the characteristic red cell distribution 'print-out' seen with certain modern-generation blood cell counters. It is also important to confirm that the direct antiglobulin (Coombs) test is negative, otherwise an autoimmune process is more likely.

b) *Autohaemolysis test*. This is another example of a test which is rarely performed nowadays. Typically, in conditions such as spherocytosis or pyruvate kinase deficiency there is increased destruction of red cells with incubation which can be partly corrected by the addition of glucose. The test has been superseded by more specific assays.

c) *Screening test for glucose-6-phosphate dehydrogenase deficiency (G-6-PD)*. G-6-PD deficiency is the commonest haemolytic anaemia associated with a red cell enzyme deficiency. There are three basic types. Firstly the 'negro' type which is seen in about 10% of blacks but where haemolysis only occurs on exposure to oxidant drugs, and antimalarials in particular. In the 'mediterranean' form chronic haemolysis may be a feature, as well as neonatal jaundice, and brisk haemolysis with ingestion of fava beans. The third or 'oriental' type may show chronic haemolysis and neonatal jaundice but favism is not a feature.

d) *Assay for red cell pyruvate kinase deficiency*. This is the second commonest red cell enzyme deficiency but nevertheless for every case of PK deficiency there are over 500,000 cases of G-6-PD deficiency. A marked reticulocytosis may be present, particularly following splenectomy.

e) *Heinz body test*. This test is based on the demonstration of typical red cell inclusions with supravital staining. Heinz bodies are typically seen in association with abnormal and unstable haemoglobins.

f) *Quantitation of other red cell enzymes and metabolites in the glycolytic pathway*. Having excluded the more common red cell enzyme deficiencies, it may be necessary to go on and assay other defects in the glycolytic pathway. These tests usually require the help of specialist laboratories.

g) *Haemoglobin F and A_2 levels*. These are particularly useful in the diagnosis of thalassaemia minor. Children with hypochromic microcytic anaemias and normal ferritin levels may be affected. The total red cell count may be disproportionately raised and there may be a characteristic red cell 'print-out'. In β thalassaemia minor the majority of patients have a raised Hb A_2 level and about 50% also have a raised HbF level. If both of these are normal then thalassaemia minor is more likely.

h) *Haemoglobin electrophoresis.* The demonstration of an abnormal haemoglobin band on electrophoresis is particularly important in the diagnosis of qualitative haemoglobin abnormalities such as sickle cell haemoglobin (HbS). It is of much less help in the diagnosis of quantitative haemoglobin disorders such as thalassaemia minor, as the rise in HbA_2 and HbF is in the order of only 2 or 3% and therefore will not be visible as a strong band on electrophoresis.

i) *Screening tests for Haemoglobin S.* These tests are based on the altered solubility of sickle cell haemoglobin when compared to adult haemoglobin. This is the basis of the 'sickledex' and is a useful screening test for the presence of sickle cell haemoglobin, although it does not differentiate between trait and disease. However, patients with sickle cell disease are much more likely to be anaemic, have a raised reticulocyte count and sickle cells on the blood film.

j) *Tests for unstable haemoglobins.* These include heat stability and isopropyl alcohol stability tests. Specialist haemoglobin electrophoresis and molecular genetic tests are usually necessary to confirm the diagnosis.

k) *Test for Haemoglobin H.* This is based on supravital staining of red cells and is a very tedious method of identifying the rare but typical inclusions seen in haemoglobin H disease, or alpha thalassaemia minor.

2) Where an autoimmune haemolytic anaemia is suspected

a) *Direct Coombs test* (antiglobulin test). A positive DCT indicates the presence of antibody or at least complement on the surface of the patient's own red cells. In the so-called 'warm' autoimmune haemolytic anaemias (AIHA) the red cells are coated with IgG, IgG and complement, or complement alone. The sensitised red cells are then removed by the reticuloendothelial system. The antibody reacts better at body temperature (37°C). In 'cold' AIHA the antibody is usually IgM and binds to red cells better at room temperature or lower temperatures.

Warm type AIHA in children may be idiopathic or secondary, when it is particularly associated with autoimmune conditions such as SLE. Cold type AIHA may also be idiopathic but may be seen in *Mycoplasma pneumoniae* or other infections.

b) *Donath–Landsteiner test.* This test is not often used in children. It is associated with paroxysmal cold haemoglobinuria, which is a rare syndrome of intravascular haemolysis after exposure to the cold in patients with the Donath–Landsteiner antibody, which binds to red cells in the cold but causes lysis with complement in warm conditions. Syphilis is now very rare in children but viral infections can produce the same effect.

c) *Quantitation of cold agglutinins.* Antibodies which react particularly in the cold can be quantitated. Samples must be kept warm before testing and examination of the blood film for autoagglutination may be equally informative.

3) Where drug-induced haemolysis is suspected

a) *Screening tests for G-6-PD deficiency.*

b) *Heinz-body stain.* Heinz bodies can only be recognised with supravital staining (e.g. methylene blue) and are red cell inclusions of denatured oxidised haemoglobin. They may be detectable in drug-induced haemolysis and unstable haemoglobins.

c) *Blood spectroscopy for abnormal haemoglobin pigments.* Free haemoglobin or methaemoglobin (oxidised haemoglobin) may be detectable in serum. The latter is particularly associated with drug or chemical oxidation of haemoglobin. Sulphaemoglobin may also be present.

d) *Urine examination for haemoglobin.* Intravascular haemolysis may result in the release of free haemoglobin into the plasma and hence into the urine. Chronic intravascular haemolysis may also result in increased levels of haemosiderin in the urine.

4) In cases of otherwise undiagnosed haemolysis

a) *Ham's test (acidified serum lysis test).* This is the diagnostic test for paroxysmal nocturnal haemoglobinuria. This very rare condition can present as either haemolytic or hypoplastic anaemia or recurrent thromboses. PNH is diagnosed by demonstration of red cell lysis at low pH when there is activation of complement by the alternative pathway.

Directed investigations and haemolytic anaemia

Hereditary spherocytosis

Anaemia and reticulocytosis
Negative Coombs test
Spherocytes on the blood film
Family studies
Increased osmotic fragility

Most cases of HS are easily diagnosed by the reticulocytosis and blood film changes. Modern generation blood counting machines may also identify a characteristic red cell pattern. A positive DCT excludes the diagnosis and raises the possibility of AIHA. It is important to remember that in about 25% of cases no abnormality can be detected in another family member. The auto-haemolysis test is now not often performed.

Hereditary elliptocytosis

Similar investigations are applicable to those in HS, although the diagnosis is nearly always based on blood film appearances only.

Red cell enzyme disorders

G6PD screening test
Pyruvate kinase test

Having performed these screening tests most laboratories will be dependent on referral of the patient, or more likely blood samples, to a specialist reference laboratory for quantitative assays of red cell enzymes or metabolites.

Haemoglobinopathies

FBC, red cell indices, blood film examination
Haemoglobin A_2 and F estimation
Haemoglobin electrophoresis (cellulose acetate and agar gel).

It is important to remember that Hb electrophoresis is only useful when significant quantities of abnormal haemoglobins are present. For example, in sickle cell trait about 40% of the haemoglobin present is likely to be HbS and easily recognisable on electrophoresis, whereas in β thalassaemia minor the raised HbA_2 and HbF levels are in the order of only a few percent and may not be easily visible on electrophoresis, and may therefore require specific quantitation.

Sickle cell screening test

These tests do not reliably differentiate between sickle cell disease (HbSS) and other sickle cell conditions such as sickle cell trait (HbAS), Haemoglobin SC disease, or Haemoglobin S/β thalassaemia. Other laboratory and clinical features are necessary.

Sickle cell preparation

Sickle cells and some target cells are seen on the blood film in sickle cell disease. Features of splenic atrophy (e.g. Howell–Jolly bodies) may also be present.

Haemoglobin H preparation

In the alpha thalassaemia syndromes, supravital staining of the blood film reveals multiple fine, deeply staining deposits ('golf ball' cells) due to β globin chain precipitation. They are plentiful in Haemoglobin H disease but seen very scantily in alpha thalassaemia minor.

Heinz body test

Heinz bodies are only seen with supravital staining and represent oxidised denatured haemoglobin. They may be identified in association with unstable haemoglobins.

Molecular genetics

Over the past few years the techniques and genetic probes available for the identification of the thalassaemia syndromes have increased dramatically (see Table 3.16). This technology is however highly specialised and requires the help of specialised laboratories.

Immune haemolytic anaemia

Direct Coombs test (including monospecific Coombs reagents)
Screening investigations for the presence of free antibodies in the serum
Presence of cold antibodies
Quantitative immunoglobulins and immunoglobulin electrophoresis
Other autoantibody tests (e.g. ANF, anti-DNA antibodies)
Complement levels
Monospot and Paul–Bunnell test.

Table 3.16 The genetic classification of thalassaemia		
Type	**Heterozygous, trait, minor**	**Homozygous, major**
α-thalassaemias		
α°	MCV, MCH low	Hydrops fetalis
α^{+}	MCV, MCH minimally reduced	As heterozygous α°-thalassaemia
β-thalassaemias		
β°	MCV, MCH low ($HbA_2 > 3.5\%$)	Thalassaemia major (HbF 98%, HbA_2 2%)
β^{+}	MCV, MCH low ($HbA_2 > 3.5\%$)	Thalassaemia major or intermedia (HbF 70–80%, HbA 10–20%, HbA_2 variable)
$\delta\beta$ and hereditary persistence of fetal haemoglobin	MCV, MCH low (HbF 5–20%, HbA_2 normal)	Thalassaemia intermedia (HbF 100%)

Microangiopathic haemolysis

Blood film
Coagulation screening tests and fibrinogen level
Fibrin degradation products, fibrin monomers, D-dimers
Serum urea and creatinine

Infections

Bacterial, viral and rickettsial cultures
Blood film examination for malarial parasites
Blood film examination for filamentous parasites
Bone marrow examination for Kala-azar.

Leukoerythroblastic anaemia

This is the term used for the presence of white cell precursors (myelocytes and metamyelocytes) and red cell precursors (normoblasts or nucleated red cells) in the peripheral blood. Associated anaemia is not mandatory. White cell counts may be normal or high. With advanced involvement, thrombocytopenia and neutropenia may also occur.

It is important to remember that a normal blood picture does not rule out the possibility of marrow infiltrative disease. Likewise white and red cell precursors may be seen in the blood in patients with regenerating bone marrow (e.g. following cytotoxic chemotherapy) or in association with severe infection, severe anoxia, or acute reactive states.

The total white cell count in leukoerythroblastic anaemia is seldom greater than $50 \times 10^9/l$.

Leukoerythroblastic anaemia is typically associated with marrow infiltrative disease. This includes conditions such as disseminated neuroblastoma, leukaemia, and less commonly rhabdomyosarcoma or other marrow secondary deposits. The association of leukoerythroblastic anaemia, hypercalcaemia, splenomegaly, and reduced visual and auditory acuity raises the possibility of osteopetrosis. Storage diseases such as Gaucher's disease and Niemann–Pick disease can infiltrate the bone marrow with storage cells resulting in leukoerythroblastic changes.

Leukaemoid reaction

This is a reactive and increased leukocytosis characterised by the presence of immature white cell precursors in the peripheral blood. These include myelocytes, metamyelocytes and promyelocytes. As expected there are similarities between leukaemoid reactions and leukoerythroblastic anaemia. Leukaemoid reactions may be particularly marked in children. Causes include acute and chronic infections (e.g. whooping cough), severe haemolysis (e.g. haemolytic uraemic syndrome) or marrow infiltrative disease. Leukaemoid reactions uncommonly result in white cell counts above $50 \times 10/^9l$, and very rarely above $100 \times 10^9/1$. The presence of a large number of white cell precursors together with splenomegaly should raise the possibility of chronic myeloid leukaemia either of the adult type (Philadelphia positive) or juvenile myelomonocytic leukaemia.

Microangiopathic haemolytic anaemia (MAHA)

The presence of fragmented red cells in the peripheral blood (schistocytes) is characteristic but not pathognomonic of this condition. The abnormal shaped red cells and red cell fragments are the result of physical damage on abnormal surfaces (e.g. prosthetic heart valves or grafts) or as a result of red cells passing through fibrin strands in DIC or through damaged small vessels as in HUS, thrombotic thrombocytopenic purpura or meningococcaemia.

These red cell changes are frequently, but not invariably, associated with variable degrees of thrombocytopenia and haemolysis. The thrombocytopenia is due to peripheral platelet destruction and consumption.

The presence of microangiopathy with schistocytes, fragmented red cells and microspherocytes should prompt a platelet count and coagulation screen as well as fibrin degradation products (or D-dimers). The presence of thrombocytopenia does not necessarily mean that a consumptive coagulopathy is also present, but this should be excluded.

Secondary anaemia (anaemia of chronic disorders)

Chronic systemic disease in children is frequently associated with anaemia which is usually mild or moderate. It is typically normochromic/normocytic, but not infrequently may be hypochromic and somewhat microcytic. The causation of secondary anaemia is multifactorial but includes mechanisms such as reduced red cell survival, impaired marrow response to anaemia, and impaired utilisation of marrow storage iron. Some of the features of secondary anaemias are listed in Table 3.17.

Table 3.17 **Features of secondary anaemias**

ESR or plasma viscosity frequently raised
Mild or moderate anaemia
Typically normocytic (sometimes microcytic)
Normochromic or hypochromic
Normal or slightly raised reticulocytes
Low serum iron together with low iron binding capacity and reduced saturation
Serum ferritin slightly or moderately raised
Increased bone marrow storage iron, but reduced iron utilization (reduced iron granules in red cell precursors)

The secondary anaemias associated with inflammatory disease include:
    Juvenile chronic arthritis
    Systemic lupus and other collagen vascular disorders
    Inflammatory bowel disease
    Cystic fibrosis
    Chronic infections (including renal infection, osteomyelitis, tuberculosis, bronchiectasis, infective endocarditis)

Anaemia of chronic renal disease

The anaemia is usually normochromic and microcytic with reticulocytopenia, except where the marrow is able to respond effectively to the anaemia. The haemoglobin level is not necessarily proportional to the degree of uraemia. The pathogenesis includes impaired renal erythropoietin production and metabolism resulting in reduced marrow erythroid activity, associated microangiopathic anaemia, and iron deficiency due to blood loss associated with haemorrhage or dialysis.

Anaemia of liver disease

Red cell survival is often reduced in liver disease and there is an element of chronic haemolysis. Red cell fragmentation ('spur-cell anaemia') may be seen in cirrhosis. Portal hypertension may result in hypersplenism with a moderate pancytopenia. Iron deficiency may follow chronic blood loss from bleeding oesophageal varices. Wilson's disease may result in chronic haemolysis due to red cell copper accumulation. Viral hepatitis can be associated with severe hypoplastic anaemia.

Neonatal anaemia

Anaemia in the neonatal period is usually the result of one of three mechanisms:

Haemorrhage—either acute or chronic
Haemolysis—usually associated with jaundice
Hypoplasia or decreased red cell production.

Haemorrhage

Prenatal blood loss may be transplacental, retroplacental, or the result of a twin-to-twin transfusion. The Kleihauer test is useful in identifying a transplacental haemorrhage, as it identifies the presence of cells in the maternal circulation which contain fetal haemoglobin which can be assumed to be of fetal origin. The test is based on the fact that red cells containing HbF are more resistant to acid elution than cells containing HbA. Examination of maternal blood films subjected to acid elution and then counterstained will reveal intact cells containing HbF amongst a larger population of cell 'ghosts' from which the HbA has been lost. It is possible to make a very crude calculation of the magnitude of the transplacental bleed using the following formula:

$2400 \times$ ratio fetal:maternal cells = transplacental haemorrhage (in ml).

The Kleihauer test may be influenced by other factors: a) certain conditions may result in a raised HbF level (e.g. thalassaemia, sickle cell anaemia, or hereditary persistence of fetal haemoglobin), b) up to 10% of fetal cells do not stain properly, and c) ABO incompatibility between mother and baby may result in rapid destruction of fetal cells.

Haemolysis

Neonatal haemolytic anaemia is nearly always associated with unconjugated hyperbilirubinaemia and a reticulocytosis. The majority of childhood haemolytic anaemias may present in the neonatal period but there are important exceptions such as β thalassaemia major and sickle cell disease where the early preponderance of HbF delays the development of symptoms for a few months.

Figure 3.3. gives test features of neonatal anaemia and reticulocytosis. The neonatal haemolytic anaemias can be subdivided into a) congenital red cell defects, and b) acquired red cell defects.

Congenital red cell defects

1) Infantile pyknocytosis is characterised by the presence of small distorted red cells on the blood film, hyperbilirubinaemia and splenomegaly. It is usually the result of vitamin E deficiency.
2) Heinz-body anaemia. Heinz bodies are red cell inclusions which are only visible on blood films stained with supravital stains.
3) Thalassaemia in the newborn. Because of the presence of HbF, β thalassaemia does not manifest itself in the neonatal period and only presents at the time when HbF levels are decreasing but are not replaced with HbA. The most severe form of alpha thalassaemia (Bart's hydrops fetalis syndrome) results in intrauterine death or demise shortly after delivery. The less severe form of alpha thalassaemia, haemoglobin H disease in later life, may present in the neonatal period with mild anaemia, haemolysis, and up to 25% Hb Bart's (gamma 4).

Acquired red cell defects These may present as haemolytic anaemia in the neonatal period with jaundice, and may be immune (Coombs test positive) or non-immune (Coombs test negative).

Immune causes:

Rhesus isoimmunisation.

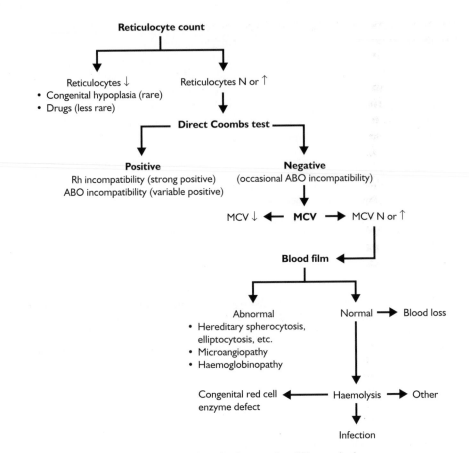

Fig. 3.3 **Neonatal anaemia and reticulocytosis: differentiating causes.**

Although Anti-D is the most important and usually the most severe, it is important not to forget other antibodies, e.g. anti-C, e, E
ABO isoimmunisation
Other blood group antibodies, e.g. anti-Kell, anti-Duffy.

Non-immune causes:

Infections, e.g. CMV, toxoplasmosis, rubella, herpes simplex
Vitamin E deficiency
Drugs and chemicals (with or without prematurity or G-6-PD deficiency).

Failure of red cell production (Diamond–Blackfan anaemia)

This congenital condition usually presents in the first year of life, and should be expected in the neonate when there is anaemia (normochromic/normocytic) and reticulocytopenia associated with a normal platelet and white cell count. The condition is confirmed by the marked reduction of red cell precursors in the bone marrow. Approximately one third of cases have other associated congenital abnormalities.

NON-MALIGNANT DISORDERS OF GRANULOCYTES AND MONOCYTES

Neutrophils (polymorphs), eosinophils and basophils together are called granulocytes. Together with monocytes they make up the blood phagocytes.

Neutrophil morphology

Some rare hereditary conditions are associated with abnormal granulocyte morphology:

May–Hegglin anomaly. An autosomal dominant condition where the neutrophils contain dense cytoplasmic inclusions. Giant platelets and mild thrombocytopenia may be associated features.

Pelger–Huet anomaly. This is associated with bi-lobed neutrophils. Inheritance is autosomal dominant.

Alder–Reilly anomaly. An autosomal recessive condition: dark purple granules are found in granulocytes, lymphocytes and monocytes.

Chediak–Higashi syndrome. In this autosomal recessive condition there are giant granules in the granulocytes and lymphocytes together with neutropenia, thrombocytopenia, hepatosplenomegaly and partial albinism.

Mucopolysaccharide disorders.

These may be associated with abnormal white cell granulation or vacuolation (e.g. Hurler's syndrome).

Neutrophilia

A rise in the neutrophil count above $8 \times 10^9/l$ is a commonly-seen change in the full blood count. Some of the more common causes are listed in the information box. Associated features include a) toxic granulation in the neutrophil cytoplasm and Döhle bodies, and b) a 'shift to the left' with the presence of less segmented neutrophils and sometimes myeloid precursors.

CAUSES OF NEUTROPHIL LEUKOCYTOSIS

1. Infections, particularly bacterial
2. Metabolic conditions, including uraemia, diabetic ketoacidosis
3. Acute inflammatory conditions, e.g. juvenile arthritis, haemolytic uraemic syndrome, Kawasaki's syndrome
4. Paediatric malignancy
5. Marrow infiltrative disease
6. Corticosteroid therapy
7. Acute haemorrhage or haemolysis
8. Myeloproliferative disorders

Neonatal neutrophilia

Neutrophil counts in the first day of life range from 8 to $15 \times 10^9/l$. By the age of 3 days they should have fallen to between 1.5 and $5.0 \times 10^9/l$. This early physiological neutrophilia is often associated with a few myeloid precursors in the peripheral blood. Persistent neonatal neutrophilia is often the result of persisting bacterial infection. The stress of severe infection in the newborn can easily exhaust the supply of marrow granulocytes and result in secondary neutropenia.

Eosinophilia

Eosinophils are proportionately reduced during the neonatal period. They also exhibit diurnal variation, showing higher levels during the evening.

The causes of eosinophilia are extensive, but can be considered under the following headings: allergic, parasitic, drugs, haematological conditions, skin disorders, and others.

Allergy

This is probably the commonest cause of eosinophilia in the western world. Over 75% of asthmatic children have an eosinophil count of greater than $0.6 \times 10^9/l$ at some point in their illness. Eosinophilia occurs in other allergies such as eczema, urticaria and angioneurotic oedema.

Parasitic

Helminthic infections are the commonest cause of eosinophilia in the third world. Eosinophilia due to parasitic infection cannot be excluded on the basis of normal faecal examination, and similarly, parasitic infection cannot be dismissed because of a lack of eosinophilia in blood.

Drugs

Antibiotics (penicillin, ampicillin, nitrofurantoin, cephalosporins), antituberculins (para-amino salicylic acid), antiepileptic (phenytoin), and antihypertensives (hydralazine) are just some of the drugs associated with eosinophilia.

Haematological disorders

Hodgkin's disease may be associated with a very marked eosinophilia. Other associations include Non-Hodgkin's lymphoma, chronic myeloid leukaemia (often with a basophilia), and malignant histiocytosis.

Skin disorders

Skin disorders include atopic dermatitis (eczema), urticaria, drug reactions and dermatitis herpetiformis.

Other conditions

Juvenile idiopathic arthritis, infected ventriculoperitoneal or ventriculopleural shunts, chronic peritoneal dialysis, disseminated malignancy, chronic liver disease, and other collagen vascular disorders are also included.

Basophilia

As basophils are the least common of the granulocyte series they are subject to the greatest counting error. The presence of a leukocytosis, together with a leukaemoid reaction and basophilia, is suggestive of chronic myeloid leukaemia (usually of the adult type), which is confirmed by identifying the Philadelphia chromosome in the marrow or peripheral blood. Other conditions associated with basophilia include Hodgkin's disease, cirrhosis, chronic haemolysis, ulcerative colitis, post irradiation and post splenectomy.

Monocytosis

These cells usually account for fewer than 10% of the blood granulocytes. Conditions particularly associated with monocytosis include: chronic bacterial infections, such as tuberculosis, brucellosis, typhoid; malignant conditions, particularly myelomonocytic leukaemia, and lymphomas. Other conditions include inflammatory bowel disease, collagen vascular disorders, and recovery from previous marrow suppression such as following cytotoxic chemotherapy or bone marrow transplantation.

Infectious mononucleosis

Typically glandular fever is associated with the presence of atypical mononuclear cells in the peripheral blood. A leukocytosis is usually seen in the febrile phase of the illness. The total WBC is rarely above normal. If more than 25% atypical mononuclears are seen on the blood film then the diagnosis is usually glandular fever. If fewer than 25% atypical mononuclears are seen, then other conditions such as CMV, toxoplasmosis, viral hepatitis or pneumonia, and other viral illnesses should be considered. An infectious mononucleosis-like syndrome may also be associated with drugs such as phenytoin, dapsone, and para-aminosalicylic acid.

The Paul–Bunnell test detects the presence of heterophile antibodies in the serum of affected patients. It is positive in about 80% of cases. False negatives may occur early in the disease, or due to a slow or low-titre antibody response. The commercial Monospot test has the advantage of being a 2-minute whole blood slide procedure.

Lymphocytosis

An absolute lymphocytosis is most commonly seen in acute infectious lymphocytosis, pertussis, tuberculosis and related infections including CMV and other viral infections.

A relative lymphocytosis may be seen in conditions where there is an associated granulocytopenia. This includes many viral illnesses such as mumps, measles and rubella. Chronic infectious lymphocytosis is characterised by a moderate leukocytosis and a preponderance of lymphocytes.

Aspects of lymphocytosis, mononucleosis and leukaemia are compared in Table 3.18.

PURPURAS

The presence of clinical purpura should raise the possibility of either a quantitative or qualitative platelet disorder. There are of course other causes such as trauma or vasculitis, but a platelet count and blood film are vital initial investigations.

Table 3.18 **Lymphocytosis, mononucleosis, and leukaemia**

	Acute infectious lymphocytosis	**Glandular fever**	**Acute leukaemia (lymphoblastic)**
Age	First decade	First 3 decades	First 2 decades
Lymphadenopathy	Absent	Present	Often present
Fever	Present	Usually present	Often present
Splenomegaly	Absent	Often present	Often present
Anaemia	Absent	Uncommon	Often present
Thrombocytopenia	Absent	Uncommon	Often present
Lymphocyte type	Small	Atypical	Often lymphoblasts
Paul–Bunnell	Negative	Usually positive	Negative

Purpura associated with thrombocytopenia

Idiopathic immune thrombocytopenia (ITP)

This condition is the commonest cause of acute thrombocytopenia without associated anaemia or leukopenia. The absence of splenomegaly or other obvious causes of low platelets is important. In the past much emphasis has been put on the identification of platelet antibodies in the serum. There is however no ideal test for the presence of antibodies in the serum and hence free antibody may not be present in a significant percentage of cases. The demonstration of platelet-bound antibody (equivalent to a positive direct antiglobulin test) is more specific.

Secondary thrombocytopenic purpura

This can be sub-divided into 1) reduced platelet production and 2) increased platelet consumption.

Table 3.19 lists the causes of thrombocytopenia.

Table 3.19 **Causes of thrombocytopenia**

Reduced platelet production	**Increased platelet consumption**
Cytotoxic drugs	Idiopathic (autoimmune)
Marrow hypoplasia	Drugs
Leukaemia	Collagen-vascular disorders
Marrow infiltration	Infections, e.g. malaria, HIV, EBV
Myelodysplasia	Post-transfusion purpura
HIV	DIC

Purpura associated with a normal platelet count

a) The typical rash, normal platelet count, bleeding time and coagulation screen, together with the gastrointestinal and renal symptoms (in some cases) are typical of Henoch–Schönlein purpura. The tourniquet fragility test (Hess's test) may be abnormal.
b) Hereditary haemorrhagic telangiectasia presents much more commonly in later life but the characteristic skin lesions may occasionally be recognised in children.
c) Infections, particularly meningococcal septicaemia, rubella and Coxsackie.
d) Ehlers–Danlos syndrome, where an abnormality of collagen can result in abnormal platelet function, easy bruising, poor wound healing and purpura.

Purpura associated with a high platelet count

Thrombocytosis usually means a platelet count above $400{\times}10^9/l$. Platelet counts above $1000 \times 10^9/l$ may be associated with haemorrhagic or thrombotic complications. Thrombocytosis can be subdivided into defective increased platelet production (e.g. chronic myeloid leukaemia) and reactive thrombocytosis (e.g. malignant states, inflammatory conditions, acute blood loss, and post-splenectomy).

Neonatal and infantile thrombocytopenia

Thrombocytopenia in the young child and neonate can present specific diagnostic problems. Unlike most haematological parameters, platelet counts in neonates and premature babies are not significantly different from older children and adults.

Normal or increased marrow megakaryocytes

a) Immune thrombocytopenia of maternal origin. This results from the passive transfer of maternal antibody across the placenta which has specificity against fetal platelets. This is associated particularly with maternal ITP or SLE. The thrombocytopenia is not usually very severe in the baby if there is a reasonable maternal platelet count.
b) Isoimmune neonatal thrombocytopenia. This condition is confirmed by the presence of severe thrombocytopenia in the foetus or newborn and the detection of antibodies in the maternal serum which are directed against the baby's platelets. These are usually anti HPA Type 1. Further confirmation is based on the demonstration of a platelet antigenic difference between mother and baby. First pregnancies can be affected in over 50% of cases and the level of thrombocytopenia and haemorrhagic complications can be dramatic.
c) Disseminated intravascular coagulation. Any of the many neonatal causes of DIC may be associated with thrombocytopenia. Neonatal sepsis is a common cause, due to a variety of infections both congenital and acquired. In the syndrome of giant haemangioma and thrombocytopenia (Kasabach–Merritt syndrome), vascular anomalies result in platelet and fibrinogen consumption in the lesion with or without evidence of a generalised DIC.
d) Inherited thrombocytopenia.

1) Wiskott–Aldrich syndrome. This condition is associated with thrombocytopenia, small platelets, normal marrow megakaryocytes, low levels of plasma isoagglutinins, generalised eczema, and X-linked inheritance.
2) Pure X-linked and autosomal recessive thrombocytopenia.
3) May–Hegglin anomaly consisting of thrombocytopenia, giant platelets and abnormal neutrophil granules.

Reduced marrow megakaryocytes

♦ Thrombocytopenia and absent radii (TAR syndrome)
♦ Thrombocytopenia and microcephaly
♦ Congenital rubella and other viral and congenital infections
♦ Rarely, with immune neonatal thrombocytopenia.

The investigation of platelet function

Abnormal bleeding associated with a prolonged bleeding time but a normal coagulation screen and platelet count may be the result of a platelet functional abnormality.

The investigation of platelet aggregation in response to a variety of aggregating agents is an important aspect of the investigation of a child for a possible platelet functional abnormality. In essence, platelet-rich plasma is warmed to 37°C and continually mixed in a plastic tube inside a platelet aggregometer, which monitors light transmission through the plasma. The addition of aggregating agents results in the formation of platelet clumps, allowing increased light transmission and a fall in optical density which is monitored by a chart recorder.

The commonly-used platelet aggregating agents include ADP, collagen, adrenaline, ristocetin and arachidonic acid. Table 3.20 sets out platelet responses to these agents.

Defects of platelet function may be the result of deficiency of platelet membrane glycoproteins (e.g. in Glanzmann's thrombasthenia where there is a defi-

Table 3.20 Platelet aggregation responses					
	ADP	**Collagen**	**Adrenaline**	**Ristocetin**	**Arachidonic acid**
Thrombasthenia (Glanzmann's)	AbN	AbN	AbN	N or AbN	AbN
Bernard–Soulier syndrome	N	N	N	AbN	N
von Willebrand's disease	N	N	N	AbN	N
Storage pool disease	N	AbN	AbN	N	N
Aspirin defect	N	AbN	AbN	N or AbN	AbN

ciency of glycoproteins IIb and IIIa, or the Bernard–Soulier syndrome where there is a deficiency of glycoprotein Ib) or a deficiency of platelet enzymes. In the storage pool defect there is a deficiency of platelet granules. In the Grey Platelet syndrome there is a virtual absence of alpha-granules and in the more common Delta-storage pool disease there is a deficiency of dense granules. As a result there is no secondary wave of platelet aggregation as there is no storage pool of ADP to be released and initiate secondary aggregation.

In von Willebrand's disease the abnormality is the result of a deficiency of plasma von Willebrand factor rather than a specific platelet defect.

When performing platelet function tests it is important to remember that patients must not have ingested aspirin for at least 10 days, and that samples are taken promptly into plastic tubes using citrate anticoagulant and tested without delay.

COAGULATION DISORDERS

Normal blood coagulation is dependent on the interaction of circulating coagulation factors, platelets, and the vascular endothelium. A stable fibrin clot is the endpoint of the coagulation cascade; children deficient in coagulation factors may form a primary haemostatic plug which is largely platelet-dependent, but these may be unstable, and delayed bleeding and subsequent poor wound healing are characteristic features of patients with coagulation abnormalities.

It is impractical to initiate a comprehensive barrage of coagulation tests on every patient with a suspected bleeding disorder. Rather it is more logical to perform a set of screening tests and then go on to further specific assays if indicated.

Screening tests for haemostasis

The screening tests used most often in the initial investigation of coagulation disorders are the prothrombin time (PT), partial thromboplastin time (PTT, APTT, or PTTK), and the thrombin time (TT). Coagulation screening tests are summarised in Table 3.21.

Prolonged prothrombin time

Common causes include:

♦ oral anticoagulant therapy
♦ liver disease (particularly with low factor VII levels)
♦ haemorrhagic disease of the newborn.

Table 3.21 Summary of coagulation screening tests			
PT	**PTT**	**TT**	**Interpretation**
N	AbN	N	Deficiency of factors VIII, IX, XI, XII
AbN	N	N	Deficiency of factor VII
AbN	AbN	N	Deficiency of factors X, V, II or multiple
AbN	AbN	AbN	Heparin (normal reptilase), DIC, abnormal fibrinogen

Less common causes include:

♦ malabsorption (vit K deficiency)
♦ congenital factor II, V, VII or X deficiency
♦ hypofibrinogenaemia or dysfibrinogenaemia; heparin therapy.

Prolonged partial thromboplastin time

The PTT is most useful in the detection of haemophilia A or B but cannot be used to differentiate between the two.

The PTT is also useful in monitoring intravenous heparin therapy, and an otherwise unexplained prolongation of the PTT should raise the possibility of heparin contamination of the sample.

The PTT is not usually prolonged unless the level of the intrinsic coagulation factor deficiency is less than 25% of normal. Female haemophilia carriers, who have a factor VIII level typically of 50%, usually have a normal PTT. Patients with mild von Willebrand's disease may also have a normal PTT.

Prolonged thrombin time (TT)

Common causes:

● heparin therapy
● fibrin degradation products (FDPs)
● hypofibrinogenaemia.

Less common causes:

● dysfibrinogenaemia
● liver or renal disease (the result of abnormal fibrin polymerisation).

Thrombin time using reptilase   Reptilase (or other snake venoms, e.g. Atroxin) can be used as part of the thrombin time and has the advantage that it is not influenced by the presence of heparin. A prolonged thrombin time but normal reptilase time is highly suggestive of heparin. The reptilase time is less prolonged than the thrombin time in the presence of FDPs, but is more prolonged when there is congenital or secondary dysfibrinogenaemia.

Specific coagulation tests

Quantitation in plasma of a specific coagulation factor may be necessary:

1) To make the diagnosis of a specific coagulation disorder
2) To assess the laboratory severity of the disorder
3) To monitor therapy
4) To aid in the detection of female carriers.

As indicated in Table 3.22, a prolonged partial thromboplastin time in conjunction with a normal prothrombin time is highly suggestive of a defect in the intrinsic pathway. Correction (mixture) experiments can be performed using adsorbed plasma and aged normal serum. However, it is often quicker to go straight on and perform specific assays. As factor VIII deficiency is the commonest cause this should be performed first and then followed by factors IX, XI, and

Table 3.22 **Laboratory features of haemophilia and von Willebrand's disease**

	Haemophilia A	Christmas disease	von Willebrand's disease
Platelet count	Normal	Normal	Normal
Bleeding time	Normal	Normal	Usually prolonged
Prothrombin time	Normal	Normal	Normal
PTT	Prolonged	Prolonged	Prolonged or normal
Factor VIII:c	Markedly reduced	Normal	Reduced
Factor IX	Normal	Markedly reduced	Normal
VWF:Ag	Normal	Normal	Reduced
Ristocetin-induced platelet aggregation (VWF:RiCo/VW:Act)	Normal	Normal	Impaired

XII as indicated. Other very rare defects in the intrinsic pathway can cause an isolated prolongation of the PTT but require specialist laboratory help.

Most congenital coagulation factor deficiencies are classified as mild, moderate or severe on the basis of the factor level. For example, in classical haemophilia, severe corresponds to a factor VIII level of <2%, moderate between 2 and 10%, and mild >10%.

Specific coagulation assays are necessary in assessing factor replacement therapy when clinical response is suboptimal, and also to evaluate the potency of coagulation concentrates. This only really applies to haemophilia A and B. For other coagulation deficiencies where specific concentrates are not available, monitoring the PTT is probably adequate.

Where the inheritance pattern suggests the possibility of an asymptomatic carrier of a coagulation deficiency, then factor assays are an important part of genetic counselling.

The laboratory investigation of haemophilia

The factor VIII molecule is made up of 2332 amino acids and has distinct functional and antigenic properties.

The functional properties include the procoagulant activity (FVIII:c) which is absent in affected haemophiliacs and present in factor VIII concentrates. The higher the purity of the concentrate, the higher the ratio of factor VIII to other non-specific proteins. Another functional property in the factor VIII molecule is von Willebrand factor (VWF), which is necessary for the adhesion of platelets to the vascular endothelium (and hence correction of the prolonged bleeding time) and platelet aggregation in response to Ristocetion (RiCoF/vW:Activity). This activity is reduced in patients with von Willibrand's disease but normal in haemophilia.

The factor VIII molecule also has antigenic properties. Antigenic sites are present which react with heterologous (e.g. rabbit) antibodies to factor VIII. These antigenic sites are present on von Willebrand factor and are another method of assaying VWF.

Table 3.22 highlights some of the main laboratory features of the more common hereditary bleeding disorders.

Haemophilia carriers and antenatal diagnosis

For many years carrier detection and antenatal diagnosis were based on measuring the ratio of factor VIII:c and VWF:Ag in plasma. Typically the female carrier has a 50% factor VIII:c level and a normal VWF level, giving a ratio of 0.5. However, the wide range in normal factor VIII levels and random inactivation of the X chromosome in female carriers (Lyonisation) makes accurate carrier detection difficult in many females. Recently, genetic methods using restriction length polymorphisms or specific gene probes have made diagnosis much more accurate but this depends on at least one affected patient being present in the kindred. These genetic techniques can be extended to first-trimester antenatal diagnosis on DNA samples obtained from chorionic villus biopsies.

Haemophilia B (Christmas disease) is diagnosed on the basis of a prolonged PTT and a low factor IX (procoagulant) level. Definitive carrier detection and antenatal diagnosis are dependent on molecular techniques.

Von Willebrand's disease

This condition combines abnormal platelet adhesion with reduced factor VIII activity. The laboratory features which make up a diagnosis include:

1) A prolonged bleeding time (although this is not always present and is not essential for the diagnosis)
2) Reduced levels of factor VIII:c
3) Reduced levels of VWF — a) measured immunologically as VWF:Ag, and b) defective platelet aggregation with ristocetin using a ristocetin-treated donor 'pool' platelet assay, VWF:RiCoF/VW:Act.

The laboratory parameters in mildly affected patients can very considerably and the diagnosis may not be definite despite repeated testing. Several sub-types have been described based on the multimeric structure of the factor VIII molecule. In Type I there is an overall quantitative reduction in the multimeric bands. In Type II there is a qualitative change in the multimeric bands and in the Type III (homozygous) form the bands are virtually absent. Multimeric factor VIII analysis requires specialist laboratory facilities.

CLINICAL ASSESSMENT AND DIAGNOSIS OF PAEDIATRIC SOLID TUMOURS

Without wishing to over-simplify the problem, it is usually the case that the diagnosis of paediatric oncological lesions is dependent upon the history and clinical examination followed by sophisticated imaging and surgical biopsy. Tables 3.23 and 3.24 list the chief presenting complaints and clinical signs and symptoms relating to the majority of paediatric malignancies.

A small percentage of paediatric tumours can however present in an unusual fashion. This has implications for subsequent investigations before a final diagnosis is made. Table 3.25 lists only a few of these unusual modes of presentation, if only to illustrate the many diverse ways in which childhood malignancy can present.

Table 3.23 **Common symptoms of childhood malignancy**	
Symptom	**Likely malignancy**
Fever and bone pain	Leukaemia, Ewing's sarcoma
Morning headache and vomiting	Brain tumour
Increasing localised lymphoma	Hodgkin's or non-Hodgkin's lymphadenopathy
Abdominal mass and swelling	Wilms tumour, neuroblastoma, hepatoma
Limp	Osteosarcoma or other bone tumour
Bone pain	Leukaemia, Ewing's sarcoma, neuroblastoma
Eye protrusion	Neuroblastoma, lymphoma, histiocytosis
Pallor and fatigue	Leukaemia and lymphoma
Vaginal bleeding	Rhabdomyosarcoma, yolk sac tumour
White dot in eye	Retinoblastoma
Swelling of face and neck	Lymphoma, Leukaemia
Chronic ear discharge	Histiocytosis, rhabdomyosarcoma

Table 3.24 **Differential diagnosis of the more common paediatric malignancies**		
Signs or symptoms	**Differential diagnosis**	**Malignancy**
Lymphadenopathy	Infection	Lymphoma
Bone pain	Trauma, infection	Bone tumour, leukaemia
Headache and vomiting	Sinusitis, migraine	Brain tumour
Mediastinal mass	Infection, cysts	Lymphoma
Abdominal mass	Renal cyst, constipation, bladder	Wilms tumour hepatoma
Bruising and bleeding	Coagulation and platelet disorders	Leukaemia

Table 3.25 **Unusual presentation of paediatric malignancy**

Malignancy	Uncommon presentation
Hodgkin's disease	Pruritus Eosinophilia Dermatomyositis
Non-Hodgkin's lymphoma	Hepatitis 'Transient' intra-cranial mass Superior mediastinal obstruction
Thymoma	Myasthenia gravis
Hepatic tumours	Thrombocytosis Erythrocytosis Inferior vena caval thrombosis
Wilms tumour	Beckwith syndrome WAGM syndrome
Rhabdomyosarcoma	Bronchial cysts Pericardial effusion
Brain tumours	Diencephalic syndrome
Ewing's sarcoma	Acute inflammatory syndrome Superior vena caval syndrome
Neuroblastoma	Skin nodules Hypertension Recurrent diarrhoea Lymphadenopathy
Acute lymphoblastic leukaemia	Juvenile arthritis Hypercalcaemia Acute renal failure Hypoplastic anaemia Haemophagocytic syndrome Myelofibrosis Cyclical neutropenia Bone marrow necrosis Skin nodules Pericardial effusion
Acute myeloid leukaemia	Chloroma Myelofibrosis Pericarditis Ovarian mass
Chronic myeloid leukaemia	Priapism

Imaging investigations in paediatric malignancy

Over the past few years the technological explosion in the field of diagnostic imaging has made the assessment of tumour size and spread much more accurate. Not all modalities are appropriate for each malignancy.

Imaging procedures and their merits The plain X-ray continues to play an essential role in the evaluation of children with malignant disease. It is fast, easy and relatively inexpensive, and requires no sedation. A plain chest X-ray is the first-line investigation for diagnosing thoracic lesions such as mediastinal masses, pulmonary metastases and pulmonary infections. Likewise, although abdominal X-rays will often be followed by CT scans, the plain film often reveals calcification and abnormal gas patterns, and may lead to a specific diagnosis.

CT and MRI scanning have to a large degree replaced barium studies, particularly as primary malignant involvement of the gastrointestinal tract is relatively uncommon in children (except possibly for non-Hodgkin's lymphoma).

Radioisotope bone scans may be positive before changes appear on skeletal films, but by the time patients become symptomatic changes are usually visible on plain X-rays.

The value of imaging methods is examined in Table 3.26.

CT and MRI scanning have become the backbone of neurological investigation. MRI is particularly useful for diagnosing intracranial lesions and also abnormalities of the spinal cord and meninges.

Biological markers and their applications in paediatric malignancy

The development of assays for determination of tumour markers has become increasingly important in the diagnosis, staging and follow-up of paediatric malignancies.

Neuroblastoma Dopamine and its metabolites VMA and HVA are often excreted in high amounts in neuroblastoma. The vast majority of patients show raised levels. In general, the more differentiated the tumour the lower the catecholamine levels. Although the prognostic value of the initial level is questionable, there is evidence that the speed of return to normal levels correlates with disease response.

Table 3.26	**Imaging methods and their value**				
	Plain X-ray	**Isotope**	**Ultrasound**	**CT**	**MRI**
Thoracic	3	1	1	7	6
Abdominal	2	4	5	8	7
Skeletal	3	5	1	6	7
Intracranial	1	3	1	7	7
Intraspinal	1	1	1	6	7

Scores on a scale of 1–10. Scores based on a composite evaluation of sensitivity, complication risk and cost.

The serum ferritin is also a useful marker in neuroblastoma. Levels at diagnosis are closely related to long-term prognosis. High levels are associated with active disease except in children with stage IVs disease who have normal levels.

Neurone-specific enolase is also a good marker, particularly in children with stage III and IV disease.

Amplification of the tumour oncogene N-myc appears to be relatively specific for neuroblastoma, and high-level amplification is more often seen in advanced cases.

Wilms tumour

The mucopolysaccharide hyaluronidase is raised in the serum of many patients with Wilms tumour. The concentration decreases rapidly with effective treatment. Many patients also show deletions of the short arm of chromosome 11. This is particularly seen in patients with aniridia.

Germ cell tumours

In children, the germ cell tumours as a group are embryonal carcinoma, yolk sac tumour, teratocarcinoma, choriocarcinoma, and mixed tumours. Alpha fetoprotein (AFP) is a useful marker. Levels may be grossly increased and a persistence of the protein with treatment is often associated with a suboptimal response. The degree of elevation of the serum AFP in different types of germ cell tumours depends on the extent of the yolk sac carcinoma element.

Human chorionic gonadotrophin (HCG) may be raised in embryonal tumours, and about 90% of children with non-seminomatous germ cell tumours, such as embryonal carcinoma, chorioncarcinoma and yolk sac tumours, have raised levels.

Hepatoblastoma/hepatocellular carcinoma

Hepatoblastoma, the commonest liver tumour in children, is nearly always associated with a raised AFP. Levels fall progressively with effective treatment, although there may be a transient small rise associated with hepatocyte regeneration after surgical resection. Serum ferritin levels are also raised in the majority of children with liver tumours, but measurement is probably of more use in monitoring therapy.

Biological markers have a definite role in paediatric oncology in both diagnosing and monitoring therapy. New markers are constantly being introduced but their value needs to be continually assessed. The newer molecular techniques relating to cytogenetics and tumour oncogenes may offer the greatest opportunity for more accurate tumour definition.

Conclusion

The investigation of children with haematological and oncological disorders has many similarities and also many differences when compared to adults, not least due to the fact that the spectrum of disease is very different. Over the past few years there have been major advances in diagnostic techniques, particularly in molecular genetics and imaging, but these must be used in parallel with more traditional methods. Finally it is vital that the tests suggested in this chapter are not used in isolation but in conjunction with all the appropriate diagnostic armamentarium available.

FURTHER READING

Oliveri, N.F. (1997) Thalassaemia. In: David T. (ed.) *Recent Advances in Pediatrics*. New York: Churchill Livingstone.
Wood, A.J.J. (1999) Management of sickle cell disease. *NEJM* 340: 1021–1030.

4
Endocrinology
P Bareille and R Stanhope

Normal physiology

THE ANTERIOR HYPOTHALAMIC – PITUITARY AXIS

To recognise and investigate clinical endocrine problems, it is essential to understand the complex physiological interrelations with and between endocrine organs. Figure 4.1 illustrates the interactions between the hypothalamus, the anterior pituitary gland and the peripheral (target) glands. The caption to Figure 4.1 describes the interactions in more detail.

POSTERIOR PITUITARY

The posterior pituitary releases two hormones: vasopressin (ADH) and oxytocin. Only ADH is clinically important in childhood. It plays a central role regarding water balance by causing the kidneys to retain water adequately in order to maintain plasma osmolarity constant.

Lack of ADH results in failure of the kidneys to concentrate urine appropriately (diabetes insipidus). The same phenomenon occurs when the kidneys fail to respond to ADH (nephrogenic diabetes insipidus).

THE ADRENAL GLANDS

Figure 4.2 illustrates the adrenal steroid biosynthetic pathway.

THE PARATHYROID GLAND

The parathyroid gland responds to changes in plasma calcium levels by adjusting its synthesis and release of PTH. Ionised calcium acts through a G protein-coupled receptor: the calcium sensing receptor.

PTH (parathyroid hormone) raises plasma calcium concentration directly by augmenting bone osteoclastic activity and tubular resorption of calcium, and indirectly by increasing synthesis of calcitriol (1–25(OH)D) by the kidneys. Calcitriol in turn stimulates absorption of calcium and phosphate in the intestine. Vitamin D hormone also plays an important role in the modelling of bones, and at high concentration augments osteoclastic activity.

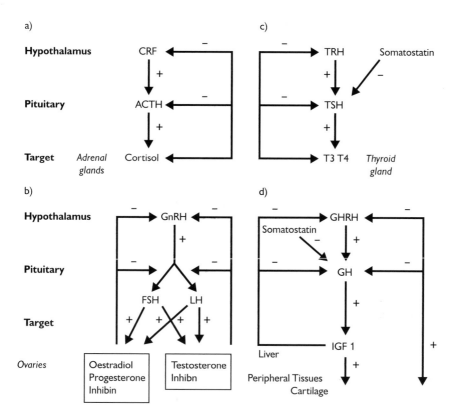

Fig. 4.1 **Schematic and simplified representation of the interactions between the hypothalamus, the anterior pituitary gland and the peripheral (target) glands. a) Hypothalamic-pituitary adrenal axis: CRF (corticotrophin-releasing hormone) stimulates the release of ACTH (corticotrophin) which stimulates cortisol secretion. Cortisol, in turn, exerts an inhibiting effect on ACTH and CRF secretion. b) hypothalamic-pituitary gonadal axis: GnRH (gonadotrophin-releasing hormone) stimulates LH and FSH release, which stimulate the gonads. Gonadal hormones in turn inhibit gonadotrophin and GnRH release. c) Hypothalamic-pituitary thyroid axis: TRH (thyrotrophin-releasing hormone) stimulates TSH (thyrotrophin) release, which stimulates thyroid hormones (T3, T4). Thyroid hormones in turn inhibit TSH and TRH release. Somatostatin inhibits TSH release. d) Somatotroph axis: GHRH (growth hormone-releasing hormone) stimulates GH production, which stimulates IGFI secretion by the liver. IGFI mediates part of the action of GH. IGFI inhibits GH and GHRH release. GH inhibits its own secretion and GHRH release. Somatostain inhibits GH release.**

MALE SEXUAL DIFFERENTIATION

Figure 4.3 and its caption illustrate the process of male sexual differentiation.

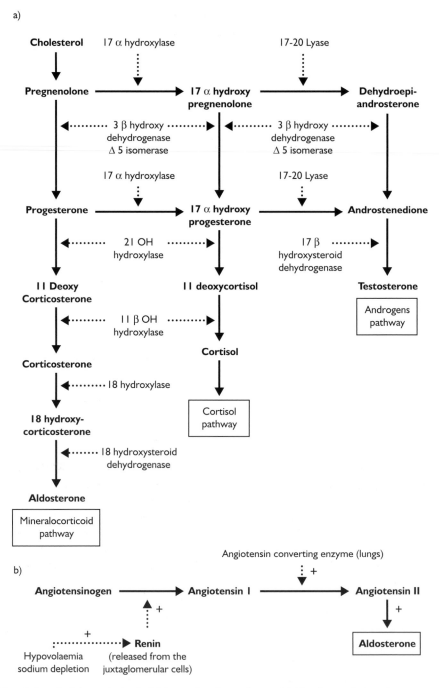

Fig. 4.2 **a) Adrenal steriod biosynthetic pathway. b) Renin-angiotensin system. Aldosterone secretion is stimulated by angiotensin II (ACTH plays a minor role) whose production is stimulated by the release of renin from the juxtaglomerular cells. + = stimulation.**

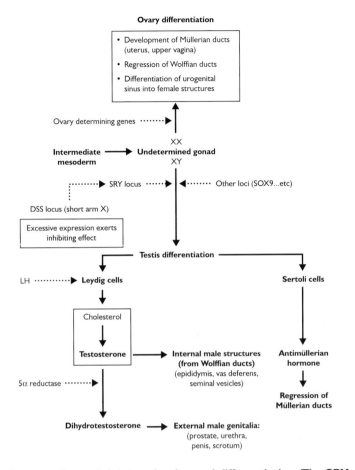

Fig. 4.3 **Process of gonadal determination and differentiation. The SRY gene
(Y chromosome) expressed in the undertermined gonad (probably in
coordination with other factors) causes differentiation of the testis. The testis, in
turn, produces testosterone (from Leydig cells) and antimüllerian hormone
(AMH) from Sertoli cells) which establish maleness. The differentiation of Leydig
cells might require LH, although the initial step seems to be gonadotrophin-
independent. AMH causes regression of müllerian structures (which otherwise
develop into fallopian tubes, uterus and upper vagina). Testosterone is
responsible for internal male structure development from Wolffian ducts. It is
converted into Dehydrotestosterone (DHT), a more potent androgen which
causes the development of external genitalia (prostate, urethra, penis, scrotum).
This differentiation can be disrupted at any level. Testosterone synthesis requires
several enzymes. Any of these enzymes can be deficient, thereby impairing
testosterone production. Testosterone conversion into DHT can be affected by
deficiency in the converting enzyme. Mutations of the androgen receptor gene
(located on the X chromosome) bring about androgen resistance. Duplication of
the short arm of the X chromosome (without the rest of the X chromosome) can
also be implicated in the absence of male differentiation (dosage-sensitive sex
reversal).**

List of tests

LABORATORY AND TOLERANCE TESTS

Somatotroph axis
    Growth hormone tests for deficiency
        Single measurement
        12- or 24-hour physiological
           secretion
        Urinary GH excretion
        Provocative test
        IGF1
        IGFBP3
    Growth hormone tests for excess
        Single measurement
        24-hour measurement
        Dynamic tests
        IGF1, IGFBP3

Adrenal function (cortex)
    Hypofunction
        Insulin tolerance test
        Synacthen tests
    Hyperfunction
        ACTH measurement
        Dexamethasone suppression
           tests
        CRF test

    CRF + DDAVP
    Metapyrone
Gonadotroph function
    Basal LH and FSH
    LHRH test
    HCG tests

Thyroid function
    Thyrotropin (TSH)
    T4 and T3
    THRH
    Thyroglobulin

Anterior pituitary
    Combined pituitary function test

Posterior pituitary
    Diabetes insipidus tests

IMAGING

X-rays
    Bone age
    Skeletal survey
MRI/CT scan
Thyroid scan
Uptake and perchlorate discharged tests

ABBREVIATIONS USED IN THIS CHAPTER

ACTH — adrenocorticotrophic hormone
ADH — vasopressin
AMH — antimüllerian hormone
CAH — congenital adrenal hyperplasia
CRF — corticotrophin releasing hormone
CS — Cushing syndrome
DHT — dehydrotestosterone
FHH — familial hypocalciuric hypercalcaemia
GHD — growth hormone deficiency
GHRH — growth hormone releasing hormone
GnRH — gonadotrophin releasing hormone

LMBS — Lawrence–Moon–Biedl syndrome
MEN — multiple endocrine neoplasia
MIBG — ^{131}I meta-iodobenzyl-guanidine scintigraphy
NSH — neonatal severe hyperparathyroidism
PP — precocious puberty
PRA — plasma renin activity
PTH — parathyroid hormone
PWS — Prader-Willi syndrome
SRY gene — Sex determining region Y chromosome
TRH — thyrotrophin releasing hormone
TSH — thyrotrophin stimulating hormone

Tests

LABORATORY AND TOLERANCE TESTS

When a high level of hormone is suggested a **suppression test** should be used, whereas a **stimulation test** is used in suspected low values.

A. Somatotroph axis

Growth hormone deficiency (GHD)

a) GH

- *Single measurement:* May be meaningless because of the pulsatile secretion but a high value excludes GHD.
- *12- or 24-hour physiological secretion*: It requires blood sampling every 15–20 min. The analysis evaluates GH concentration (mean of all GH measurements), the mean peak pulse amplitude, the frequency of pulsatile GH secretion and integrated secretion (area under the GH curve). The pattern of 24-hr GH secretion can be helpful in a short child with subnormal growth velocity but normal response to provocative tests. Nevertheless, there is significant overlap between the lower range of normal subjects and values reported in growth hormone deficiency. Hence, study results have been contradictory and have failed to establish a clear correlation between 24-hr secretion and auxological parameters.
- *Urinary GH excretion*: Not very useful for diagnosis, partly because there is considerable variability in urinary GH excretion over time.
- *Provocative test (see protocol)*: These are potentially dangerous and should be conducted by an experienced unit. They explore the ability of the pituitary gland to respond to an intercurrent stress event. The principle is to induce GH secretion by causing metabolic changes (e.g. hypoglycaemia) which usually occur in response to specific metabolic events.

A large number of stimuli are used in clinical practice and are usually pharmacological. Insulin-induced hypoglycaemia, glucagon, arginine, clonidine, L-dopa are some of the commonest tests used in practice. GHRH test may allow the clinician to distinguish between hypothalamic and pituitary defects. In patients at risk of hypoglycaemia and in young children the insulin test should be avoided. For young children, the glucagon test is an alternative, but possible rebound hypoglycaemia may occur because glucagon is a potent stimulant of insulin secretion.

GH secretion is particularly low in early puberty with poor response to provocative tests. At this age sex steroid priming may increase GH responsiveness and sensitivity of the tests. The cut-off limit of adequate response depends on the assay used to measure plasma GH. These tests are considered as the gold standard for diagnosing GHD. Nevertheless, they are not without flaws: they may not reflect the physiological endogenous secretion; the development of different immunoassays of GH coupled with many different tests of various degrees of reliability makes interpretation unclear; their reproducibility is uncertain; and the threshold value between GHD and normal response is purely empirical. Two or more tests in sequence or in combination may improve reliability.

b) IGFI

Low values suggest a growth disorder, not only GHD. For example, values reported in hypothyroidism, malnutrition, and even normal young children overlap with those found in hypopituitarism. Low IGF1 with elevated GH suggest GH resistance (Laron syndrome, anorexia nervosa).

c) IGFBP3

IGFBP3 is the major carrier protein for IGF1. It reflects GH status and is less dependent on other factors (e.g. age, thyroid hormones, nutrition) than IGF1 but is affected by liver failure. Nevertheless, it seems to be more specific than sensitive. It has been proposed as a screening test for GHD (in combination with IGF1) but further evaluation is necessary. IGFBP3 levels are low in GH insensitivity.

GH excess

a) GH

- *Single measurement*: A random high value may be seen in a normal subject if the sampling coincides with a GH pulse, and thereby is of limited interest. Non-detectable GH excludes the diagnosis.
- *24-hour measurement*: Can demonstrate persistently high levels. Pulsatile secretion may be exaggerated or blunted. This procedure is not usually conducted in clinical practice.
- *Dynamic tests*: The glucose tolerance test (see protocol) may be utilised in practice for investigating tall stature. Nevertheless, some patients with renal failure or diabetes may exhibit unsuppressed GH levels. It has also been suggested that the TRH test may be used for diagnostic purposes. Indeed, a paradoxical GH response is shown in pituitary gigantism. This test, however, lacks specificity as the response may be identical in some normal children during puberty.

b) IGFI and IGFBP3

High values usually correlate with excessive secretion of GH.

B. Adrenal function (cortex)

General points

- There is diurnal variation in plasma cortisol concentration with highest values in the morning (peak around 06.00 hours) and lowest values at night (trough around midnight). Hence, random measurement is not of great interest. Nevertheless, this circadian variation does not exist before the age of 3–6 months.
- 95% of cortisol is normally bound to protein (transcortin) and very little free cortisol is excreted. Augmentation of cortisol production causes increased free cortisol excretion because the capacity of transcortin is rapidly exceeded. Hence, 24-hr urinary free cortisol level is a sensitive means of detecting Cushing's syndrome.
- All steroid treatments other than dexamethasone or betamethasone cross-react with cortisol (in the assay); hydrocortisone therapy should therefore have been

stopped for at least 12 hours prior to the tests and prednisolone or prednisone for at least 3 days. Dexamethasone can provide steroid cover.

Hypofunction

Insulin tolerance test: the cortisol response to hypoglycaemia is the only test of adrenal function validated against the response to surgical stress. It tests the whole hypothalamo–pituitary–adrenal axis.

Synacthen tests (see protocols)**:** they explore the ability of the adrenal glands to respond to a high dose of exogenous ACTH. Three synacthen tests can be performed: standard short, modified (physiological), and prolonged. They are indicated in suspected adrenal insufficiency (primary and secondary) and in suspected CAH.

- The short test will not detect minor degrees of adrenal suppression.
- The modified test using a lower dose (of ACTH) can reveal more subtle variation of adrenal impairment.
- The long test is particularly indicated if secondary adrenal failure is suspected. It explores the ability of the dormant (more or less atrophic) adrenal gland to be reactivated by repeated ACTH stimulation.

Hyperfunction

ACTH measurement: demonstrates a distinction between corticotrophin-independent Cushing's (adrenal tumour) and corticotrophin-dependent Cushing's (Cushing's disease and ectopic Cushing's syndrome).

Dexamethasone suppression tests (see protocols)**:** dexamethasone is a synthetic glucocorticoid which normally suppresses ACTH release and thereby cortisol secretion.

CRF test: evaluates the ACTH and cortisol response to CRF. It is useful for discriminating between ectopic ACTH (no response since the tumour has no CRF receptor) and Cushing's disease (normal or exaggerated response).

CRF + DDAVP: a variant of the CRF test. DDAVP may increase CRF reaction in Cushing's disease.

Metapyrone: blocks the conversion of 11 deoxycortisol which in turn causes ACTH stimulation. The response leads to elevated plasma 11 deoxycortisol and increased urine 17 hydroxycorticosteroid excretion. Typically a positive response is observed in Cushing's disease and no response in ectopic and adrenal tumours. The test is hazardous (risk of acute adrenal failure) and not technically easy.

C. Gonadotroph function

Basal LH and FSH: can discriminate between primary (high values) and secondary gonadal failure (low values).

LHRH test (see protocol)**:** It tests the ability of the pituitary gland to secrete FSH and LH in response to LHRH. It is indicated in precocious puberty and delayed sexual maturation. It is of limited value in hypopituitarism, ambiguous genitalia, bilateral cryptorchidism. This test is valueless between the ages of 6 months and 10 years except in premature sexual maturation.

HCG tests (see protocol)**:** To evaluate the secretion of testosterone by the testis, *two tests can be performed*: 3 days stimulation test (short test) and 3 weeks stimulation test (long test). They are indicated in the circumstances in which testis function may be affected: cryptorchidism, ambiguous genitalia, delayed puberty, testosterone biosynthetic defect, 5α reductase deficiency. The long test is more specifically indicated in hypogonadotrophic hypogonadism with bilateral cryptorchidism. It may also be used for facilitating the descent of the testis (this point is however controversial) or increasing the size of the phallus.

D. Thyroid function

Thyrotropin (TSH): Thyrotropin is probably the most sensitive marker of *primary* thyroid dysfunction; in primary hypothyroidism it is the first marker to be disturbed with raised values before detection of a decrease in T4. However, after commencing substitutive treatment TSH may take longer than thyroid hormones to normalise. This phenomenon is probably due to a higher negative feed-back set point. Subsequently when it has returned to normal, TSH is a reliable detector of inadequate treatment. Sensitive assays can detect very low levels (<0.5 μU/L) characteristic of hyperthyroidism.

T4 and T3: Free hormone levels need to be measured instead of total hormone levels; total thyroid hormone concentration is too dependent upon binding protein concentrations which are affected in numerous pathological or physiological situations. However, one should remain aware that the measurement of free hormones may be technically problematic. Usually fT4 is a more sensitive marker of hypofunction than fT3, which can be normal in mild hypothyroidism. Free T3 is on the other hand sensitive in detecting hyperthyroidism and can in some cases be the only hormone elevated (T3 thyrotoxicosis). In severe illnesses or malnutrition, there is reduced conversion of T4 to T3. T4 is normal (but may become low as well as TSH) whilst fT3 is low. The disturbance is termed the 'euthyroid sick syndrome'. Values vary according to age. In the premature or in low birth-weight syndrome the levels are lower than in term infants. Figure 4.4 illustrates variations in T4, T3, rT3 and TSH concentrations in relation to age.

TRH test (see protocol)**:** tests the ability of the pituitary gland to secrete TSH. It is indicated in suspected hypopituitarism (secondary hypopituitarism) and in equivocal hyperthyroidism (e.g.: normal fT3/fT4 and low TSH). It may allow the clinician to distinguish between hypothalamic (tertiary) and pituitary (secondary) hypothyroidism.

Thyroglobulin: detection of plasma thyroglobulin in congenital hypothyroidism demonstrates the presence of thyroid tissue. It is also useful in the monitoring of differentiated thyroid cancer, post total thyroidectomy.

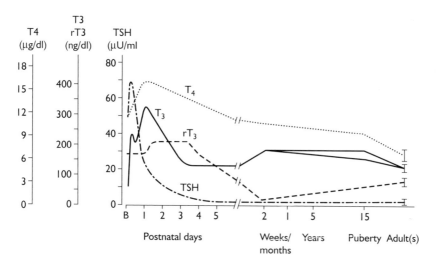

Fig. 4.4   Variations in thyroid hormones (T4, T3, rT3 and thyrotrophin stimulating hormone (TSH) concentrations in relation to age. Reproduced with permission from Ranke (1992).

E. Anterior pituitary

Combined pituitary function test: The assessment of GH and cortisol secretion (ITT or glucagon) is combined simultaneously with TRH and LHRH test. The ITT and glucagon test the hypothalamo–pituitary–peripheral axis, whereas the TRH and LHRH tests evaluate the pituitary–peripheral axis. The detailed procedures of each of these tests are described separately in the relevant sections. It should be stressed that patients with suspected hypopituitarism cannot cope appropriately with hypoglycaemia. Hydrocortisone IV 100 mg should be prepared before testing and kept by the patient's bed ready for injection. High concentrations of glucose (25% or more) should NOT be used for resuscitation.

F. Posterior pituitary

Diabetes insipidus is characterised by failure to adequately concentrate the urine. A single urine morning sample coupled with a blood sample may often suffice for the diagnosis: if the urine osmolality:plasma osmolality ratio > 1.5 or urine osmolality >750 mosm/kg, diabetes insipidus is excluded.

Otherwise a water deprivation test is indicated under careful surveillance (see protocol) followed by DDAVP administration to distinguish between nephrogenic and hypothalamic diabetes insipidus. DDAVP should not be given if the child has concentrated his urine normally. If the results are equivocal, measurements of plasma ADH coupled with plasma osmolality can be useful for establishing the diagnosis. Before any assessment of posterior pituitary function, cortisol deficiency should be sought and adequately replaced as cortisol is needed to excrete a water load.

IMAGING

X-rays

Bone age

Routinely used in paediatric endocrinology, the bone age is measured on a simple X-ray of the left hand and wrist. It is based upon the appearance and the maturity of the epiphyseal centres compared to the metaphysis. Bone age is aimed at providing an estimation of the growth potential and thereby predicting final stature at the time of assessment. Different methods have been established: the methods of Greulich and Pyle, and of Tanner and Whitehouse are the most widely used. Subsequently, prediction is based on either the Bailey and Pinneau or Tanner–Whitehouse methods, each having its advantages and disadvantages. The Tanner method is more precise and the method of choice in the UK, although it may not be reliably applicable in some pathological or extreme situations, notably in disorders such as skeletal dysplasia or Turner syndrome. Long-term high doses of glucocorticoid treatment can produce an artefact which leads to underestimation of the bone age and consequently an over-estimation of final height. Bone age is particularly useful in premature sexual maturation, at the time of diagnosis and for the follow-up (excessive advancement of the bone age indicates inadequacy of the treatment). In short and tall stature the estimation of bone age is important but the final height prediction may not always be reliable.

Skeletal survey

Skeletal survey is essentially indicated when there is suspicion of skeletal dysplasia (disproportionate short stature), rickets, pseudohypoparathyroidism and McCune–Albright syndrome. Unfortunately subtle skeletal dysplasia can be difficult to diagnose, especially at a very young age when most of the skeleton is not ossified; the survey may therefore need to be repeated.

MRI/CT-scan

To scan the hypothalamo–pituitary region, the MRI-scan provides the most accurate information. The CT is a satisfactory alternative if the MRI cannot be performed. They are chiefly aimed at excluding the presence of a tumour. Structural and morphological abnormalities are also sought which can be isolated or associated with other brain anomalies, notably mid-line defects. Optic nerves and chiasma hypoplasia, absent septum pellucidum and pituitary aplasia are typical of the septo–optic dysplasia syndrome. Holoprosencephaly and dysplasia of the cerebellum are some other examples of malformations associated with hypopituitarism. The presence of a small pituitary gland (measurable by MRI) may support the diagnosis of growth hormone insufficiency when the test results are equivocal.

Thyroid scan

Technetium-99m pertechnetate (^{99m}-Tc) is the common radio-isotope utilised to visualise the thyroid gland. It is concentrated by the thyroid but is not incorporated into thyroid hormone. Radio-iodine, ^{131}I, however, is utilised in hormonogenesis and will demonstrate dyshormonogenesis.

Uptake and perchlorate discharged tests

These tests are indicated when an inborn error of hormonogenesis is suspected. The first step consists of the administration of radio-iodine (^{131}I) to study thyroid iodide uptake over time, early and late uptake corresponding to iodide trapping followed by iodide organification and release. Mean 24-hour uptake is variable, usually 15%–30%, with half of this in the first 6–8 hours. Subsequently oral perchlorate, an I-competitor, is given which blocks iodide uptake. Normally less than 10% of the total radio-iodine measured at the time of perchlorate administration is released. In dyshormonogenesis there is rapid and excessive uptake followed by considerable discharge after perchlorate. In iodide transport defect there is no radio-iodine uptake and therefore the perchlorate test should not be performed.

Clinical problems

I. GROWTH FAILURE

Growth failure is defined as persistently slow growth velocity for age over a period of one year or more, or loss of the normal relationship between growth acceleration and puberty.

Important points

1. Investigations should be guided by the clinical study of the child, auxological criteria and the family history.
2. Any chronic disease or ill-treatment can cause growth failure.
3. Short stature is a prominent feature of common syndromes, e.g. Turner syndrome, Noonan syndrome, Russel–Silver syndrome, Prader–Willi syndrome, Down syndrome and other chromosomal abnormalities.
4. Unless there is an obvious disorder, careful documentation of growth velocity over a period of at least 6 months should be obtained before prompting investigations. Growth rate deceleration is a better indicator of an ongoing disorder than short stature in itself. Thus, a child who is short but growing at a normal rate should NOT be tested for GHD whereas a child whose height is within the normal range but with subnormal growth velocity may have GHD.
5. A healthy child who is short but with a normal growth rate is likely to have constitutional short stature, especially if there is retarded bone age (delay in growth) and/or short parents (familial short stature). Apart from a bone age, no further investigations are necessary. The predicted final height is usually in line with the target height.
6. Children affected with constitutional delay in growth and puberty usually exhibit subnormal growth velocity at the normal age for puberty. No investigations are needed.
7. Very short parents (below 3SD) should be referred to an adult endocrinologist to be investigated as well.

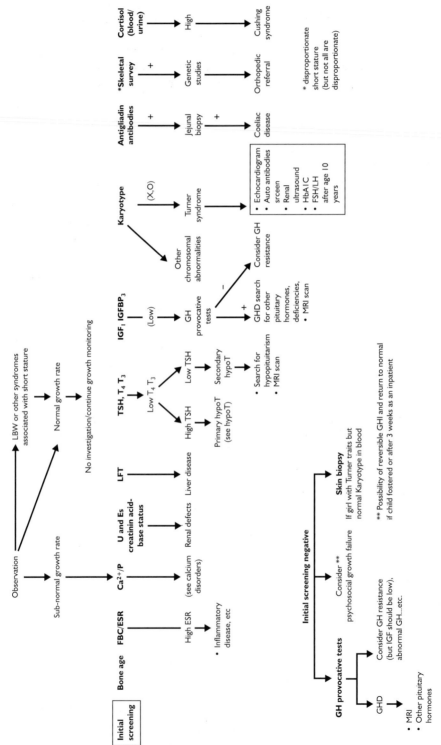

Fig. 4.5 **The route of investigations in short stature. + = positive findings.**

8. History of cranial irradiation and/or other pituitary hormone deficiencies and/or visual field defects accompanying subnormal growth velocity strongly suggest GHD.

9. The diagnosis of GHD is usually based on subnormal growth rate associated with a stunted response to a provocative test. When GHD has been identified, imaging studies of the hypothalamo–pituitary region (MRI or CT scan) must complete the investigations.

The route of investigations into short stature is illustrated in Figure 4.5.

2. TALL STATURE

Important points

1. Constitutional tall stature is by far the commonest cause of tall stature.
2. Otherwise tall stature is more often due to an underlying syndrome (e.g. Marfan's syndrome, Soto's syndrome or homocystinuria) than an endocrinopathy.
3. Investigations are performed when clinically appropriate or there is need to exclude:
   - pituitary gigantism: can be either isolated or part of a complex syndrome as MENI or McCune–Albright syndrome
   - thyrotoxicosis
   - precocious puberty
   - others: Marfan's homocystinuria, Soto's.

Investigations in tall stature are listed in the information box.

INVESTIGATIONS IN TALL STATURE

- IGFI, IGFBP3: elevated values in pituitary gigantism
- Oral glucose tolerance test
- Thyroid function
- PRL: may be high in pituitary gigantism
- Karyotype for XXY or XXX (if suspected)
- If pituitary gigantism suspected: search for other hormonal anomalies
- Hand X-ray: for metacarpal index (Marfan's syndrome)
- MRI scan (brain) if pituitary gigantism
- Echocardiography and ophthalmic examination if suspicion of Marfan's syndrome: look for aortic root dilatation and other cardiac abnormalities as well as dislocated lens or spherophakia
- If appropriate: LHRH, testosterone, oestradiol, 170 hydroxyprogesterone
- DNA studies (McCune–Albright syndrome).

---

3. PREMATURE SEXUAL MATURATION

Premature sexual maturation is defined as the onset of secondary sexual characteristics before the ages of 8 years in girls and 9 years in boys.

Important points

1. Clinical examination and history are highly informative and investigations should be aimed at:
   - demonstrating puberty (pubertal levels of testosterone in boys and of oestrogen in girls, values according to pubertal stage) and thereby excluding adrenarche or thelarche (points 4 and 5).
   - distinguishing between gonadotrophin-dependent precocious puberty or PP (pubertal response to LHRH with increase in LH/FSH) and gonadotrophin-independent precocious puberty (LH/FSH suppressed). (The latter can also trigger onset of the former.)
   - identifying the underlying aetiology (points 2 and 3).
2. Gonadotrophin-dependent PP is usually caused by an underlying intracranial pathology in boys whilst often idiopathic in girls.
3. Gonadotrophin-independent PP results frequently from constitutive activation of Gsα protein (McCune–Albright syndrome, combined PP and pseudohypoparathyroidism Ia) or of the G-protein dependent receptor (familial male PP).
4. In thelarche (isolated premature breast development) FSH levels may be elevated but LH levels are low with a prepubertal response to LHRH. Pelvic ultra-

---

INVESTIGATIONS IN PREMATURE SEXUAL MATURATION

- Bone age
- Basal testosterone and oestradiol (testosterone should be measured in the middle of the night and oestradiol after breakfast)
- 17OHP, androstenedione, and dehydroepiandrosterone. Short synacthen test if equivocal results to diagnose atypical CAH
- LHRH test
- Pelvic ultrasound
- MRI scan (brain): obligatory in boys (and very young girls before 2–3 years of age) with gonadotrophin-dependent PP. Search for intracranial pathology, especially tumours
- DNA studies: when gonadotrophin-independent PP (see point 3 above)
- In gonadotrophin-independent PP a further investigation should seek other disorders linked to the G protein pathway, notably other neuroendocrine abnormalities (e.g. in McCune–Albright syndrome: thyrotoxicosis, acromegaly, Cushing's syndrome; in combined PP and hypoparathyroidism, hypocalcaemia, hypothyroidism).

sound may show isolated ovarian cysts and a uterus which is slightly enlarged. There is no significant advancement of bone age.

5. The isolated development of pubic hair, axillary hair and body odour (all the more where there is associated excessive virilisation) suggests excessive androgen secretion. Investigations should be performed with a view to excluding CAH or an androgen-secreting tumour, although in most cases it is merely premature adrenarche. In the latter case bone age can only be slightly advanced and growth rate is not significantly accelerated.

Investigations in premature sexual maturation are listed in the information box.

4. DELAYED SEXUAL MATURATION

Defined as the absence of the onset of pubertal development (breast stage 2 in girls and testis volume ≥ 4 ml in boys) at 2 SD from the timing of normal puberty.

Important points

1. On average puberty starts at around the age of 11 years in girls and 12 years in boys but the 'normal' range can extend up to the ages of 13.5 years in girls and 14 years in boys. Usually, apart from a bone age, there is no need for intervention or investigations before these ages unless there is an associated disorder (e.g. Turner's syndrome, GHD, etc.). Nevertheless, in practice the adolescent or the parents may exert pressure to intervene earlier for psychological reasons. It may be necessary to trigger the first pubertal changes or accelerate the natural process if puberty has started but with slow progress, by giving a small amount of sex steroid for 6 months to 1 year. If no response, or if after stopping the treatment no further progress occurs, investigations should be performed.

INVESTIGATIONS IN DELAYED SEXUAL MATURATION

- Bone age
- Olfaction assessment (panels of various odours available) for Kallman syndrome
- Thyroid function tests
- LHRH test
- hCG test
- Karyotype: genetic sex, Turner's syndrome, Klinefelter's, XYY syndrome...
- Pelvic ultrasound (in girls)
- MRI scan
- DNA studies: Kallman syndrome, X-linked adrenal hypoplasia congenita, etc.

---

2. Investigations are aimed at
   - distinguishing between primary gonadal failure (hypergonadotrophic hypogonadism with high FSH/LH) and defects at the hypothalamo–pituitary level (hypogonadotrophic hypogonadism with low FSH/LH)
   - identifying the underlying aetiology.
3. It may be difficult to discriminate definitely between delayed puberty and hypogonadotrophic hypogonadism, although generally in the latter case there is no response to LHRH whereas there is a blunted response in the former. The hCG test may be helpful.
4. Delayed puberty may reveal intersex conditions (e.g. androgen insensitivity) or late presenting (partial) enzyme deficiencies (e.g. 17α hydroxylase deficiency, 17β-hydroxysteroid dehydrogenase deficiency) or Turner's syndrome.

Investigations are listed in the information box.

5. GENITAL AMBIGUITY

Important points

1. The diagnosis and management of a disorder of sexual differentiation is extremely complex; the affected child should be referred to a specialised centre for a multidisciplinary approach.
2. The sex of rearing and the subsequent management ought to take into account the genetic, gonadal and phenotypic sex, which are established in three sequential steps.
   - Genetic sex → Sex chromosomes, SRY → Karyotype, DNA studies
   - Gonadal sex → Testicles, ovaries, ovotestis → Ultrasound, laparoscopy, biopsy
   - Phenotypic sex → External and internal genitalia → Clinical examination, ultrasound, genitography, laparoscopy.
3. The route of investigations to follow is determined by the above findings. A defect can occur at any level (see figure 4.3).
4. Female pseudo-hermaphroditism (excessive masculinisation in the presence of ovaries) initially suggests congenital adrenal hyperplasia.
5. A male XY with micropenis and small/undescended testis may suffer from hypopituitarism (see Hypopituitarism).

Investigations are given in the information box.

INVESTIGATIONS IN GENITAL AMBIGUITY

- Careful examination (in search of palpable gonads), a karyotype, a pelvic ultrasound (to look for gonads and Müllerian structures), 17OH progesterone (when virilised female) and an hCG test (if suspicion of testicular tissue) are usually sufficient initially. Hypopituitarism should be excluded in an XY male with micropenis and/or undescended testis (see Hypopituitarism).

- Subsequent investigations will be determined by the results of the above tests.

6. Obesity

Important points

Investigations are performed with two objectives:

— differentiating 'idiopathic' obesity from secondary obesity, notably Cushing syndrome, Prader–Willi syndrome (PWS), Lawrence–Moon–Biedl syndrome (LMBS) and hypothalamic obesity
— seeking complications, e.g. non-insulin-dependent diabetes.

Investigations are listed in the information box

INVESTIGATIONS IN OBESITY

- Cushing's syndrome screening: diurnal plasma cortisol and 24-hr urine cortisol excretion

- Thyroid function tests

- Glucose tolerance test with measurement of insulin levels

- DNA studies (analysis of chromosome 15 for Prader–Willi syndrome)

- Hypothalamo–pituitary imaging if suspicion of hypothalamic obesity

- Ophthalmology, gonadal function in LMBS

- In PWS: look for associated GHD and LHRH/hCG tests to assess gonadal function

- Energy expenditure (indirect calorimetry).

---

7. Goitre

Important points

1. A goitre may be accompanied by normal as well as hypo or hyper function of the thyroid.
2. A congenital goitre
   - is present in dyshormonogenesis or iodide trapping defects
   - may be the consequence of antithyroid drugs or iodides taken during the pregnancy
   - is rarely the consequence of thyrotropin receptor mutations.
3. Endemic goitres are seen in countries with poor natural source of iodine and no salt supplementation.
4. A sporadic goitre
   - is usually induced by an autoimmune disorder: it is diffuse, firm with an irregular surface and can be asymmetric
   - can be induced by excessive iodine intake or goitrogens
   - rarely can be acute or subacute after bacterial or viral infection, followed by complete regression after treatment or spontaneously (acute bacterial thyroiditis and subacute non suppurative thyroiditis)

- can be purely isolated ('idiopathic' or 'colloid'). It is soft, small and homogeneous
- A multinodular goitre is rare in childhood; sometimes seen in McCune–Albright syndrome
- Should point to the suspicion of malignancy if single nodule and in families affected with MEN 2 (medullary thyroid carcinoma).

Investigations in goitre are given in the box.

INVESTIGATIONS IN GOITRE

- fT3, fT4 and TSH

- Ultrasound and thyroid scan (Technetium or ^{131}I), indicated when a tumour is suspected

- Needle biopsy when (isolated) cold nodule

- In families affected by MEN: plasma calcitonin, DNA analysis (RET gene). (Screening biochemical tests are beyond the scope of this book.)

- Urinary 24-hr iodine if suspicion of insufficient or excessive iodine intake.

See for further details section on hypo- and hyperthyroidism.

---

8. Hypoglycaemia

Hypoglycaemia is defined as a blood glucose below 2.4 mmol/l regardless of age.

Important points

1. The metabolic pathways of energy production and utilisation are hormone-controlled processes closely co-ordinated in order to maintain glucose haemostasis. Hypoglycaemia occurs when key enzymes involved in these pathways are deficient or defective or when the close balance between gluco-regulatory hormones is disturbed.
2. Infants and young children are at high risk of having problems with fasting because their energy needs are particularly high, and several key enzymes involved in the energy pathways have reduced activity at this age.
3. The commonest endocrine and metabolic reasons for hypoglycaemia in children are: hyperinsulinism, hypopituitarism and liver disease. However, failure to identify a precise cause is common; many of these cases (because of the laboratory findings) are labelled as 'ketotic hypoglycaemia'.
4. Clinical data and family history may initially narrow the investigations down. For example, presence of a micropenis and a cleft palate suggest hypopituitarism, hepatomegaly suggests a defect in gluconeogenesis, glycogenesis or galactosaemia, etc.
5. The diagnosis requires measurement of hormones and metabolite intermediates at the time of hypoglycaemia.

Investigations in hypoglycaemia are listed in the information box.

INVESTIGATIONS IN HYPOGLYCAEMIA

- Initially *24-hr glucose profile*. Blood glucose measurements hourly and if chemical symptoms related to hypoglycaemia. If hypoglycaemia, collect blood specimens for metabolites and hormones (same as fast test if possible). At least GH, cortisol, insulin, ketones, NEFA (free fatty acid) should be measured. A urine specimen ought also to be collected (first urine output following the hypoglycaemic episode) and assayed for organic acids, galactose, fructose and ketones.

- A diagnostic *provocative fast* (see protocol) is the next stage if spontaneous hypoglycaemia cannot be documented. A fast procedure necessitates careful surveillance and strict guidelines. It should ONLY be performed in a specialist unit, for safety reasons. The test is particularly hazardous in β oxidation defects. Analysis of blood acylcarnitines prior to fasting may detect these defects, avoiding fasting tests in this situation. In addition to providing information regarding aetiology, a fast test may allow the clinician to determine how long the child can fast without danger.

- The *glucagon provocation test* may be useful in glycogen storage diseases and hyperinsulinism. An appropriate response to glucagon requires adequate glycogen stores, and glucagon stimulates insulin secretion. In glycogenesis there is no increase in glucose level whereas in hyperinsulinism there is an excessive hyperglycaemic response followed by an exaggerated rebound hypoglycaemia. Other tolerance tests to assess other (rare) defects (e.g. fructose-1,6 diphosphatase, etc.) are beyond the scope of this chapter.

- *Imaging studies, enzyme assays (on biopsies)* and *DNA studies* are performed according to the suspected diagnosis.

9. GYNAECOMASTIA

Gynaecomastia is enlargement of the male breast.

Important points

1. The commonest form is pubertal gynaecomastia, which can affect more than 60% of boys. When isolated in a healthy pubertal boy, it does not require any investigation, only reassurance. There is usually spontaneous regression.
2. It may be associated with genital ambiguity and can reveal some intersex conditions such as 17α hydroxylase deficiency.
3. Gynaecomastia occurs frequently in hypogonadism. Notably it is a common feature of Klinefelter's syndrome.
4. On the other hand, it can accompany conditions associated with excessive androgen production by interstitial cell tumours of the testis (hCG secreting tumours which in turn stimulate Leydig cells) or adrenal disorders.
5. Gynaecomastia can be the consequence of feminising adrenal tumours or oestrogen-secreting tumours of the testis.

6. The condition can be induced by several medications (e.g. ketoconazole, spironolactone), exogenous androgens or oestrogens.
7. A non-endocrine tumour of the breast is usually unilateral.

Investigations are set out in the information box.

INVESTIGATIONS IN GYNAECOMASTIA

- Screening

  — Thyroid function (thyroid dysfunction can be associated with gynaeco-mastia)
  — FSH, LH, testosterone, oestradiol, dehydroepiandrosterone
  — PRL (rarely directly involved)
  — hCG measurement
  — Karyotype
  — Ultrasound (if unilateral)

- Further investigations determined by screening results.

---

10. CALCIUM DISORDERS

Maintenance of calcium homeostasis is due to the co-ordinated action of hormones (PTH, vitamin D and calcitonin) interacting with target organs (bones, kidneys, parathyroid and intestine). Defects affecting these hormones (PTH or vitamin D but apparently not calcitonin), or impairment in the target organs' function (kidneys and parathyroid) lead to disruption of calcium homeostasis (hypo or hypercalcaemia). Only the ionised fraction of calcium is active. Total plasma calcium level should be corrected according to the albumin level.

1. if [albumin] <40 g/l. Corrected calcium (mmol/ml) = [ca] + 0.02 × {40−[alb]}
2. if [albumin] >45. Corrected calcium = [ca] − 0.02 × {[alb] − 45}

Hypocalcaemia (calcium level <2.25 mmol/l or ionised calcium <1.2 mmol/l)

Important points in hypocalcaemia
Hypocalcaemia is commonly caused by hypoparathyroidism, vitamin D deficiency and renal impairment. Primary hypomagnesaemia and isolated calcium deficiency can also bring about hypocalcaemia.

1. *Hypoparathyroidism* may be isolated or part of a complex syndrome. It can be inherited with various patterns of inheritance. It can be caused by
   - Glandular failure (developmental defects, autoimmune disorders, mitochondrial disorders, post thyroidectomy damage): low calcium, high phosphate, low PTH, normal 25(OH)D, normal or low 1,25 (OH)$_2$D.
   - PTH deficiency (absence of *or* abnormal PTH of genetic cause): low calcium, high phosphate, low PTH, normal 25(OH)D, normal or low 1,25(OH)$_2$D.
   - PTH resistance (pseudohypoparathyroidism): low calcium, high phosphate, high PTH, normal 25(OH)D, low or normal 1,25(OH)$_2$D.

- Calcium-sensing receptor gene mutation: Low calcium, normal or high phosphate, inappropriately normal PTH.

2. *Vitamin D deficiency* causes rickets. It can be caused by:
   - Insufficient intake (dietary, malabsorption, insufficient exposure to sunlight): Vitamin D-deficient rickets. Normal or low calcium, low phosphate, high PTH, low 25(OH)D, normal or low or high (due to secondary hyperparathyroidism) 1–25(OH)$_2$D.
   - Vitamin D metabolism disorders: 1α hydroxylase deficiency in vit D-dependent rickets type 1. Low calcium, low phosphate, high PTH, normal 25(OH)D, low 1,25(OH)$_2$D. Disorder of 1α hydroxylase in renal impairment (see Chapter 5 nephrology). 25 hydroxylase deficiency (same biology as in deficient rickets).
   - Vitamin D resistance: Vit D-dependent rickets type 2. Low calcium, low phosphate, high PTH, normal 25(OH)D, high 1,25(OH)$_2$D.
   - Hypophosphataemia: X-linked hypophosphatemic rickets, phosphate deficiency, renal tubular disorders. Usually: low phosphate, normal calcium, normal 25(OH)D, normal or low 1,25(OH)$_2$D, normal PTH. Other rare forms of familial autosomal hypophosphatemic rickets are associated with hypercalciuria.

3. *Isolated calcium deficiency* can cause rickets. Normal 25(OH)D and high 1,25(OH)$_2$D, low calcium.

4. Neonatal hypocalcaemia is common. Early transient neonatal hypocalcaemia characteristic of premature infants is the commonest form. Investigations are not necessary. Late neonatal hypocalcaemia (within the first 2 months) is usually due to transient hypoparathyroidism.

Key points in calcium disorders

1. 25(OH)D measurement is more useful than 1,25(OH)$_2$D for distinguishing between hypoparathyroidism (normal value) and rickets (low value). 1,25(OH)$_2$D is only necessary and useful for the diagnosis of rickets type 2.

2. High PTH with low plasma calcium concentration demonstrates secondary hyperparathyroidism (rickets or renal failure).

3. Alkaline phosphatase activity is usually normal in hypoparathyroidism and always increased in rickets.

Hypercalcaemia (calcium level >2.75 mm/l or ionised calcium >2.4 mm/l)

Hypercalcaemia is chiefly due to primary hyperparathyroidism. Cancer is a rare cause in children.

Important points

1. Excessive production of PTH by parathyroid tumours or parathyroid hyperplasia. It is characterised by: high calcium, low P, high PTH and cAMP, normal 25(OH)D and normal or high 1,25(OH)$_2$D. The disorder can either be isolated or more frequently be part of a multiple endocrine neoplasia syndrome (MEN). These conditions are mostly inherited with an autosomal dominant pattern. It can also be part of a complex malformative syndrome.

INVESTIGATIONS IN CALCIUM DISORDERS

General screen

— Renal function, albumin, assessment of renal tubular function

— Calcium, phosphate, magnesium: plasma and urine

— Alkaline phosphatase activity

— Intact PTH

— Vitamin D: 25(OH)D, (1,25(OH₂D)

— Skeletal survey (for rickets and pseudohypoparathyroidism)

— Chest X-ray (to look for thymus)

— Urine cAMP: high in rickets, low in hypo and pseudohypoparathyroidism

— Autoimmune screening

— Cortisol (plasma, urine)

Specific investigations (conducted in a specialist unit)

- In pseudohypoparathyroidism: PTH infusion test. Distinguishes between pseudohypoparathyroidism I (no rise in cAMP and urinary P) and pseudo-hypoparathyroidism II (elevated basal and post stimulation cAMP and no rise in P). In pseudohypoparathyroidism I, search for associated hormonal dysfunctions (thyroid, glucagon, gonadotrophins, etc.)

- In DiGeorge syndrome: echocardiography, immune function and DNA studies (usually deletions of the proximal long arm of chromosome 22)

- Relating to the specific syndrome (e.g. association of hypoparathyroidism, deafness and renal dysplasia — skeletal survey and ophthalmologic assessment in Kenney–Caffey syndrome, etc.)

- In isolated hypoparathyroidism: DNA studies (PTH gene, X-linked para-thyroid gene, calcium-sensing receptor gene, etc. with familial screening)

- In autoimmune hypoparathyroidism: look for Addison, hypothyroidism, per-nicious anaemia, etc., as well as DNA analysis

- In rickets: DNA studies (Vitamin D receptor in rickets type 2), renal tubular function

---

2. Mutations of the calcium-sensing receptor are responsible for familial hypocalciuric hypercalcaemia (FHH) and neonatal severe hyperparathyroidism (NSH). FHH is the heterozygous form, is asymptomatic and is characterised by: moderate hypercalcaemia, low urine calcium excretion and inappropri-ately normal PTH. NSH is the homozygous form, is fatal if untreated and is characterised by very high PTH and calcium levels.

3. Hypercalcaemia in cancers may be due to extensive bone destruction or caused by secretion by the tumour of vitamin D- or PTH-related protein. Abnormal synthesis of vitamin D can also occur in sarcoidosis.
4. Moderate hypercalcaemia can be seen in thyrotoxicosis and Addison's disease, or may be idiopathic.
5. Iatrogenic hypercalcaemia may be due to vitamin D treatment, thiazide diuretics, theophylline, aluminium intoxication. Vit D intoxication is characterised by: high calcium, normal P, low PTH, high 25(OH)D and low, normal or high $1,25(OH)_2D$.

INVESTIGATIONS IN HYPERCALCAEMIA

— Calcium, phosphate, magnesium in plasma and urine

— Plasma albumin

— Alkaline phosphatase activity

— Urea and electrolytes, plasma creatinine

— Plasma 25(OH)D

— Intact plasma PTH

— Tubular resorption of phosphate

— DNA studies (MEN, calcium-sensing receptor)

— In primary hyperparathyroidism: look for other tumours (e.g. phaeochromocytoma, thyroid tumour)

— Skeletal survey

Common endocrine disorders

I. HYPOTHYROIDISM

Important points

1. *Congenital hypothyroidism*
   - in 2/3 of cases, caused by agenesis or dysgenesis of the thyroid gland. In approximately half of these cases the location of the gland is ectopic, mainly sublingual.
   - in 15% of cases caused by inborn defects of thyroid hormone synthesis. They are transmitted in an autosomal recessive pattern and are usually characterised by the presence of a goitre. Associated severe deafness characterises Pendred syndrome.
   - more rarely caused by resistance to TSH or thyroid hormones, or by hypothalamo–pituitary deficiencies.
2. *Acquired hypothyroidism* (See also Hypopituitarism) is mainly caused by an autoimmune disorder. The presence of auto-antibodies may precede by

several months or years the onset of thyroid dysfunction. In autoimmune thyroiditis they are rarely undetectable when a sensitive assay is used and both microsomal and anti-thyroglobulin antibodies are measured. Iodine deficiency is a rarer aetiology in western countries. Congenital defects can be missed by the initial screening, particularly in mild enzymatic defects, thyrotropin or thyroid hormone resistance, and may be expressed and revealed later in life.

INVESTIGATIONS IN HYPOTHYROIDISM

- In all cases: serum free T4, serum free T3, TSH

- In secondary (pituitary) or tertiary (hypothalamic) hypothyroidism: *TRH test*. Not necessary with a low fT4 associated with low TSH.

- In congenital hypothyroidism:
  * Ultrasound to search for the presence of a thyroid gland in normal or ectopic positions. If abnormal, a radio-isotopic scanning (^{99m}-Tc) is useful to confirm the findings.
  * If dyshormonogenesis is suspected, ^{123}I uptake will be assessed, followed if positive by the discharged perchlorate test. DNA studies (thyroglobulin, thyroid peroxidase genes) should complete the investigations and later, hearing assessment for Pendred syndrome.

- In acquired hypothyroidism:
  * Autoantibodies (anti-thyroglobulin, anti-microsomal, anti-adrenal and anti islet cells).
  * An ultrasound or a scintigraphy may complement the laboratory investigations but are not necessary unless there is a suspicious nodule.
  * Biopsy is rarely performed unless there is a cold nodule.
  * HLA typing (not routinely)

- In thyroid hormone or thyrotropin resistance: DNA analysis and familial screening

- Urinary iodine excretion if suspicion of iodine deficiency.

---

2. HYPERTHYROIDISM

Important points

1. Congenital hyperthyroidism is chiefly caused by transplacental passage of maternal thyroid-stimulating antibodies. The disorder is transient. Persistence of hyperthyroidism suggests a mutation of the thyrotropin receptor.
2. Acquired hyperthyroidism is mainly due to an autoimmune disorder (Graves' disease). Acquired activating mutation of Gsα can occur in McCune–Albright syndrome. TSH-secreting tumours are extremely rare.

INVESTIGATIONS IN HYPERTHYROIDISM

- Serum free T3, serum free T4, TSH

- Autoantibodies (anti-microsomal, antithyroglobulin, thyroid receptor stimulating antibodies, and also anti-adrenal and anti-islet cells)

- Ultrasound or radio-isotopic scanning are not necessary in typical Graves' disease (an isolated toxic nodule is extremely rare in childhood)

- TRH test in equivocal cases

- Ophthalmology assessment if suspicion of infiltrative ophthalmopathy associated with Graves' disease

- DNA studies (for TSH receptor or Gsα)

3. HYPOPITUITARISM

Important points

1. Congenital hypopituitarism is often a feature of a developmental disorder with anomalies of the midline structures of the brain. Septo–optic dysplasia is the most frequent developmental disorder. It is characterised by the association of hypoplasia of the optic nerves (so visual impairment), agenesis of the septum pellucidum and panhypopituitarism. The latter is an evolving process, and therefore investigations should be repeated over time to detect hormonal deficiencies which may appear later in life. More frequently, however, congenital hypopituitarism is isolated. In this case, it may also be an evolving process.
2. The onset of hypopituitarism later in life points to the suspicion of a tumour. In childhood, craniopharyngioma is the most frequent peri-pituitary tumour.
3. Diabetes insipidus may be isolated and may precede by several months or years the discovery of the causal lesion (mainly tumour and histiocytosis).

INVESTIGATIONS IN HYPOPITUITARISM

- Combined pituitary function test. The LHRH test is valueless between 6 months and 10 years of age. The TRH test is not necessary if TSH is low with low thyroid hormone levels

- Posterior pituitary assessment

- Imaging studies (obligatory): MRI scan (or CT scan)

- Ophthalmology (visual fields, fundus, optic discs, etc.)

- Karyotype and DNA studies

- In congenital hypopituitarism: search for associated malformations, notably other brain anomalies, liver disease, heart defects and renal abnormalities

Thus, unless familial diabetes insipidus, neuro-imaging studies must be repeated approximately once a year for many years. The onset of anterior pituitary defects suggests an intracranial lesion.

4. CONGENITAL ADRENAL HYPERPLASIA

1. 21 hydroxylase deficiency represents 95% of patients with CAH
2. Unrecognised, a salt-losing crisis is fatal. It usually occurs during the second week of life and is often confused with a gastro-enteritis, especially in boys. The diagnosis is rarely missed in girls, alerted by the excessive virilisation at birth.

5. CUSHING'S SYNDROME (CS)

DIAGNOSTIC AND FOLLOW-UP INVESTIGATIONS IN CONGENITAL ADRENAL HYPERPLASIA

— 17 OH progesterone: basal early morning sample, basal DHEA and andro-stenedione. High values confirm the diagnosis.

— Electrolytes (plasma and urine): Low plasma levels/high urine excretion of Na. Elevated plasma K level is often the prelude of a salt-losing crisis.

— Plasma renin activity (PRA) and aldosterone for identifying salt-losers (high PRA and low aldosterone).

— Synacthen test (short standard): useful in non-classical CAH and hetero-zygous forms. 17OHP, DHEA, androstenedione and cortisol should be measured.

— Other steroid metabolites should be measured if another form of CAH than 21 hydroxylase deficiency is suspected, using steroid gas liquid chromoto-graphy.

— Pelvic ultrasound (in girls).

— Karyotype (when in doubt about the genetic sex).

— DNA for genotype. The genotype does often correlate with the phenotype (albeit not always) and therefore is essential for genetic counselling.

Follow-up investigations

— Clinical examinations, bone age and growth velocity should be at the fore-front to detect signs of inappropriate steroid dose or poor compliance. PRA needs to be measured at intervals to assess adequacy of mineralocortoid replacement. It may also be necessary to measure androgens, 17OHP and hydrocortisone as a 24 hour profile for adjusting the treatment regimen.

The differential diagnosis of Cushing's syndrome is often difficult.

Important points

1. Iatrogenic Cushing's (due to chronic corticosteroid treatment) is the commonest cause of CS in childhood.
2. The main causes of endogenous Cushing's syndrome in children are adrenal tumours (benign or malignant) and Cushing's disease. Adrenal tumours cause corticotropin-independent tumours and represent the majority of CS in young children (before 5 years). These tumours may secrete androgens as

---

INVESTIGATIONS IN CUSHING'S SYNDROME

- Initially, the diagnosis should be made by demonstration of high cortisol secretion.

  Daily urinary cortisol excretion: Elevated urine free cortisol is a sensitive indicator of Cushing syndrome. Nevertheless, 24-hour specimens are required for reliability, which is not easy in children. Furthermore, because cortisol excretion may fluctuate from day to day in CS, specimens should be collected for 2–3 successive days. Incomplete collection cannot be reliably corrected by expressing the cortisol excretion as a fraction of the urinary creatinine, because in contrast to creatinine, cortisol is excreted episodically.

  Plasma cortisol (8am and midnight): loss of diurnal variation with raised values indicates pathological over-production provided the patient is resting, asleep for the midnight sample, and is not stressed. A low nocturnal value excludes the diagnosis. However, there is no physiological diurnal variation before the age of 3–6 months.

  Overnight and 48-hour low-dose dexamethasone suppression tests—see protocol.

- The second stage is aimed at establishing the cause.

  ACTH measurement: to discriminate between corticotropin-dependent and corticotropin-independent Cushing's. Ideally this should be measured at night coupled with cortisol level. High values demonstrate corticotropin-dependent Cushing's syndrome.

  High-dose dexamethasone suppression test: helps distinguish between Cushing disease, an adrenal tumour and ectopic corticotropin syndrome. Partial suppression strongly suggests Cushing's disease (high specificity) but failure of suppression is less conclusive (lower sensitivity).

  CFR/CRF + Desmopressin: typically a positive response suggests Cushing's disease.

- Imaging procedures (MRI/CT scan) are the final step to determine the source of ACTH (corticotropin-dependent Cushing's) or cortisol (corticotropin-independent Cushing's). They may be completed by further investigations (biopsies, catheterisation) which are beyond the scope of this chapter.

well. Cushing disease is due to a pituitary adenoma secreting corticotropin, and accounts for 2/3 of CS in older children.

3. Ectopic corticotropin tumours and primary adrenal nodular hyperplasia are extremely rare in children. The latter may be part of McCune–Albright syndrome with constitutional activation of G protein (see premature maturation).
4. Pseudo-Cushing syndrome can occur in severe depression. In this case the evening cortisol level usually remains low and cortisol secretion is easily suppressed by dexamethasone.

6. ADRENAL HYPOFUNCTION

Important points

1. Inherited congenital defects in steroid synthesis (notably CAH) are the most frequent cause of adrenal insufficiency in young children.
2. Auto-immunity is the commonest cause in older children and adolescents.
3. Hypopituitarism with ACTH deficiency needs to be considered.
4. In boys, adrenoleukodystrophy and X-linked adrenal hypoplasia congenita should be excluded.
5. Tuberculosis is a rare cause (the size of the adrenal gland is increased, calcified).
6. Abrupt termination of long-term corticosteroid treatment ought to be considered. Some drugs (e.g. ketoconazole, cyproterone acetate) can inhibit adrenal enzymes and then cause renal failure.
7. Isolated familial glucocorticoid resistance or deficiency is rare.

INVESTIGATIONS IN ADRENAL HYPOFUNCTION

- Cortisol profile
- ACTH, PRA, plasma aldosterone
- Standard short synacthen test
- When the diagnosis has been established, other investigations may be required (e.g. autoantibodies screen, MRI, tuberculin skin and Mantoux tests, neurological assessment, etc.)
- In boys, DNA studies coupled with LHRH and hCG tests (after the age of 10 years or if delayed puberty) should be performed in order to exclude X-linked adrenal hypoplasia congenita. VLCA plasma coupled with DNA studies should also be considered to rule out adrenoleukodystrophy

---

7. PHAEOCHROMOCYTOMA

Important points

1. Very rare in children.
2. Can be a component of two disorders with autosomal dominant inheritance: multiple endocrine neoplasia type 2 and Von Hippel Lindau disease. These syndromes are often associated with high morbidity and mortality.

3. Early detection of phaeochromocytoma and other associated tumours in affected families may be life-saving.

INVESTIGATIONS IN PHAEOCHROMOCYTOMA

Biochemical screening. Plasma and/or 24-hr urine: catecholamines or meta-nephrines. Excellent sensitivity (above 95%) and specificity (above 90%). Plasma metanephrines are the most sensitive test. Some drugs interfere with the assays. Vanillyl mandelic acid (VMA) measurement, because of poor sensitivity and specificity, should be abandoned.

Pharmacological tests. The glucagon stimulation test and the pentolinium or clonidine suppression tests are rarely useful and not without false negatives and positives. They are only performed in equivocal cases or in renal insufficiency. The glucagon test is hazardous. These tests can only be performed after careful consideration in centres which are accustomed to the assessment of such patients.

Imaging studies. Abdominal ultrasonography, CT scan, MRI with T2-weighted images, MIBG scintigraphy.

DNA studies and family screening.

Final checklist

A FEW IMPORTANT POINTS TO REMEMBER IN PAEDIATRIC ENDOCRINOLOGY

- Careful history and documentation of the growth pattern, combined with the bone age and the pubertal staging, can alert the paediatrician to most endocrine disorders.
- The diagnosis and management of genital ambiguity are difficult and the management should be discussed urgently with a paediatric endocrinologist.
- Some endocrine disorders can be induced by drugs: long-term corticosteroid treatment (Cushing syndrome), abrupt termination of chronic corticosteroid treatment (adrenal failure), excessive intake of vitamin D (hypercalcaemia), oestrogens (gynaecomastia and isolated thelarche), etc.
- Some tests are hazardous and must be conducted in experienced centres with medical and nursing staff dedicated to the procedure: insulin tolerance test, glucagon and fasting tests.
- The diagnosis of growth hormone insufficiency may be difficult and rests on auxological data combined with provocative tests. Serum IGF1 and IGFBP3 may be useful screening tests.

Protocols Tables 4.1 to 4.9 gives practical details of tests.

INSULIN TOLERANCE/GLUCAGON TESTS

Table 4.1	Insulin tolerance/glucagon tests	
	ITT (after 10 years of age)	**Glucagon**
Contraindications	Epilepsy, hyperinsulinism	Phaeochromocytoma, hyperinsulinism, primary adrenal insufficiency
Protocol	Insulin: 0.10–0.15 IU/kg IV Sampling every 30 min for 2 h for BM stix/glucose/ cortisol/GH	Glucagon: 100 µg/Kg IV Sampling every 30 min for 3 h for BM stix/glucose/ cortisol/GH

Indication: Assessment of GH and cortisol secretion.
Warning: These tests are hazardous. They should only be conducted in experienced centres, under strict conditions of surveillance and safety. Insulin-induced hypoglycaemia should never be caused in young children.

Sex steroid priming:

In a prepubertal girl with a bone age of more than 10 years; in a prepubertal boy with bone age more than 11 years or in early puberty prior to the onset of the growth spurt.

These tests are performed in the morning, the child fasting from midnight. If glucose concentration less than 2.4 mm/l, neither glucagon nor insulin should be administered.

If glucose level below 2.2 mm/l during the test (usually at times 20–30 min with insulin and 90–120 min with glucagon) give oral glucose. If the child does not tolerate it commence glucose IV (dextrose 10%: 2 ml/kg over 3 min then glucose infusion at a rate of 5–10 mg/kg/min) and continue taking blood samples. Dextrose 50% is contraindicated (risk of hyperosmolar coma).

- At the end of the test: do not remove the cannula if the child is vomiting and before the child has had a meal and BM stix above 4 mm/l.

- Interpretation: GH cut off values depend on the assay used. Cortisol: increment: at least 2-fold from the basal value; peak: above 450 nm/l.

- In congenital adrenal hyperplasia, a normogram plotting baseline serum 17 OH progesterone (OHP) against ACTH-stimulated 17 OHP has been constructed using data from individuals of various 21OH deficiency genotypes. It helps interpret the results, notably in heterozygous forms and atypical CAH.

Table 4.2 Synacthen tests

Short test	Physiological test	Long test
Procedure 9 am insert cannula, inject synacthen IM or IV: 62.5 µg < 6 months 125 µg 6–24 months 250 µg > 2 years	12 am bed rest, inject synacthen IM or IV: 500 ng/1.73 m^2	9 am, inject synacthen IM or IV for 3 days: 250 µg < 6 months 500 µg 6–24 months 1 mg > 2 years
Sampling 0–30–60 min	Every 5 min from + 10 to ± 45 min	Before test and after last injection
Normal Results Peak cortisol > 500 nm/L or increment > 200 nm/L above baseline	Rise >200 nm/L above baseline	Cortisol to rise by more than 3 × or > 600 nm/L

Table 4.3 Dexamethasone (DX) tests in Cushing syndrome (CS)

	Overnight test	Low dose test	High dose test
Indication	Screening test for suspected CS	Differentiating hypersecretion from obesity	Elucidating cause of CS
Protocol	At 12 pm: DX: 0.3 mg/m^2 oral At 8 am: plasma cortisol	DX: 0.5 mg 6-hourly oral for 48 hrs Plasma cortisol + ACTH before and 48 hrs after commencement of test	DX: 2 mg 6-hourly oral for 48 hrs Same as low dose test
Results	Normal: < 50 nm/l False positives in obesity or stress.	*Before test:* Cortisol 170–700 nm/l. *After test:* Cortisol < 50 nm/l No suppression in CS (in vast majority of cases)	Cortisol drops to 50% or less of the basal value in Cushing's disease. No suppression in ectopic ACTH tumour or adrenal Cushing's.

Table 4.4   LHRH test

Protocol
LHRH 25 µg/m2 IV bolus
Sampling at 0, 20 and 60 min for FSH and LH

Interpretation
- Useful < 3–6 months or after 10–12 years or in premature maturation
- Normally: rise at 20 min and decrease at 60 min. Values vary according to pubertal stage/depend on assays utilised
- No rise indicates hypogonadotropic hypogonadism but may be seen in very delayed puberty
- Elevated basal values with exaggerated response in gonadal failure
- Pubertal response in gonadotrophin-dependent precocious puberty
- Total suppression in gonadotropin-independent precocious puberty
- LH at 60 min > LH at 20 min suggests hypothalamic defect.

Table 4.5   hCG tests

Protocol	hCG	500 U < 1 year
		1000 U 1–10 years
		1500 U > 10 years

Injection IM once daily for 3 days (short test), twice weekly for 3 weeks (long test)

Testosterone (and other androgens or DHT if appropriate) before and after the injections

Results Normally the testosterone level increases to 8–10 nmol/l or greater. Helps to confirm dyshormonogenesis defects such as 5α reductase

Table 4.6   Fast provocation (investigation of hypoglycaemia)

Warning	This test is potentially dangerous and should ONLY be conducted in centres which regularly perform this test. Good venous access is essential.
Protocol	Duration: according to age.
	Maximum times recommended:

0–6 months	8 h
6–8 months	12 h
8–12 months	16 h
1–2 years	18 h
2–8 years	20 h
> 8 years	24 h

This time should be adapted individually and reduced according to the duration of fast the child will tolerate.

What to measure?

This list is not exhaustive but should allow the clinician to detect the main causes of hypoglycaemia provided the measurements coincide with an acute hypoglycaemic episode.

Blood: BM stix, glucose, insulin, GH, cortisol, triglycerides, pyruvate, lactate, 3OH butyrate, alanine, NEFA, free carnitine, total acylcarnitine, specific acylcarnitine.

Urine: urine organic acids (dicarboxylic acids, glycine conjugates, carnitine esters ...), ketones.

When to measure?

BM stix every hour or with increased frequency if rapid fall of glucose levels. Blood samples every 2 hours and if hypoglycaemia or symptoms related to hypoglycaemia.

End of the test

When hypoglycaemia (glucose < 2.4 mm/l) or intolerance (sweating, drowsiness, pallor, etc.) immediately after collecting the blood specimens. Even if no hypoglycaemia occurs, the tests should NOT exceed the times mentioned above. The test must also be interrupted if venous access is lost.

Give IV glucose if hypoglycaemia or symptoms (start with 2 ml/kg of 10% dextrose over 3 min then glucose infusion at a rate of 5 mg/kg/min). In all cases a meal should be given and the cannula not withdrawn before complete recovery.

Table 4.7   Oral glucose tolerance test

Indications
- Tall stature with suspicion of pituitary gigantism
- Hypoglycaemia
- Insulin resistance (obesity, acanthosis nigricans, family history of insulin resistance)

Protocol
— On the morning after fasting from midnight. The child should have had a normal diet during the week prior to the test.
— Insert cannula
— **Oral glucose load** given at a dose of 1.75 g/kg to a maximum of 75 g (e.g. of a preparation: Hycal: 2.75 ml/kg = 1.75 g/kg of glucose to dilute in water).
— **Sampling** before glucose and every 30 min for 180 min afterwards, for glucose and insulin. GH should be measured in suspected pituitary gigantism. *C. peptide* is useful in suspected hyperinsulinism.

Interpretation:
- **Normally:** peak glucose <8.9 mm/l and at 120 min glucose <6.1 mm/l. GH levels drop to undetectable levels within 60 min.
- **Tall stature:** pituitary gigantism: persistently high levels of GH or even paradoxical response.
- **Insulin resistance:** exaggerated insulin response. The peak glucose can be elevated.

Table 4.8 **Water Deprivation Test (DDAVP)**

Indication:
Suspicion of diabetes insipidus. Exclusion of psychogenic polydipsia. The DDAVP is performed at the end of the deprivation test to distinguish between nephrogenic diabetes insipidus and hypothalamic diabetes insipidus.

Warning:
This test is potentially hazardous (risk of dehydration during the test and of water intoxication after DDAVP) and should be conducted during the day under careful surveillance. Supervision is also crucial to prevent surreptitious drinking.
Cortisol deficiency should be appropriately replaced.

Protocol:
Overnight prior to the test: the child should drink and eat normally apart from tea and coffee.
An intravenous cannula should be inserted.
Light breakfast with no fluids.
Start fluid fast after voiding bladder.
Hourly: weight, blood pressure, urine output and osmolality.
At 30 min, then every 2 hrs: blood sample for plasma osmolality and Na.
At the end of the test: If urine fails to concentrate administer DDAVP
either spray 10 μg intranasally (or IM 1 μg < 2 years and 2 μg >2 years). The patient is allowed to drink but not more than the previous hour's output. Careful weight and BP monitoring should be pursued. Collect urine over the next 4 hours and a blood sample at the end for Na and osmolality.

End of tests:
Deprivation: When weight loss >5% or patient clinically dehydrated.
　　　　　　　When urine osmolality >750 mOsmol/kg or plasma osmolality
　　　　　　　>300 mOsmol/kg.
　　　　　　　After 7 hours if criteria above not met.
DDAVP:　　　After 4 hours
　　　　　　　Or urine osmolality >750 mOsmol/kg.

Interpretation:
Deprivation: *Normal response:* urine osmolality >750 mOsmol/kg
　　　　　　　Ratio urine osmolality/plasma osmolality >1.5
　　　　　　　Diabetes insipidus: urine osmolality <300 mOsmol/kg
　　　　　　　Plasma osmolality >295 mOsm/kg with no adequate concomitant rise in urine concentration. Intermediate values are in favour of partial diabetes insipidus. Measurement of plasma ADH may be useful in this situation.
DDAVP:　　　Hypothalamic diabetes insipidus if urine osmolality/plasma osmolality > 1.5 or urine concentrates.
　　　　　　　Nephrogenic diabetes insipidus if no response.

Interpretation

Hyperinsulinism: Inappropriately high insulin level (>5 µU/ml), low ketones, low NEFA

β oxidation defects: high NEFA, low ketones relative to the NEFA levels, reduced total carnitine concentration (low free carnitine and increased amount of acyl-carnitine), presence of specific acylcarnitine and characteristic organic aciduria.

Ketotic hypoglycaemia: appropriate surge in NEFA and ketones and low insulin.

Inborn errors of gluconeogenesis, glycogenolysis or glycolysis: high pyruvate, lactate, alanine and glycerol. Usually appropriate rise in NEFA and ketones, low insulin.

GHD and cortisol deficiency: appropriate rise in NEFA and ketones, low insulin.

For further details: Soltesz, G., Aynsley-Green, A. (1992) Approach to the diagno-sis of hypoglycaemia in infants and children. In Ranke, M.B. (ed.) Functional endocrinologic diagnostics in children and adolescents. 168–83.

Table 4.9 TRH Test

Indication:
- Investigation of patients with hypothalamo–pituitary lesions
- Diagnosis of equivocal hyperthyroidism
- Assessment of prolactin secretion
- Pituitary gigantism.

Safety:
Major reactions to TRH have been reported (e.g. pituitary apoplexy, bronchospasm, hypertension) but are exceptional. Minor reactions (nausea, flushing, headache, abdominal pain) are more common but benign.

Protocol:
— Insert IV cannula
— Slow IV injection of TRH: 7 µg/kg up to 200 µg
— Sampling at 0, 20 and 60 min for TSH. GH and prolactin are measured if indicated.

Results:
Normally there is an initial surge in TSH with an increment from 3 to 20 mU/L (peak more than twice the basal value) at 20 min. There is a significant decrease in TSH at 60 min. GH levels remain low.
Prolactin increases by at least 4-fold at 20 min and then diminishes.
In secondary hypothyroidism (pituitary disease): absence or stunted response regarding TSH and prolactin.
In hypothalamic hypopituitarism: typically delayed response with TSH at 60 min > TSH at 20 min.
In thyrotoxicosis: TSH levels suppressed throughout the test.
In pituitary gigantism: paradoxical surge in GH.

FURTHER READING

Atkinson, A.B., Kennedy, A.L., Carson, D.J., Hadden, D.R., Weaver, J.A., Sheridan, B. (1985) Five cases of cyclical Cushing syndrome. *British Medical Journal Clinical Research* 291: 1453–1457.

Burke, C.W. (1992) The pituitary megatest (and comment). *Clinical Endocrinology* 36: 133–139.

Dunkel, L., Perheentupa, J., Virtanen, M., Maenpa, J. (1985) Analysis of the influence of a combination of gonadotropin-releasing hormone and HCG tests in the differential diagnosis of male delayed puberty. *American Journal of Diseases of Children* 139: 494–498.

Hibi, I., Tanaka, T. (eds) (1996) Sexual differentiation and maturation. *Frontiers in Endocrinology*, Vol. 17.

Krakoff, L.R. (1995) Searching for phaeochromocytoma: a new and better test? *Annals of Internal Medicine* 123: 150–151.

Marx, S.J. (1995) Calcium sensing comes full circle. *Nature Genetics* 11: 357–358.

Miller, W.L. (1994) Clinical review: genetics, diagnosis and management of 21-dehydroxylase deficiency. *Journal of Clinical Endocrinology and Metabolism* 78: 241–246.

Morris, A.A.M., Thekekara, A., Wilks, Z., Clayton, P.T., Leonard, J.V., Aynsley-Green, A. (1996) Evaluation of fasts for investigating hypoglycaemia or suspected metabolic disease. *Archives of Disease in Childhood* 75: 115–119.

Ranke, M.B. (ed.) (1992) Functional endocrinologic diagnostics in children and adolescents. Mannheim: J&J Verlag.

Rosenfeld, R.G., Albertsson-Wikland, K., Cassoria, F. et al. (1995) Diagnostic controversy: the diagnosis of childhood growth hormone deficiency revisited. *Journal of Clinical Endocrinology and Metabolism* 80: 1532–1540.

Savage, M.O., Woods, K.A. (1996) The investigation of growth hormone insensitivity. *Clinical Endocrinology* 45: 257–260.

Shah, A., Stanhope, R., Mattew, D. (1992) Hazards of pharmacological tests of growth hormone secretion in childhood. *British Medical Journal* 304: 173–174.

Shane, E. (1993) Hypocalcaemia: pathogenesis, differential diagnosis and management. In: Favus, M.J. (ed.) *Primer on the Metabolic Bone Diseases and Disorders of Mineral Metabolism*, 2nd edn, pp 188–209. New York: Raven Press.

Shenker, A., Weinstein, L.S., Moran, A. et al. (1993) Severe endocrine manifestations of the McCune–Albright syndrome associated with activating mutations of stimulatory G protein Gs. *Journal of Pediatrics* 123: 509–518.

Takashima, S., Nomura, N., Tanaka, H., Itoh, Y., Miki, K., Harada, T. (1995) Congenital hypothyroidism: assessment with ultrasound. *American Journal of Neuroradiology* 16: 1117–1123.

5

Renal Disease

A Turner and G Haycock

Part I — Introduction and basic physiology

THE PHYSIOLOGICAL BASIS OF RENAL FUNCTION

The central function of the kidney is homeostasis: the regulation of the volume and composition of the extracellular fluid (the internal environment). With the important exception of carbon dioxide, the unwanted products of metabolism are eliminated by the kidney and form about half of the solute excreted in the urine in most circumstances. Urea is quantitatively the most important of these. The remainder of the urinary solute consists of dietary minerals ingested in excess of body needs and non-renal losses. The most important of these are sodium (Na), potassium (K) and chloride (Cl). In the adult (that is, non-growing) individual, virtually all the ingested minerals are eliminated in the urine: the urinary excretion rate of these substances is determined by dietary intake, not by renal function. In the child, and especially the young infant, dietary Na, K and Cl, as well as other minerals such as calcium, inorganic phosphorus and magnesium, are retained in proportion to the amount of new tissue and body fluid being laid down in the growth process. It follows that a much smaller proportion of the ingested amount of these substances is left over for excretion, which explains in part why the very young thrive on a level of renal function that would constitute significant renal insufficiency in an adult, even if corrected for differences in body size. The same applies to the need to excrete urea. On a physiological diet, nearly all the protein consumed by an infant is incorporated into new tissue and only a small proportion of the protein nitrogen is converted to urea. In contrast, the adult needs only enough dietary protein to replace losses due to protein turnover, and any excess generates urea (and other products) that must be excreted.

COMPONENTS OF RENAL FUNCTION

The glomerulus

The first step in the formation of urine is glomerular filtration. The glomeruli, of which the average human has a mean of 1,250,000 (range about 700,000 to 1,900,000), are microscopic plexuses of highly specialised capillaries that are highly permeable to water and small solutes but virtually impermeable to molecules of the size of albumin (69,000 daltons) and above. Blood enters each glomerulus via an afferent arteriole and leaves it via an efferent arteriole. Afferent and efferent arterioles are resistance vessels, differential constriction and dilatation of which control very precisely the hydrostatic pressure in the glomerular microcirculation. Normally about 20% of the volume of plasma entering via the afferent arteriole is removed from the circulation and enters the proximal tubule as glomerular filtrate. It is conventional to correct measures of renal function to a body surface area of 1.73 m^2, that of a putative 'normal' or 'average' adult. Such an individual produces the prodigious amount of 180 litres of glomerular filtrate daily, nearly all of which (obviously) is returned to the venous blood by tubular reabsorption. All 'downstream' processes whereby the tubule modifies the composition of glomerular filtrate to turn it into urine are to some extent dependent on the provision of an adequate volume of filtrate, which is why the estimation of glomerular filtration rate (GFR) is such an important aspect of measurement of renal function.

The proximal tubule

The proximal tubule is a high-capacity 'sponge' that reabsorbs two-thirds of the volume of glomerular filtrate. Proximal tubular reabsorption is isotonic: the osmolality of the fluid leaving this segment is the same as that entering it, and therefore the same as that of plasma. Clearly, there would be no point in producing and then reabsorbing this huge volume of fluid unless its composition was also altered by its passage through this tubule segment, as is indeed the case. Nutritionally valuable solutes such as bicarbonate, glucose and amino acids are reabsorbed virtually completely, and about 90% is reclaimed of minerals (e.g. inorganic phosphate) that are filtered in amounts greatly exceeding the amount needing to be excreted. Low molecular weight proteins such as retinol binding protein and various microglobulins are also salvaged in the proximal tubule, as is the small amount of albumin that is filtered. By contrast, toxic metabolites and other waste products are not actively reabsorbed in the proximal tubule, so that they are concentrated by a factor of about three by the point at which the late proximal tubule becomes the descending limb of the loop of Henle. Detailed methods exist to measure specific aspects of proximal tubular function (e.g. reabsorption of glucose or specific amino acids), but these are rarely necessary in clinical medicine. In practice, abnormalities of proximal tubular reabsorption can be recognized either because the substance in question is present in the urine in measurable amounts at a normal blood concentration (e.g. renal glycosuria and cystinuria), or because the tubular 'leakage' of the substance leads to the plasma concentration of the substance being below its normal range (e.g. familial hypophosphataemic rickets and proximal renal tubular acidosis). Generalised failure of proximal tubular reabsorption leads to reduced reabsorption of all the substances normally reclaimed, with excessive amounts being lost in the urine and multiple biochemical abnormalities in the blood (the Fanconi syndrome).

The loop of Henle

The descending and ascending limbs of the loop of Henle, with the associated microvasculature of the renal medulla, form the system of countercurrent multiplication and exchange that underlies the ability to produce urine more osmotically concentrated than plasma. Unlike the proximal tubule, reabsorption of water and solute are here dissociated. The only part of the loop thought to engage in active transport is the thick segment of the ascending limb (TAL), in which electrolyte (mainly Na and Cl) is absorbed without water. Thus, the fluid leaving the TAL and entering the distal convoluted tubule is always hypotonic to plasma, irrespective of whether concentrated or dilute urine is being produced at the time. The salt reabsorbed in the TAL is recycled by the countercurrent system and accumulates in the medullary interstitium, leading to an osmotic gradient ascending from isotonicity (about 300 mOsmol/kg H_2O) at the corticomedullary junction to maximal hypertonicity (about 1,200 mOsmol/kg H_2O) at the papillary tip. Urea is also recycled in the medulla and contributes about half of the total osmolality observed. About 25% of filtered salt is reabsorbed in the loop, so interference with this process due to inborn abnormalities of the transport processes (Bartter's syndrome) or drugs that inhibit it (loop diuretics such as furosemide) cause a large sodium diuresis and potentially severe salt depletion and electrolyte imbalance. Large amounts of calcium and magnesium are also reabsorbed in the loop of Henle, probably in the TAL. Direct testing of loop of Henle function is difficult and is not part of the clinical repertoire.

The distal convoluted tubule (DCT)

About 7% of filtered sodium and chloride is reabsorbed in this segment. In the absence of antidiuretic hormone (ADH), salt reabsorption takes place without water and the tubular fluid becomes progressively more dilute as it passes through. Inborn errors of the DCT NaCl transporter (Gitelman's syndrome), and diuretics that block it (thiazides), produce salt loss and electrolyte imbalance similar to that found in Bartter's syndrome and loop diuretic use, but less severe because the amount of salt reabsorbed in the DCT is much less than that reabsorbed in the loop.

The collecting duct (CD)

By the time what began as glomerular filtrate reaches the CD, it has diminished in volume from 180 litres daily to a few litres, and only 2–3% of the filtered Na has escaped reabsorption in more proximal segments. It is here that the volume and composition of the final urine is determined. The main processes that take place in the CD are excretion of potassium (K), excretion of metabolically-generated hydrogen ions (H^+) and the regulation of the osmotic concentration of the urine. The secretion of both K and H^+ depends on the active reabsorption of Na through channels that are opened by aldosterone. Since Na is a cation (positively charged), its transport across the tubule epithelium leads to the establishment of an electrical gradient (voltage) with the outer (basolateral) surface of the tubule positively charged with respect to the inner (apical) membrane. This voltage facilitates the countermovement of K and H^+, both cations, into the tubular fluid. K diffuses passively through channels in the apical membrane. The H^+ is actively secreted in this part of the tubule by a transport system (H^+-ATPase or proton pump), but the process is greatly enhanced by the favourable electrical voltage generated by Na reabsorption. Various tests of the acidifying (H^+ secreting) capacity of the tubule are referred to in this chapter.

If the osmolality of the plasma is below a threshold value (about 286 mOsmol/kg H_2O), this implies water excess. The secretion of ADH is therefore suppressed, and the whole of the nephron distal to the TAL (the DCT and CD) remains impermeable to water. This results in the production of a large volume of dilute urine and the excretion of the excess water. The capacity of the kidney to dilute the urine is very large: an adult can produce 10–20 litres of urine daily under maximal water diuresis — rarely achieved in normal clinical circumstances. When the plasma osmolality rises above this threshold, implying water depletion, ADH is progressively released and makes the CD permeable to water. As the fluid passes through the medullary section of the CD, it traverses the hypertonic medullary interstitium generated by the countercurrent concentrating mechanism (see above). Water is osmotically absorbed to equilibrium, and in maximal anti-diuresis urine about 4 times more concentrated than plasma (1,200 mOsmol/kg H_2O) can be produced by the healthy adult kidney. At average rates of urinary solute generation, this allows homeostatic function to be maintained with a urine output of as little as about 750 ml. However, on a high-solute diet or in conditions of catabolic stress the increased rate of solute generation may need propor-tionately more urinary water for its excretion, a fact that needs to be remembered when dealing with sick patients, especially infants in whom the capacity to con-centrate the urine is less well developed than in adults. Methods of assessing urinary concentrating and diluting capacity are described later in this chapter.

List of tests

BLOOD TESTS

URINE TESTS

Urine microscopy and culture
Urine osmolality and specific gravity
Urine proteins
Urine amino acids
Urine glucose
Urine electrolytes

TESTS OF TUBULAR FUNCTION

Glucose reabsorption
Amino acid reabsorption
Phosphate reabsorption
Sodium reabsorption
Tests of renal excretion of non-volatile acid
  Urine pH
  Urine anion gap
  Acid (ammonium chloride) loading test

  Sodium bicarbonate loading test
  Urine PCO_2
Tests of concentration and dilution of urine
  Early morning urine osmolality
  Water deprivation test

IMAGING

Ultrasound scanning
Plain abdominal X-ray
Investigations using contrast
  Excretory urography
  Contrast cystourethrography
  Video urodynamic studies
Nuclear medicine tests
  DMSA scan
  Dynamic radioisotope scans
CT scanning
MRI scanning
Renal angiography

RENAL BIOPSY

ABBREVIATIONS USED IN THIS CHAPTER

ADH — antidiuretic hormone
ARF — acute renal failure
CD — collecting duct
CFU — colony-forming units
DCT — distal convoluted tubule
DI — diabetes insipidus
DMSA — dimercaptosuccinic acid
DTPA — diethylenetriamine-pentaacetate
ECF — extracellular fluid
GFR — glomerular filtration rate
IVU — intravenous urogram
LMWPs — low molecular weight proteins
MAG3 — mercapto acetyl triglycine

MCUG — micturating cystourethrogram
MIBG — meta-iodobenzylguanidine
PCT — proximal convoluted tubule
RTA — renal tubular acidosis
SG — specific gravity
SIADH — syndrome of inappropriate antidiuretic hormone secretion
TAL — thick (segment of) ascending limb, loop of Henle
TPN — total parenteral nutrition
TRP — tubular reabsorption of phosphate
VUR — vesicoureteric reflux

Part 2 — Tests

URINE TESTS

In certain cases a good deal can be learned from careful examination of the urine. Some tests can be performed by the clinician at the bedside whilst others require delivery of a suitable specimen of urine to the laboratory.

Urine dipstick testing

The universal availability of multipurpose dipsticks makes routine 'urinalysis' a simple and instantaneous matter. The sticks are impregnated with chemicals which interact with various constituents of urine, leading to a colour change. Dipstick testing for blood and protein should be carried out in all children suspected of having renal tract pathology. Glucose, pH, specific gravity, ketones, nitrites and leucocytes can also be detected by dipstick.

Blood The dipstick test for haematuria relies on the peroxidase-like activity of haemoglobin to catalyse the oxidation of a chromogen contained in the test paper, in the presence of hydrogen peroxide, thereby causing a colour change (green). The test depends on the presence of free haemoglobin. In practice this is not a problem since whenever significant bleeding into the urine occurs there is some cell lysis and free haemoglobin will be present. The test also detects haemoglobinuria following intravascular haemolysis, and myoglobinuria, e.g. after rhabdomyolysis. False positive results may be obtained in the presence of urine infection. The colour takes a little time to develop and the result should be read exactly one minute after applying the specimen to the test strip.

Protein The stick is impregnated with tetrabromophenol blue. With increasing protein concentrations the colour changes from yellow through to green and

Table 5.1 Causes of misleading results in dipstick screening for proteinuria	
False positives	**False negatives**
Very concentrated urine	Very dilute urine
Alkaline urine	Acid urine
Contamination with antiseptics	Non-albumin proteinuria
Drugs e.g. phenazopyridine	Sticks out of date
Gross haematuria	
Bacteriuria/pyuria	

then green – blue. This provides a rough quantitative assessment with concentrations as low as 10–15 mg/dl being detected and the highest reading being reached at concentrations >1000 mg/dl. The dipstick method binds albumin much better than other proteins and therefore reflects albuminuria rather than non-selective proteinuria. Causes of misleading dipstick results are shown in Table 5.1. Unlike the test for blood, the colour change appears immediately after contact with the specimen.

Leucocytes and nitrite A dipstick is available for testing for two markers of infection, leucocyte esterase and nitrites. Leucocyte esterase is an enzyme present in neutrophils, the presence of which indicates pyuria, whilst nitrites are produced in the urine from breakdown of dietary nitrates by urinary pathogens. Most organisms are able to reduce nitrates, other than some *Pseudomonas* species and group B streptococcus. Specimens that are positive for both leucocyte esterase and nitrite are almost certainly infected: specimens negative for both are probably not infected. If one test is positive and the other negative the result is equivocal and the result of a urine culture should be awaited (see below).

Urine microscopy
Microscopy of a fresh urine sample can reveal red and white blood cells, organisms, casts and crystals.

Indications for urine microscopy All children with suspected renal tract pathology, in particular:

- suspected urinary tract infection (UTI)
- haematuria
- suspected glomerulonephritis
- renal stone disease.

Red blood cells It is normal for a few red cells to pass through the glomerular barrier into the urine. In uncentrifuged urine there should be less than 5 red cells per ml of urine. Red cells are easily visualised when abundant, but when scanty may be overlooked. Since rapid haemolysis occurs when urine is left standing, especially if dilute, it is essential that the sample is fresh. Lower counts of red cells can be more easily identified in a centrifuged urine sample, but quantification then becomes more difficult with great variability in results between different technicians and laboratories. There are no accepted standards for an abnormal number of red cells in a centrifuged urine specimen. The Addis count, semi-quantitative counting of the red cells in a 24-hour urine specimen, is now rarely performed.

The morphology of urine red cells may help to determine the site of bleeding. Red blood cells that have passed through the glomerulus become distorted and have a variable haemoglobin content. An experienced observer can usually distinguish these from red cells lost by bleeding into the lower urinary tract. The use of a phase contrast microscope improves the reliability of interpretation of urine red cell morphology, but such machines are not routinely available.

White blood cells In normal urine there should be less than 10 white blood cells per ml. A higher number is suggestive of urinary tract infection or other inflammatory conditions of the kidney, and can also be seen with fever. Pyuria is present in most cases of UTI but its absence does not exclude the diagnosis. Pyuria that is not accompanied by bacterial growth on conventional urine culture should raise the suspicion of tuberculosis of the kidney or urinary tract.

Casts Casts are structures formed within the renal tubules from cellular debris mixed with Tamm–Horsfall protein. They are cylindrical in shape, reflecting the shape of the tubule, and are named after the cellular component within. Types include red cell, white cell and epithelial cell casts as well as granular casts in which no specific cellular component can be identified, and hyaline ('glass-like') casts. Occasional hyaline and granular casts may be present in normal urine.

The presence of red blood cell casts is always pathological and indicates glomerular bleeding. As red cell casts disintegrate they become granular in appearance and the presence of more than a few granular casts may also suggest glomerular bleeding or inflammation.

Epithelial cell casts, formed from tubular desquamated epithelial cells, may accompany red cell or white cell casts and often indicate tubular injury.

White blood cell casts occur in inflammatory conditions of the kidney such as pyelonephritis and tubulointerstitial nephritis.

Organisms The presence of organisms on urine microscopy correlates well with urinary tract infection. It is not necessary to stain the specimen to detect the presence of bacteria. If the light source is reduced to the minimum, such that particulate matter is just visible down the microscope, bacteria can be seen as tiny rods or cocci exhibiting Brownian motion. None are visible in normal, uncentrifuged urine.

Crystals Uric acid, phosphates, cystine and oxalate are among the compounds that may crystallise in the urine. Sometimes their characteristic shapes are recognisable to the experienced observer, but biochemical identification of the causative substance must be undertaken in every such case.

Urine culture Semiquantiative urine culture should be performed on all children suspected of having a urinary tract infection. A calibrated loop is used to transfer a known volume (usually 10 μl) of freshly voided urine onto a culture plate. Each organism in the specimen gives rise to a colony, which is visible to the naked eye after 24 hours' incubation. A pure growth of $>10^5$ colony forming units (CFU) per ml from a midstream or clean catch specimen strongly suggests a urinary tract infection. However, if there is no accompanying pyuria or if the child is not acutely ill it must be remembered that contamination is common and the test should be repeated. A positive culture from a bag specimen should always be repeated since contamination is statistically more likely than infection. Infants who are clinically septic should have a specimen obtained by suprapubic bladder aspiration or by urethral catheterisation before antibiotic treatment is started: bag specimens are a waste of time and a distraction in this context. Any growth from a sample obtained by suprapubic aspiration is likely to be clinically significant whilst a growth of $>10^4$ CFU/ml from a catheter specimen confirms infection. A mixed growth suggests contamination of the specimen and does not exclude infection. Urine collection should therefore be repeated.

Urine osmolality and specific gravity

Both osmolality and specific gravity (SG) provide a measure of the concentration of urine, the former being the more accurate.

Osmolality The urine osmolality is a function of the total number of discrete particles dissolved in a given quantity of water and is expressed as milliosmoles per kg of water (mOsm/kg H_2O). Quantatively the most important constituent is urea, which contributes 40–50% of the total osmolality, while the major electrolytes are sodium, potassium, ammonium and chloride. Urine is usually hyperosmotic to plasma with a normal range of 300–800 mOsm/l, although a healthy child may show a urine osmolality of <100 mOsm/l after drinking large amounts of fluid, or up to 1400 mOsm/l when dehydrated. Fixed isosthenuria (the inability to alter urine osmolality significantly in either direction from that of plasma, about 300 mOsm/l), is a feature of advanced renal insufficiency.

Indications

- Suspected diabetes insipidus
- Syndrome of inappropriate ADH secretion (SIADH)
- Distinguishing established intrinsic acute renal failure, where the urine and plasma osmolality will be similar, from prerenal acute renal failure, where the urine osmolality will be high.

Specific gravity The specific gravity (SG) indicates the number and weight of solute particles in the urine. It overestimates osmolality in the presence of proteinuria. It can be measured in the laboratory by urometry and refractometry but more often is measured at the bedside using a solid phase reagent strip. A refractometer, a device like a small telescope that gives an accurate estimate of SG on a single drop of urine, can also be used in the ward or clinic. The results obtained from the strip method have been shown to correlate well with laboratory methods of SG measurement and, outside the neonatal period, with urine osmolality. A urine SG of 1.010 is approximately equal to an osmolality of 300 mOsm/l, 1.020 to 700 mOsm/l, and 1.030 to 1,100 mOsm/l. The strip method is affected by urine pH with overestimation of SG when the pH is less than 6.5 and understimation when the pH is above 7. A rough correction can be made by adding 0.005 when the pH is above 7. The usual range for urine SG is 1.010 to 1.022, although as with osmolality this depends on fluid intake and can fall as low as 1.001 and rise to as high as 1.030.

Indications

- As a simple alternative to urine osmolality for the indications above
- When interpreting dipstick proteinuria — urine with an SG > 1.025 may be falsely positive for protein, while conversely a dilute urine with an SG < 1.002 may be falsely negative
- Home monitoring to assess adequate hydration in patients with nephrolithiasis (SG > 1.012 is a risk factor).

Urine proteins

In normal circumstances high molecular weight plasma proteins, e.g. albumin (molecular weight about 70 kd), cross the glomerular barrier in low concentrations, whilst low molecular weight proteins (LMWPs, < 40 kd) are freely filtered. The majority of the protein in the glomerular filtrate is then reabsorbed by pinocytosis by the cells of the proximal convoluted tubule (PCT), where it is digested and returned to the blood as its constituent amino acids. Protein is added to the filtrate in the thick ascending limb of the loop of Henle in the form of uromucoid Tamm–Horsfall protein which makes up about 40% of the final urine protein. The remainder is composed of around 40% albumin, 15% α_1 and α_2 globulins and very low concentrations of other low molecular weight proteins.

The simplest method of assessment of proteinuria is by dipstick. Where a positive result is obtained, quantification should be performed. An excellent alternative, and somewhat more reliable (if less convenient) than dipsticks, is to add 1 ml of a solution of 3% sulphosalicylic acid to 10 ml of urine in a standard test tube. If protein is present a precipitate appears instantly and its density correlates with the concentration of protein in the specimen. Some nephrologists still prefer this method to dipsticks for home monitoring of proteinuria in children with relapsing nephrotic syndrome. A variety of methods are available in the laboratory, the most commonly used being a turbidometric method in which protein is precipitated out at acid pH and the reduction in light transmission measured, in order to enable calculation of the protein concentration. Traditionally this is performed on a urine specimen collected over a defined time period, usually 12 or 24 hours. A level of > 4 mg/m² body surface area/hour is regarded as significant. In children, and especially in infants, timed urine collections are often inaccurate and impractical and measurement of urine albumin: creatinine ratio ($U_A:U_{Cr}$) in a spot sample has been shown to correlate well with 24 hour albumin excretion. $U_A:U_{Cr}$ < 20 mg albumin per mmol creatinine is normal.

Glomerular proteinuria Increased albumin excretion may be due to increased glomerular permeability, reduced tubular reabsorption, or both. However, because in normal circumstances only small quantities of albumin pass through the glomerulus, large increases in albuminuria reflect increased glomerular permeability. Measurement of $U_A:U_{Cr}$ on a spot urine sample, preferably obtained immediately on rising in the morning, or measuring the albumin excretion rate in a timed urine specimen, is used to assess glomerular proteinuria.

The protein–selectivity ratio The protein–selectivity ratio compares the clearance of a high molecular weight and a low molecular weight protein, usually IgG and albumin or IgG and transferrin. This test was fashionable at one time in an attempt to distinguish minimal change, steroid-responsive nephrotic syndrome from other more serious forms of the disease. However, the overlap between the two groups is such that it adds little to the diagnosis and management of glomerular disease and should not be recommended in the modern day.

Tubular proteinuria Since LMWPs are freely filtered by the glomerulus and almost completely reabsorbed by the proximal convoluted tubule, LMWP excretion in the urine represents a sensitive index of proximal tubular function. Two proteins are measured in clinical practice, β_2 microglobulin (β_2M) and retinol-binding protein (RBP). RBP is the more useful of the two since it is stable in acid urine, unlike β_2M.

Measurement of a further protein, N-acetyl-β-D glucosaminidase (NAG) is also useful. This is a lysosomal enzyme present in proximal tubular cells, which is released into the urine when cellular damage occurs, providing an index of proximal tubular necrosis.

Tubular proteinuria can be distinguished from glomerular proteinuria by urine protein electrophoresis, the two conditions having quite different electrophoretic patterns.

Electrolytes

The main electrolytes in urine are sodium, potassium, ammonium, chloride and bicarbonate. In addition small quantities of calcium, phosphate, magnesium and other trace elements are present. In clinical practice measurement of urine sodium is widely used and measurement of urinary calcium and magnesium are performed in cases of renal stone formation.

Sodium In a steady state, 24-hour urine sodium excretion reflects dietary intake. Changes in sodium intake lead to changes in extracellular fluid (ECF) volume, which in turn causes sodium excretion to increase or decrease to achieve a new steady state. In health, therefore, the sodium excretion rate is a good indicator of ECF volume. In the absence of water diuresis, a urine sodium concentration of < 10 mmol/l indicates marked ECF volume contraction. The most frequently encountered indication for this measurement is in the assessment of circulating volume in children in acute nephrotic relapse. It is an essential preliminary if intravenous albumin infusion is being considered, since serious adverse effects may ensue if albumin is given to a patient who is mistakenly thought to be volume-depleted but is actually not.

The most physiological index of renal sodium handling is the fractional sodium excretion FE_{Na}. This is the proportion of sodium filtered by the glomeruli which is excreted in the urine, and is calculated by dividing the sodium excretion rate by the sodium filtration rate. The sodium excretion rate is $(U_{Na} \times V)$, where U_{Na} is the urine sodium concentration and V is the urine flow rate in, for example, ml/min. The sodium filtration rate is $(P_{Na} \times GFR)$. If creatinine clearance is taken as equivalent to GFR, the V terms in $U_{Na} \times V$ and GFR cancel each other out, and the equation reduces to:

$$FE_{Na}\ (\%) = \frac{U_{Na} \times P_{Cr}}{P_{Na} \times U_{Cr}} \times 100$$

It is *not* necessary to obtain a timed urine collection to make this calculation: simultaneous, random blood and urine samples are all that is required. In the patient with acute renal failure a value of <1% suggests prerenal failure due to impaired renal perfusion while $FE_{Na} > 2.5\%$ suggests established acute renal failure (acute tubular necrosis).

TESTS OF TUBULAR FUNCTION

Disorders of tubular function take the form of failure of reabsorption of essential substances resulting in syndromes due to their depletion; failure of renal excretion of non-volatile acid, resulting in renal tubular acidosis; and failure of concentration of urine, resulting in diabetes insipidus.

Proximal tubule

The proximal tubule is responsible for reabsorption of glucose, amino acids, phosphate and bicarbonate, amongst other compounds. These substances are all almost completely reabsorbed below a certain plasma concentration, the renal threshold, but above this level there is no further increase in reabsorption and the amount escaping into the urine rises.

Glucose reabsorption Glycosuria is due either to an elevated blood sugar level exceeding the renal threshold or, if the plasma glucose concentration is normal, to impaired proximal tubular glucose reabsorption, renal glycosuria. This may occur in isolation or may be part of a generalised abnormality of proximal tubular function, the Fanconi syndrome.

The simplest method of detection of glycosuria is by dipstick. This utilises the glucose–oxidase/peroxidase reaction leading to a colour change in the presence of glucose. The presence of glycosuria with a normal blood sugar should prompt a search for other abnormalities of proximal tubular function, e.g. aminoaciduria, phosphaturia, bicarbonaturia.

Amino acid reabsorption In normal circumstances amino acids pass freely through the glomerular basement membrane into glomerular filtrate and are then virtually completely reabsorbed in the proximal convoluted tubule by specific active transport processes, leaving only very small amounts in the urine.

Urine amino acids are measured by thin-layer, gas or column chromatography. One-dimensional thin-layer chromatography is used to screen the urine for an abnormal amino acid pattern as is seen in the specific transport defects and inborn errors of metabolism, while two-dimensional thin-layer chromatography and high-performance liquid chromatography allow quantitative analysis of individual amino acids. Detection of generalised aminoaciduria is due to abnormal tubular function. This usually occurs as part of a generalised defect, the Fanconi syndrome, and its discovery should again prompt a search for other abnormalities of tubular function.

Increased urinary excretion of only one or a group of amino acids may be due either to abnormally high plasma concentrations of the amino acid in question, or to a defect in the specific proximal tubular transport protein responsible for its reabsorption. Measurement of the plasma amino acid concentration profile will distinguish between these two types of disease. Those in the former category are inborn errors of metabolism affecting the whole body, usually with normal renal function: maple syrup urine disease (branched chain amino aciduria) is an example. Those in the latter are specific defects of renal tubular function, often referred to as tubulopathies: cystinuria is the commonest.

Tubular reabsorption of phosphate (TRP) The plasma phosphate level is normally a little above the threshold value for phosphate reabsorption. As with sodium, urinary excretion of phosphate is ultimately determined by dietary intake (with allowance for accumulation of phosphate, mainly in the skeleton, during growth). The simplest method of assessing renal phosphate handling is by calculation of the TRP using the formula:

$$\text{TRP (\%)} = \left[1 - \frac{U_{Pi} \times P_{Cr}}{P_{Pi} \times U_{Cr}} \right] \times 100$$

where U_{Pi} and P_{Pi} represent the urine and plasma phosphate concentrations and U_{Cr} and P_{Cr} the urine and plasma creatinine concentrations. Note that this is, in essence, the same calculation as that used to estimate FE_{Na}, with Pi substituted for Na. For no very good reason, it is conventional to speak of fractional *excretion* of sodium and fractional tubular *reabsorption* of Pi. It is obvious that each is the mirror image of the other: fractional Pi excretion of 15% is the same as TRP of 85%. The normal value for TRP is > 85%.

An alternative way of expressing tubular phosphate reabsorption is by calculation of the effective renal threshold for phosphate, expressed in shorthand as TmPi/GFR. This is derived as follows:

$$\text{TmPi/GFR} = P_{Pi} - (U_{Pi} \times P_{Cr})/U_{Cr}$$

TmPi/GFR has the advantage over TRP that it is unaffected by changes in GFR, and therefore gives a 'truer' picture of how avidly the tubule is reabsorbing filtered Pi.

Distal tubule

Tests of concentration and dilution of urine

Loss of the kidneys' ability to concentrate the urine, secondary to either failure of antidiuretic hormone (ADH) production (central diabetes insipidus—central DI) or resistance of the kidney to its action (nephrogenic DI) leads to polyuria, poly-dipsia, episodes of dehydration and failure to thrive.

Early morning urine osmolality

This is a first-line screening test for suspected diabetes insipidus. In a normal child the first sample of urine passed in the morning is concentrated. A urine osmolality of >600 mOsm/l in any one of a series of early morning urine speci-mens excludes the diagnosis, while a low urine osmolality, especially in the pres-ence of a raised serum osmolality, makes the diagnosis likely. However, children may produce persistently dilute urine, even in the early morning, as a result of clandestine water drinking, and the suspicion of DI must be confirmed by a formal water deprivation test. In addition at least one random plasma sample for sodium and osmolality measurement should be obtained prior to undertaking a water deprivation test.

The water deprivation test

This test assesses the ability to produce ADH and concentrate the urine under conditions of water deprivation. In essence, the normal patient, over the period of the test, should concentrate the urine and thus maintain serum osmolality within the normal range. The patient with diabetes insipidus will fail to concentrate the urine and will therefore have a rise in serum osmolality and continue to produce dilute urine. Following the end of the initial test period the patient is given a dose of 1-desamino-8-D-arginine-vasopressin (desmopressin), a synthetic analogue of vasopressin. Patients with central DI will then be able to concentrate their urine, whereas those with nephrogenic DI will be resistant to the effects of desmopres-sion and their urine will remain dilute. The detailed protocol for the test is given in section 3.

Tests of renal excretion of non-volatile acid

The kidneys' role in acid–base homeostasis is achieved by two processes:

1. the reabsorption of filtered bicarbonate, primarily by the proximal tubules
2. the excretion of hydrogen ions, H^+, primarily by the distal nephron. This process generates an equimolar amount of bicarbonate in the renal tubular cells, which is then delivered to the blood. Hydrogen ions are buffered in the urine by HPO_4^{2-} to form $H_2PO_4^-$, and ammonia, NH_3 to form NH_4^+.

Defects in these processes lead to a group of disorders known as renal tubular acidosis (RTA). The tests used to assess and diagnose these disorders are outlined here, while a general scheme for investigation of suspected RTA is given in section 2.

The urine pH pH is the negative logarithm to the base 10 of the H^+ concentra-tion in a solution. Thus a pH of 7.4 (normal plasma) is a $[H^+]$ of $10^{-7.4}$ molar, equivalent to 40 nmol/l. The urine pH therefore reflects the concentration of free H^+ in the urine. This represents <1% of the total H^+ excreted by the kidney since most is buffered by HPO_4^{2-} and NH_3. The demonstration of an inability to lower the urine pH to <5.5 in the presence of metabolic acidosis has traditionally been used to diagnose distal RTA. The test is not however totally reliable since in some (rare) cases of distal RTA where H^+ secretion is intact but ammonium secretion is impaired, the urine pH may be below 5.5 while total acid output is much reduced.

In cases of proximal RTA, a disorder of bicarbonate reabsorption, when the plasma bicarbonate concentration falls below the renal threshold the urine pH will be acidic, since distal tubular acidification mechanisms remain intact.

The urine anion gap The urine anion gap provides an indirect index of urine ammonium (NH_4^+) excretion, which in itself is difficult to quantify. The concentration of Na^+, K^+ and Cl^- are measured and the anion gap is calculated as:

$$Na^+ + K^+ - Cl^-$$

The concentrations of the other cations, calcium and magnesium, excreted in the urine are small and the concentrations of the other anions aside from ammonium (sulphate, phosphate and organic acids) are relatively constant. The urine anion gap is therefore proportional to the negative value of the urine NH_4^+ concentration. In a patient with acidosis a positive anion gap implies inadequate ammonium secretion, while a negative anion gap implies that distal tubular acidification is adequate. Patients with proximal RTA (failure of bicarbonate reabsorption) often exhibit a negative urine anion gap, although this is not always the case. The test may therefore help to distinguish proximal and distal renal tubular acidification defects. The clinical value of measurement of the urinary anion gap is somewhat contentious. It is misleading if the urine contains large amounts of other unmeasured anions such as salicylates, ketoacids, etc.

Acid (ammonium chloride) loading test This is the definitive investigation to establish the diagnosis of distal RTA. It is performed in children in whom RTA is suspected and the urine pH is above 5.5. Since it will worsen existing acidosis it is contraindicated (and unnecessary) in the severely acidotic patient, who is already stressing his kidneys with an endogenous acid load.

A loading dose of ammonium chloride is given orally or via a nasogastric tube, in order to produce a systemic acidosis which in normal individuals will lead to acidification of the urine. The details of the test are given in section 3.

The diagnosis is excluded when:

- urine pH < 5.5 with plasma tCO_2 < 22.5 mmol/l
- urine pH < 5.0 with plasma tCO_2 < 20 mmol/l.

Fractional excretion of bicarbonate (FE_{bic}) This test is carried out to confirm suspected proximal RTA.

The patient is given sufficient oral or intravenous sodium bicarbonate to bring the plasma bicarbonate concentration into the normal range. Blood and urine samples are then taken simultaneously for measurement of bicarbonate and creatinine concentrations. The FE_{bic} is calculated as for the fractional excretion of any substance in the urine (see above) using the formula:

$$FE_{bic} (\%) = \frac{U_{bic} \times P_{Cr}}{U_{Cr} \times P_{bic}} \times 100$$

The normal FE_{bic} is <3%. FE_{bic} > 5% is diagnostic of proximal RTA with values > 15% often being reached.

Urine PCO_2 Distal tubule acidification can also be assessed by measurement of the urine: blood (U–B) PCO_2 gradient.

The principle behind the test is that CO_2 is generated in alkaline urine by formation and breakdown of carbonic acid from secreted H^+ and urinary bicarbonate. The reaction occurs slowly, largely in the bladder, since carbonic anhydrase, required to catalyse the reaction, is absent in the lumen of the distal tubule. The generated CO_2 cannot be reabsorbed from the bladder and can therefore be measured in the urine. If there is no distal H^+ secretion the reaction cannot take place and CO_2 will not be formed.

To carry out the test oral or intravenous sodium bicarbonate is administered until the urine pH is greater than the plasma pH. The blood and urine PCO_2 and bicarbonate concentration are then measured and the U–B PCO_2 calculated.

In a normal child the U–B PCO_2 gradient should rise to > 20 mmHg. If not, a failure of distal H^+ secretion is likely.

Measurement of U–B PCO_2 gradient can conveniently and usefully be combined with measurement of FE_{bic}.

IMAGING

Imaging of the renal tract has advanced greatly in recent years with less invasive tests such as ultrasound and radioisotope scans becoming widely available. A general rule when planning imaging is to select the least invasive test with the lowest radiation dose that will provide the required information.

Ultrasonography

The abdominal ultrasound scan (USS) is a simple, non-invasive study carrying no radiation burden that is available in all units. It should be the first-line investigation in all children requiring imaging of the renal tract. The USS provides anatomical detail but no information on function. In addition Doppler ultrasound scanning gives information on blood flow in arteries and veins with different colours representing blood flow towards and away from the probe. It must be borne in mind that the results obtained with ultrasonography depend upon the skill of the operator. Certain conditions are demonstrated well by USS whilst others are not clearly shown. Strengths and weaknesses of USS of the renal tract are shown in Table 5.2.

Plain abdominal X-ray

The plain abdominal X-ray (AXR) will show nephrocalcinosis and radio-opaque calculi within the renal tract. It may also reveal unsuspected anomalies of the lumbosacral spine, and reveal or confirm the presence of constipation.

Indications for plain abdominal X-ray

- any child with a confirmed urinary tract infection
- a clinical picture suggestive of renal stone disease.

Table 5.2 Strengths and limitations of renal ultrasonography

Well demonstrated	Poorly demonstrated
Renal tract dilatation	Small renal scars
Renal size	Abnormalities of renal vessels
Renal cysts/dysplastic kidneys	Functional abnormalities/VUR
Other structural abnormalities e.g. horseshoe kidney	
Bladder wall abnormalities	
Abdominal/renal masses	
Stones/nephrocalcinosis	

Excretory urography

The intravenous urogram (IVU) was once the cornerstone investigation in imaging of the renal tract. A dose of intravenous contrast is given and images are then taken as the dye is excreted by the kidneys. It provides good anatomical information, especially of the calyces, pelvis and ureter, and gives some information on function. However it carries a high radiation dose and in many cases has been superseded by the USS and radioisotope studies.

Indications for excretory urography

- investigation of renal calculi
- to provide detailed anatomical images of calyces/pelvis/ureter
- in suspected recessive polycystic disease
- for further investigation of a suspected occult duplex kidney.

Contrast cystourethrography

The micturating cystourethrogram (MCUG) provides the definitive method for investigation of the lower urinary tract, providing clear images of the bladder and urethra. It does, however, entail a high radiation dose to the gonads, especially in girls, and requires urethral catheterisation.

The test requires passage of a urinary catheter. Contrast is then instilled into the bladder via the catheter and images are taken of the bladder when full and then during and post micturition.

The MCUG will only provide information on the upper renal tract in the presence of vesicoureteric reflux (VUR).

Indications for MCUG

- first UTI in all children under 1 year of age
- thick-walled bladder on USS
- clinical picture of lower tract abnormalities, e.g. terminal haematuria
- further investigation of antenatal diagnosis of hydronephrosis

- investigation of renal failure of uncertain cause
- small kidney.

For girls with a first UTI or an abnormal DMSA scan who require exclusion of reflux a direct radioisotope cystogram (see below) can be carried out as an alternative to the MCUG and carries a much lower radiation dose. However, this is less widely available. In addition follow-up of known VUR should be by direct or indirect radioisotope cystography rather than MCUG.

Video urodynamic studies

The videourodynamic study combines a filling and voiding cystometrogram, in which pressure changes within the bladder are measured, with a simultaneous micturating cystourethrogram recorded on video. This enables correlation of intravesical pressure changes with the behaviour of the bladder neck and sphincter mechanisms. The study involves placement of a special multichannel urodynamic urethral catheter, which allows bladder filling through one port and intravesical pressure monitoring through the other. A rectal catheter is also introduced to monitor intraperitoneal pressure, which is subtracted from the simultaneously obtained intravesical pressure to give the desired information on the activity of the detrusor muscle.

Indications for video urodynamic studies

- neuropathic bladder
- wetting with a suspected associated neurological lesion
- day and night wetting in children aged over 10 years with no associated pathology.

DMSA scintigraphy

The static renal scan uses the radioisotope[99m]-Tc dimercaptosuccinic acid ([99m]-Tc DMSA) which, after intravenous injection, circulates to the kidneys and binds to the proximal convoluted tubules. It remains fixed here for many hours and thus provides images of functioning cortical mass. It has a lower radiation dose than the IVU because the radioactive half life of technetium is only about 6 hours, and gives good images of the renal parenchyma as well as an estimation of differential function of the two kidneys. The pictures are taken approximately 4 hours after the contrast injection. With experienced staff it should be possible to carry out the investigation without sedation.

The DMSA scan is indicated whenever detailed images of the parenchyma are required, for example:

- detection of renal scarring following UTI
- during the acute phase of a UTI to look for renal involvement
- detection of focal parenchymal abnormalities in renovascular disease — these may become more apparent following a dose of captopril
- detection of a second kidney if not clearly visualised on USS
- confirmation of absence of useful function, e.g. in a dysplastic kidney.

Dynamic radioisotope scans

Dynamic isotope scans provide information on renal perfusion, differential renal function and drainage of the collecting systems. The isotopes most often used are ^{99m}-Tc diethylenetriaminepentaacetate (99m Tc DTPA) or ^{99m}-Tc mercapto acetyl triglycine (^{99m}-Tc MAG3). DTPA provides information on glomerular function while MAG3 additionally is secreted by the proximal convoluted tubules (PCT) and therefore reflects both glomerular and PCT function. For this reason, MAG3 passes from the blood to the tubular system more quickly than DTPA, leading to clearer pictures at a lower total radiation dose. The MAG3 study is to be preferred to the DTPA on all grounds other than cost. This is particularly true in patients with low renal function due to disease or immaturity: in these cases the DTPA scan should be considered obsolete. Dynamic scans carry a lower radiation dose than the DMSA scan and much lower dose than the IVU. The isotope is given by intravenous injection and pictures are taken in front of a gamma camera, beginning immediately and therefore capturing the initial perfusion and subsequent excretion phases. In addition an indirect radioisotope cystogram can be carried out when most of the isotope has drained from the kidney into the bladder, typically after an hour or so. The toilet-trained child voids in front of the gamma camera. This enables detection of VUR, in which radioisotope will be seen to pass from the bladder back up the ureters to the kidneys, although grade I and possibly grade II reflux may be missed. Where urine flow rates are high, for example after administration of a diuretic, or in the obstructed system where large amounts of contrast are still present, reflux may be easily missed.

Indications for dynamic radioisotope scans are:

- assessment of differential renal function
- following a diuretic, in suspected obstruction — with good drainage the renal curve should fall to less than 75% within 10 minutes of the diuretic injection.
- following surgery to the renal pelvis/ureter
- post-transplant.

Indirect cystography is indicated in:

- the older child requiring exclusion of renal reflux
- follow-up of children with known VUR

In addition the DTPA scan can be carried out with a prior dose of oral captopril. In cases of renovascular disease this may reveal evidence of renal ischaemia not seen in the non-captopril images.

Computerised axial tomography (CT)

CT scanning is rarely needed in paediatric nephrology. The main indication is in the further investigation of renal and abdominal masses, e.g. Wilms' tumour, phaeochromocytoma. A CT scan is sometimes used for precise localisation of a percutaneous biopsy needle to ensure that tissue is sampled from the precise area of interest: this is not necessary in the routine percutaneous renal biopsy. The scan may require sedation in younger children. Images are taken pre and post contrast.

Magnetic resonance imaging (MRI)

This scan requires the child to be still for fairly long periods of time and therefore usually requires sedation, and in young children general anaesthesia. The main indication in paediatric nephrology is in the child with a neuropathic bladder with no obvious cause, in order to provide detailed imaging of the spine.

Renal angiography

Renal angiography is an invasive investigation, carrying a high radiation dose. It involves insertion of a small catheter into the femoral artery and advancement up to the renal arteries. Small doses of non-ionic contrast are then injected into the renal arteries and aorta, providing images of the renal vasculature.

Indications for renal arteriography are:

- hypertension, where a renovascular cause is thought likely
- suspected vasculitis, e.g. polyarteritis
- prior to interventional procedures such as balloon dilatation of renal artery stenosis, embolisation for AVM
- confirmation of vascular anatomy in the potential living related kidney donor.

Where arteriography is being performed to investigate hypertension, bilateral renal vein renin sampling and even segmental renal vein renin sampling can be carried out by also cannulating the inferior vena cava and from there the renal veins. A ratio of greater than or equal to 1.5 in the renin levels between the two sides suggests asymmetrical release, with the healthy kidney being suppressed by the increased release from the diseased kidney. In this situation surgery is likely to be successful in relieving the hypertension.

Renal biopsy

Percutaneous needle biopsy of the kidney was first reported in children in 1957, and has since become a widely used and safe technique. The complication rate is low in experienced hands. The procedure should therefore only be carried out in specialist centres by experienced operators.

Indications for renal biopsy

- acute nephritis of uncertain aetiology
- persistent microscopic/macroscopic haematuria
- certain cases of nephrotic syndrome, including
    failure to respond to standard treatment
    significant haematuria
    severe hypertension
    accompanying acute renal failure
- significant, persistent proteinuria
- acute renal failure of uncertain aetiology
- chronic renal failure of uncertain aetiology
- transplant kidneys with deterioration in function
- evaluation of severity of renal involvement
    systemic lupus erythematosus
    Henoch–Schonlein purpura

- evaluation of progress and treatment
  certain glomerulonephritides
  some cases of transplant rejection
  drug toxicity, e.g. cyclosporin A, tacrolimus

The procedure involves removing a tiny piece of kidney using a Trucut or similar needle. This is then examined by:

- light microscopy
- immunostaining
- electron microscopy.

List of clinical problems

URINARY TRACT INFECTION

PROTEINURIA

HAEMATURIA

RENAL TUBULAR ACIDOSIS

RENAL STONES

HYPERTENSION

ANTENATAL RENAL ABNORMALITIES

DISORDERS OF MICTURITION

RENAL FAILURE

Part 3 — Clinical problems

URINARY TRACT INFECTION

In suspected UTI a fresh uncentrifuged sample of urine should be examined by microscopy and culture. The presence of pus cells, red blood cells (RBCs) and organisms should be noted. Significant pyuria (> 10 white blood cells/μl) is suggestive of infection, as is presence of bacteria, although their absence does not exclude the diagnosis. The presence of microorganisms on microscopy correlates well with infection.

A growth of > 10^5 organisms/ml confirms a UTI. Following a confirmed UTI **ALL** children require further investigation.

Objectives

- to identify structural abnormalities of the urinary tract, e.g. obstruction, stones that predispose to infection
- to identify vesicoureteric reflux (VUR)
- to identify renal scarring.

In addition patients in the following categories should be investigated for vesicoureteric reflux with MCUG or direct or indirect radionuclide cystography:

- recurrent infections
- clinically diagnosed acute pyelonephritis

INVESTIGATIONS IN UTI

In all children under 1 year of age:

- USS of renal tract
- MCUG
- ^{99m}-Tc DMSA scan.

In all children under 5 years of age:

- plain abdominal X-ray
- USS
- ^{99m}-Tc-DMSA scanning (at least 4 weeks after infection).

- family history of VUR or reflux nephropathy (probably the strongest indication)
- scarred kidney(s) on DMSA scan.

Cystography can be safely omitted in children over 1 year of age, with unscarred kidneys, and in whom none of the other above risk factors are present.

INVESTIGATIONS IN CHILDREN OVER 5 YEARS OF AGE

- renal ultrasound scan
- plain abdominal X-ray
- If normal, 3-monthly urine checks, with follow-up for 2 years
- ^{99m}-Tc-DMSA scan if—
    recurrent infections
    acute pyelonephritis
    family history of VUR
    abnormal USS.

PROTEINURIA

In all patients with dipstick proteinuria quantification should be performed. Abnormal protein excretion is > 4 mg/hour/m^2, or on a spot sample > 20 mg protein/mmol creatinine.

Causes of intermittent proteinuria include:

- orthostatic — no protein in overnight urine collection/early morning urine
- exercise
- fever
- urinary tract infection
- some glomerulonephritides — e.g. IgA nephropathy.

When significant proteinuria is confirmed further investigation is warranted.

Baseline investigations which should be performed in all cases, along with the diagnoses suggested, are given in Table 5.3.

Table 5.3 Investigations designed to elucidate the cause of proteinuria

Investigation	Diagnosis suggested
Urine microscopy and culture	Urinary tract infection. Casts suggest glomerulonephritis (GN)
Electrolytes, urea and creatinine	Renal impairment
Serum albumin	Nephrotic syndrome
GFR	Renal impairment
Markers of streptococcal infection— ASOT, anti DNAase B	Acute post-streptococcal GN
Antinuclear antibody, anti-dsDNA	Systemic lupus erythematosus (SLE)
Complement (C3 and C4)	Acute post-streptococcal GN SLE Membranoproliferative GN

Indications for renal biopsy in asymptomatic proteinuria:

- impaired renal function
- low complement
- accompanying haematuria
- asymptomatic proteinuria for more than one year with normal investigations.

HAEMATURIA

Blood in the urine, haematuria, may be visible to the naked eye (macroscopic) or detectable only on dipstick or laboratory testing (microscopic).

It is normal for a few red blood cells to pass through the glomerular barrier into the urine. A trace reading on dipstix can therefore be safely ignored.

Macroscopic haematuria requires only a tiny quantity of blood to have entered the urine — as little as 0.1 ml per 100 ml of urine. Other causes of red urine, which must be distinguished from haematuria, are given in Table 5.4.

Table 5.4 Causes of red urine

Blood — red cells and/or haemoglobin
Myoglobin
Urates
Porphyrins
Foods — beetroot, berries, e.g. blackberries, red food colouring
Drugs, e.g. rifampicin, phenothiazines, phenolphthalein

It is usual to begin investigation of macroscopic haematuria immediately, whereas in cases of microscopic haematuria without proteinuria dipstick testing should be repeated several times over the course of a month to confirm the presence of blood before moving on to further investigations.

The collection of three urine samples, initial, mid-stream and terminal, may help identify the source of bleeding. Blood present only in the initial specimen suggests urethral bleeding, while terminal haematuria is seen in the presence of bladder pathology.

Investigation should be preceded by a careful history and clinical examination; this will often point to the diagnosis and guide investigation. Investigations can then be divided into baseline tests to be carried out in all cases and further investigations to be performed where specifically indicated. Baseline tests for the investigation of haematuria are shown in Table 5.5.

Further investigations which may be indicated:

- cystoscopy — indicated in the presence of lower urinary tract symptoms with a sterile urine culture, haematuria at onset of stream, or where there is no suggestion of a glomerular origin and no other cause apparent after appropriate imaging studies
- dipstick testing of urine of other family members
- ophthalmological examination — macular flecks and lenticonus in Alport's disease, retinal abnormalities in several syndromes with a renal component
- audiometry — high-tone sensorineural deafness in Alport's disease
- anti-streptolysin O titre, anti-DNAase B — in haematuria of < 6 months standing

Table 5.5   Initial investigations in children with haematuria

Investigation	Diagnosis suggested
Urine microscopy — red cell morphology, casts	Glomerular source of haematuria
Urine culture	Urinary tract infection
Plain abdominal X-ray	Renal calculi, nephrocalcinosis
Renal ultrasonography	Structural abnormalities, tumours, calculi, nephrocalcinosis
Full blood count, clotting ± sickle screen	Coagulation disorders, thrombocytopenia, sickle cell disease
Urine calcium:creatinine ratio	Hypercalciuria
Urine protein:creatinine ratio	Glomerulonephritides
Plasma urea, electrolytes and creatinine	Abnormal renal function, e.g. in glomerulonephritides

- C3 and C4 components of complement — as screening for other glomerulonephritides, e.g. mesangiocapillary glomerulonephritis, post-infectious glomerulonephritis, SLE
- anti-nuclear factor — screening for SLE
- anti-neutrophil cytoplasmic antibody (ANCA) — screening for systemic vasculitis.

If all these results are negative/normal the patient should be monitored.
Indications for renal biopsy in a patient with haematuria are as follows:

- accompanying significant proteinuria
- renal impairment
- results suggestive of glomerular pathology other than post-infectious GN
- accompanying hypertension
- haematuria persisting/frequently recurring over the course of one year.

RENAL TUBULAR ACIDOSIS (RTA)

1. Suspect renal tubular acidosis when there is a hyperchloraemic metabolic acidosis with a normal plasma anion gap, calculated as

$$Na^+ - (HCO_3^- + Cl^-) \qquad \text{(normal anion gap 8–16 mmol/l)}$$

This reflects loss of bicarbonate from the extracellular fluid, which may be either renal or from the gastrointestinal tract, e.g. diarrhoea, GI fistulae. In addition the administration of acidic chloride-containing salts, e.g. NH_4Cl, or chloride-containing amino acid mixtures as found in some TPN mixtures, may lead to the same picture.

2. Calculate the urine anion gap ($Na^+ + K^+ - Cl^-$) as an index of urinary ammonium excretion. A negative anion gap implies intact NH_4^+ excretion and therefore gut loss or proximal RTA, while a positive result implies that a distal acidification defect is likely (although proximal RTA is not definitely excluded).

3. If the results suggest proximal RTA, calculate the fractional excretion of bicarbonate after bicarbonate loading.

4. If the results suggest distal RTA:
i) measure the plasma K^+ to diagnose hyperkalaemic RTA
ii) measure the U–B PCO_2 gradient after bicarbonate loading
iii) perform an ammonium chloride loading test.

RENAL STONE DISEASE

Renal stone disease is uncommon in childhood, affecting 1–2 children per million population per year in Europe. Stones in children fall into the following groups:

- infective — > 80% — ammonium magnesium phosphate (struvite) mixed with calcium hydrogen phosphate (calcium apatite). Caused by infection with urea-splitting organisms, e.g. *Proteus* species, especially in the presence of urinary stasis
- calcium phosphate — 10–20% — most often due to idiopathic hypercalciuria but other causes include distal RTA, vitamin D toxicity, immobilisation, hyperparathyroidism and sarcoidosis

- cystine — 2% — due to cystinuria
- oxalate — due to hyperoxaluria type I or type II or more often to enhanced absorption or dietary load
- purines
  uric acid — may be dietary, due to inborn errors of metabolism, e.g. Lesch–Nyhan syndrome, or following chemotherapy for leukaemia/lymphoma
  xanthine oxidase — due to xanthinuria
  2,8-dihydroxyadenine — due to adenine phosphoribosyl transferase deficiency.

Strategy for investigation of renal stone disease

1. Obtain a thorough history and identify any risk factors:
   - immobilisation
   - poor fluid intake and urine output
   - history of UTI
   - ketogenic diet
   - chemotherapy
   - family history of renal calculi
   - consanguinity.
2. Plain AXR and renal USS — all stones other than purine stones are radioopaque and therefore seen on plain AXR.
3. Urine microscopy and culture — infection must be diagnosed and treated before further metabolic tests are performed. It is essential that metabolic screening is not overlooked when a diagnosis of UTI is made, since metabolic disorders and infection can coexist and in fact one may predispose to the other. In addition urine microscopy may reveal crystals, the nature of which may be determined by an experienced microscopist.
4. Blood tests — calcium, urate, phosphate and creatinine.
5. Urine analysis — the second urine sample of the morning, after an overnight fast, should be sent as a spot sample for calcium, oxalate, cystine, uric acid, creatinine and pH. Oxalate and urate excretion vary with age, whereas calcium excretion is fairly stable with a 97th centile Ca:Cr ratio of 0.69 mol:mol.

Further metabolic tests may then be indicated:

- hypercalciuria with normocalcaemia does not require further investigation. If hypercalcaemia is present, further investigation into aetiology is required
- abnormal plasma and urine uric acid levels require further investigation by an expert laboratory into a disorder of purine or pyrimidine metabolism
- urine chromatography will confirm cystinuria (excess excretion of cystine, arginine, ornithine and lysine)
- if urine oxalate is high, a sample should be sent to a specialist laboratory for investigation of glyoxylic and glyceric acids to diagnose hyperoxaluria type 1 or type 2.

HYPERTENSION

Hypertension may be defined as an average systolic or diastolic blood pressure greater than or equal to the 95th percentile for age and sex, measured on at

Table 5.6 Causes of secondary hypertension in childhood	
Renal	**Non-renal**
Renovascular disease	**Catecholamine excess**
Fibromuscular hyperplasia	Phaeochromocytoma
Renal artery aneurysm	Neuroblastoma
AV fistula	
Neurofibromatosis	**Coarctation of the aorta**
Vasculitis, e.g. polyarteritis nodosa	
	Endocrine — corticosteroid
Parenchymal	**excess**
Renal scarring/reflux nephropathy	Congenital adrenal hyperplasia
Polycystic disease	Cushing's syndrome
Glomerulonephritides	Conn's syndrome
Renal dysplasia	Iatrogenic
Haemolytic uraemic syndrome	
Chronic renal failure	
Renal tumours	

least three separate occasions. The correct technique for blood pressure measurement is vital — for advice on technique and tables of normal values for age and sex the reader is referred to the 'Update on the 1987 task force report on high blood pressure in children and adolescents' in the Further Reading List. The commonest errors in the measurement of blood pressure in children are (i) the use of too small a cuff (false high reading); (ii) incorrect application of the cuff to the arm; and (iii) failure to palpate (as opposed to auscultate) the pulse while the cuff is inflated.

The extent of investigation of hypertension in childhood depends upon the severity and persistence of the problem, with transient cases requiring monitoring only. Primary or essential hypertension is relatively uncommon before adolescence and most cases will have an underlying cause (secondary hypertension). More than 80% of this group have an underlying renal cause. Causes of hypertension in childhood are given in Table 5.6.

Investigations can be divided into baseline tests to be carried out in all children and further tests to be carried out where indicated by initial test results.

Baseline tests in hypertension

- plasma electrolytes, urea and creatinine
- urinalysis — for protein and blood
- urine MC&S
- renal USS including doppler USS of renal arteries and aorta
- ^{99m}-Tc-DMSA scan
- plasma renin, aldosterone and catecholamine measurement

- urinary catecholamine measurement (VMA, HVVA)
- chest X-ray, ECG and echocardiography
- plasma cortisol, urinary steroids.

Further investigations

- MCUG to look for VUR if evidence of renal scarring or history of UTI
- IVU to further elucidate cause of small kidney on USS
- DMSA and DTPA scans pre and post captopril
- iodine meta-iodobenzylguanidine (MIBG) scan in suspected neuroblastoma or phaeochromocytoma
- renal angiography
- bilateral renal vein/segmental renal vein renin sampling
- CT scan to further investigate mass on USS.

PRENATAL SCAN ABNORMALITIES

Most pregnant women in the United Kingdom receive a detailed scan of the fetus between 18 and 20 weeks gestation, enabling antenatal detection of many renal abnormalities.

By far the most common abnormality seen is hydronephrosis, either unilateral or bilateral. In a large study from Sweden in 1986 the incidence of antenatally-detected renal abnormalities was 0.28% of all pregnancies, with hydronephrosis accounting for approximately two-thirds of these. With continuing technological advances the incidence today is likely to be higher still, with more minor defects being detected.

Other abnormalities include:

- multicystic dysplastic kidney/other cystic disorders
- Unilateral/bilateral renal agenesis
- Unilateral/bilateral renal hypoplasia (small kidneys).

Postnatal investigation of antenatally-diagnosed hydronephrosis

Antenatal hydronephrosis is often defined as an anteroposterior renal pelvis diameter of >5 mm. However, if this measurement never exceeds 15 mm on sequential scans, serious pathology is very unlikely. (Dhillon, K.H., unpublished data). Where this abnormality is present in the fetus several other features should be assessed on the antenatal scan:

- Is the abnormality unilateral or bilateral?
- The ureters and bladder should be examined for dilatation, bladder wall thickening
- The other kidney should be studied for other abnormalities
- The fetus should be assessed for other anomalies
- The amniotic fluid volume should be assessed.

Unilateral hydronephrosis may be transient and found to have resolved on repeat scanning. In such cases a postnatal ultrasound examination should still be performed, ideally at 1–3 months postnatal age, since the hydronephrosis may recur

| Table 5.7 Differential diagnosis of renal pelvis dilatation ||
Unilateral	Bilateral
Unilateral PUJ obstruction	Bilateral PUJ obstruction
Unilateral vesicoureteric reflux	Bilateral vesicoureteric reflux
Unilateral multicystic dysplastic kidney	Bilateral multicystic dysplastic kidneys
Unilateral vesicoureteric junction obstruction	Bilateral vesicoureteric junction obstruction
	Neuropathic bladder
	Posterior urethral valves
	Other urethral problems, e.g. urethral atresia, cloacal abnormalities

when urine flow rate increases following birth. Intermittent hydronephrosis is suggestive of vesicoureteric reflux.

The strategy for postnatal investigation depends on whether the abnormality is unilateral or bilateral. Differential diagnosis is set out in Table 5.7.

Investigation of bilateral renal pelvis dilatation

An USS should be performed within a few hours of birth for the following groups:

- Bilateral hydronephrosis
- Unilateral hydronephrosis and oligohydramnios, or other kidney abnormal.

If this suggests posterior urethral valves or other urethral problems an MCUG should be performed. This should only be done in a unit accustomed to performing and interpreting the study in small infants. If this expertise is not available locally the infants should be referred to a paediatric urological/nephrological centre after placing a fine urethral catheter if the bladder is distended or there is dribbling of urine.

Investigation of unilateral renal pelvis dilatation

Providing the infant is well at birth and passes urine within the first 24 hours of life, investigations are not urgent. Prophylactic antibiotics should be commenced and the strategy for investigation depicted in Figure 5.1 followed.

DISORDERS OF MICTURITION

Nocturnal enuresis (bedwetting)

This is the commonest disorder of micturition to affect children. It is usually defined as failure to be consistently dry at night after the age of 5 years, in the absence of daytime urinary symptoms. If the history and clinical examination are

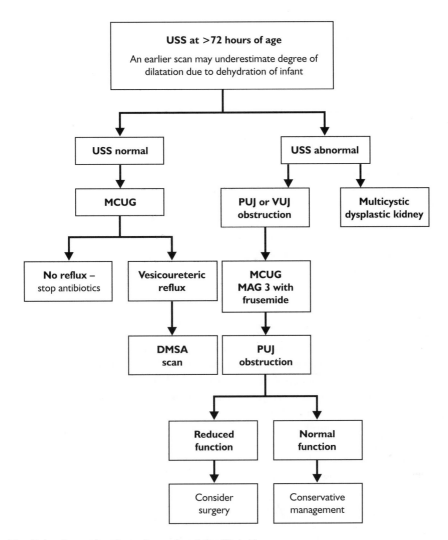

Fig. 5.1 **Investigation of renal pelvis dilatation.**

normal, and especially if there is a positive family history of enuresis, no tests are needed except a urine microscopy and culture and perhaps an ultrasound examination of the urinary tract (mainly for its reassurance value).

Daytime wetting and urgency

This is much more likely than nocturnal enuresis to be the result of either a physical or social/behavioural disorder. Careful examination of the abdomen, genitalia and back are essential, as is a thorough neurological examination of the lower limbs. In the absence of overt neurological abnormality the likeliest cause is instability of the detrusor muscle of the bladder — inability to suppress involuntary contractions, leading to frequency and especially urgency. An abdominal ultrasound examination should be performed in all cases, and it is worth asking the ultrasonographer to examine the sacrum as well. If these are normal and there are no features suspicious of a more serious abnormality, more invasive investigations are generally not indicated. If the symptoms are severe or associated with even minor neurological abnormality, or if there is no improvement with a reasonable trial of treatment, the lumbosacral spine should be examined by magnetic resonance imaging and a video-urodynamic study carried out.

A symptom of particular importance is constant, slight to moderate dampness in a child who appears otherwise to have normal bladder function, i.e. voiding normally and at appropriate intervals. This is highly suspicious of the presence of an ectopic ureter draining (usually) the dysplastic upper moiety of a duplex kidney into the urethra or the vagina, while the lower moiety ureter and that from the contralateral kidney drain normally into the bladder. There is nearly always a dilated ureter visible on ultrasonography low down behind the bladder and the examiner should be asked to take special care to look for this finding. The importance of making this diagnosis lies in the fact that it is a surgically curable condition.

RENAL FAILURE

Acute renal failure (ARF) is the clinical syndrome resulting from an abrupt reduction in GFR such that normal extracellular fluid volume and composition can no longer be maintained. In a child presenting in renal failure it is essential to urgently assess fluid, electrolyte and metabolic disturbances and to determine the aetiology, in order that reversible causes can be treated as soon as possible.

In the relatively well child presenting in renal failure it may be difficult to distinguish acute from chronic causes. Factors which may help to do this are given in Table 5.8.

ARF may be prerenal, intrinsic renal or post renal (obstructive) in nature. Causes of ARF are given in Table 5.9.

The investigations that establish the cause of ARF are given in Tables 5.10 and 5.11.

Table 5.8 Factors and investigations helping to distinguish acute from chronic renal failure

	ARF	CRF
Previous health	Good	Poor
Growth	Normal	Poor
FBC	Dilutional anaemia	Normochromic, normocytic anaemia
Renal USS	Often large kidneys	Often small kidneys
Hand/wrist X-ray, knee X-ray	Normal	Bone disease — rickets and hyperparathyroidism
PTH	Normal or high	High

Table 5.9 Causes of acute renal failure

Prerenal failure	Intrinsic renal failure	Postrenal failure
Hypovolaemia	**Acute tubular necrosis**	**Urethral obstruction**
Dehydration	Prolonged hypoxia	Posterior urethral valves
Haemorrhage	Nephrotoxins, e.g.	
3rd space loss	NSAIDs	**Neurogenic bladder**
	Aminoglycosides	
Normovolaemic	Cisplatin	**Bilateral ureteral**
hypotension	Heavy metals	**obstruction**
Reduced cardiac output	Tubular lumen obstruction	VUJ obstruction
Sepsis	Haemoglobinuria	PUJ obstruction
Vasodilator drugs	Myoglobinuria	
		Obstruction in a single kidney
	Glomerulonephritis	
	Post-infectious GN	
	MCGN	
	HSP	
	SLE	
	Others	
	Vascular	
	Haemolytic uraemic syndrome	
	Vasculitis, polyarteritis	
	Bilateral renal artery thrombosis	
	Bilateral renal vein thrombosis	
	Bilateral cortical necrosis	
	Infection	
	Pyelonephritis	
	Sepsis	
	Interstitial nephritis	
	Drug-induced	
	Idiopathic	

INVESTIGATIONS IN ACUTE RENAL FAILURE

Assessment of metabolic abnormalities
- Plasma sodium, potassium, urea and creatinine
- Venous blood gas to assess pH and bicarbonate
- Serum calcium, phosphate and PTH
- Full blood count.

Table 5.10 **Investigations to elucidate the cause of acute renal failure**

Investigation	Information obtained
Plasma and urine electrolytes and osmolality	Helps distinguish prerenal and intrinsic renal ARF (see Table 5.9)
FBC and film	Microangiopathic haemolytic anaemia in haemolytic uraemic syndrome
Glomerulonephritis screen: ASOT / anti-DNAase B Complement levels — C3 and C4 Urine microscopy — casts, cells Antinuclear antibodies Anti-GBM titre Anti-neutrophil cytoplasmic antibody	 Post-streptococcal GN Low in MCGN, SLE, APSGN Suggests glomerulonephritis SLE Anti-GBM disease ANCA-positive vasculitis
Renal ultrasound scan	Excludes obstruction. Large kidneys in acute GN, obstruction, infection, tumour. Small kidneys may indicate CRF.
Doppler renal ultrasound scan	Assesses patency of renal arteries, veins and IVC
Radioisotope studies	DTPA scan shows blood flow and parenchymal uptake
Renal biopsy	Performed where aetiology is unclear

Table 5.11 **Typical urinary indices in acute renal failure**

	Prerenal failure	Intrinsic renal failure
Urine sodium (mmol/l)	<20	>40
Urine:plasma urea	>10:1	<3:1
Urine:plasma creatinine	>20	<20
Urine osmolality (mOsmol/kg)	>500	<350
Fractional excretion of sodium	<1%	>2.5%

Part 4 — Practical details of the tests

BLOOD TESTS

The technical methods used for the various blood tests in the investigation of renal disease vary from laboratory to laboratory and, in general, need not concern the clinician. Two important exceptions are *creatinine* and the major *electrolytes*.

For many years the standard laboratory method for estimating creatinine concentration was the alkaline picrate (Jaffe) reaction, which relies on the generation of a purple colour. All samples of human plasma or serum contain other substances (non-creatinine chromogens) that interfere with the reaction, typically (but variably) leading to an overestimate of the 'true' creatinine by about 20 μmol/l. This is relatively unimportant when the creatinine is in or above the normal range for adult patients, 70–110 μmol/l, but can be seriously misleading in infants and young children with good renal function, in whom the true creatinine may be 30–40 μmol/l or even less. The error in the Jaffe reaction can be minimised by measuring the rate of generation of chromogen in the first minute or so of the reaction, but some overestimation remains. Several more recently-developed methods give much more accurate and reliable results at low creatinine concentrations, but these are not available in all laboratories. We recommend that paediatricians who regularly measure renal function in the very young should review the creatinine method available in their own hospital laboratory with the medical and scientific staff of the Clinical Chemistry department, to enable the results provided to be realistically interpreted.

Similarly, for many years the major cations (sodium and potassium) were measured using flame photometry, which estimates the amount of the ion present in a given volume of *total sample*, e.g. plasma. However, 100 ml of normal human plasma contains about 92 ml of water, the other 8 ml consisting of non-aqueous material (protein and lipid). The electrolytes are dissolved in the aqueous phase of plasma. Flame photometry has been largely replaced in routine laboratory work by the use of ion-selective electrodes, which measure the *activity* of the ion, i.e. its concentration in plasma water. Thus, a specimen of normal plasma having a sodium concentration (by flame photometry) of 140 mmol/l has a sodium activity of 152 mmol/l. Because clinicians were universally familiar with the 'old' normal ranges (say 137–147 mmol/l and 3.5–5.0 mmol/l for sodium and potassium respectively), the reports issued by most laboratories have been 'corrected' by the use of a 'fudge factor' to correspond roughly with the results that would have been obtained by flame photometry. Whether this is desirable is debatable at best. Usually it makes no practical difference, but there are exceptions to this. In the presence of greatly altered protein or lipid concentrations, the difference between the two methods can be much exaggerated (e.g. hypercholesterolaemia or myeloma). Here again, apparently anomalous electrolyte results should prompt a discussion with a clinical chemist or senior laboratory scientific officer in order to safeguard against misinterpretation.

URINE TESTS

Urine microscopy and culture

Specimen collection The ideal specimen is a clean-catch urine in an infant or a mid-stream specimen in an older child. Only social cleanliness is required and antiseptic solutions should not be used since these may contaminate the specimen and inhibit bacterial growth. In an infant, where a clean-catch specimen cannot be obtained, a bag specimen provides an alternative. The nappy should be left off and the bag should be removed as soon as urine is passed. The specimen should be transferred immediately into a sterile container. A negative result from a bag sample excludes UTI. A positive result should be confirmed on a clean-catch sample or a specimen obtained by suprapubic aspiration (see below). If a urinary catheter is in situ the specimen should be taken from this.

The urine specimen should be stored in either a plain sterile container or a container with boric acid added as a preservative, in which case the correct amount of urine must be added. Ideally the specimen should be transported immediately to the laboratory, and microscopy performed as soon as possible. Where not practical, for example out of hours, the sample may be refrigerated at 4°C for a maximum of 24 hours.

Procedure for suprapubic aspiration of urine In infants the full bladder extends out of the pelvis up into the abdomen. Urine can therefore be aspirated directly through the anterior abdominal wall.

- Simple and useful technique for obtaining urine in infants
- Carry out 30 minutes after a feed, when nappy is still dry, and hopefully bladder is full
- If ultrasound readily available, can be used to assess volume of urine in bladder before procedure (not essential)
- Lie infant supine, with assistant to hold in position
- Clean skin over lower abdomen
- Insert 21G needle attached to 10 ml syringe, vertically, in midline, 1–2 cm above pubic symphysis
- Advance needle slowly while applying gentle suction
- Urine should be obtained at a depth of 2–3 cm below the skin surface.

Complications — uncommon

- Occasional macroscopic haematuria
- Bowel perforation — this leads to contamination of the specimen, but, owing to the fine gauge of needle used, does not cause any other problems.

The water deprivation test

Prior to undertaking a water deprivation test several precautions should be undertaken:

- the child should have a normal GFR
- other causes for polyuria, e.g. diabetes mellitus, should be excluded.

Protocol for water deprivation test

- Free fluids are allowed until 0630 hours on the day of the test
- No tea or coffee is allowed from midnight the previous day
- A light breakfast can be consumed by 0630 hours
- No fluids or food are allowed during the test
- The test must be carried out in hospital.

Weigh patient at start of test then hourly throughout; stop the test if >4% of body weight is lost.

Blood should be taken at the times shown in Table 5.12, into two heparinised tubes, and sent to the laboratory immediately. The first tube is for measurement of ADH, and the second, which is less subject to dilutional errors, is for immediate measurement of plasma osmolality. The test should be stopped if the plasma osmolality exceeds 300 mOsm/l (diagnostic of DI).

At the end of the test an intranasal dose of DDAVP is given as follows:

    neonate   5 mcg
    infant   10 mcg
    older child 20 mcg

Free fluids are allowed. The urine is collected hourly for a further 4 hours.

Diabetes insipidus is diagnosed if:

    weight loss > 4% initial body weight occurs
    serum osmolality > 300 mOsm/kg
    urine:serum osmolality ratio <1.9 with serum osmo > 285 mOsm/kg

Nephrogenic DI is diagnosed if the urine does not become concentrated within 4 hours of the injection of DDAVP.

Table 5.12	Timing of samples in water deprivation test	
Time (h)	**Urine**	**Blood**
0	Discard	
0.5		Sample 1
1	Sample 1	
3	Discard	
3.5		Sample 2
4	Sample 2	
5	Discard	
5.5		Sample 3
7	Sample 3	
8	Sample 4	Sample 4

Protocol for the ammonium chloride (NH₄Cl) loading test

1. Obtain urine sample for pH measurement and venous blood gas for acid–base status.
2. Give NH_4Cl 0.15 g/kg, orally over 30–45 minutes. The tablets taste unpleasant and can be crushed and added to food or drinks.
3. The child can eat and drink normally throughout the test.
4. Collect urine hourly, or in younger children as voided.
5. At 4 hours — take venous blood sample for acid–base status and urine specimen. If the plasma CO_2 is only slightly depressed and the urine pH is still > 5.5 the test should be continued until 6–8 hours.

If acidosis is severe (plasma total CO_2 <15 mEq/l) and urine pH is still > 5.5, distal RTA is likely. In proximal RTA the urine pH may fall below 5.5, although this may only occur in the presence of severe acidosis (tCO_2 <12 mEq/l).

Percutaneous renal biopsy

Procedure Percutaneous needle biopsy of the native kidneys is carried out only after excluding contraindications (see Table 5.13) and ensuring the patient is fit for the procedure. Renal biopsy can usually be carried out under sedation, although in younger children, or difficult cases, general anaesthetic may be required. The biopsy is taken from the lower pole of either kidney with the patient lying in a prone position, the appropriate position having first been localised, traditionally fluoroscopically but more recently, and now more commonly, by ultrasound scan. A core of kidney is taken using either a trucut needle or a biopsy gun, an automated version of the trucut needle. Complications are few and are given in Table 5.14.

The specimen is examined by light microscopy and where indicated by immunofluorescence techniques and electron microscopy.

Table 5.13 **Contraindications to renal biopsy**	
General contraindications	**Renal contraindications**
Coagulation disorder	Single kidney
Thrombocytopenia	Renal neoplasm
Severe uncorrected anaemia	Gross hydronephrosis
Severe uncontrolled hypertension	Contracted, scarred, fibrotic kidney
Factors making sedation hazardous	Renal cystic disorders
	Ectopia, fusion defects and other major anatomical abnormalities

Procedure for renin/aldosterone/catecholamine measurement

1. Insert large IV cannula for multiple blood sampling, and send initial bloods as needed.

Table 5.14   **Complications of renal biopsy**

- **Haematuria** — microscopic haematuria is almost invariable and is not a problem. If a calyx has been punctured, macroscopic haematuria may occur, and may lead to clot retention and the requirement for urethral catheterisation. Rarely haemorrhage may be so severe that transfusion is required. Serious bleeding, never common, has become much less so since the introduction of the 'gun' which automates the action of the biopsy needle and the use of real time ultrasound for accurated localisation.
- **Perirenal haematoma** — a small subcapsular haematoma is probably present after most biopsies but is asymptomatic and resolves spontaneously. Less often large haematomas causing loin pain occur and very occasionally, where tearing of the capsule has occurred, exploration may be required.
- **Penetration/inadvertent biopsy of other organs** — occasionally the spleen, liver or pancreas may be mistakenly biopsied. Perforation of the bowel may also occur. Usually this is not problematic, although very occasionally laparotomy is required.
- **Anaesthetic problems** — occasionally problems relating to sedation or general anaesthetic occur.

---

2. Patient must then lie completely supine for the next 4 hours.
3. After 4 hours of lying supine, blood is taken via the cannula for catecholamines and renin and aldosterone. Both require immediate delivery to the biochemistry lab, and catecholamines require a special bottle. The test must therefore be discussed with the lab beforehand.
4. Then get the patient to stand up and walk around for 30 minutes — he/she should not sit or lie down during this time.
5. Then repeat the blood samples as in step 3, marking the tubes 'standing'.
6. Throughout the test, monitor blood pressure hourly.

FURTHER READING

Dalton, R.N., Haycock, G.B. (1999) Laboratory investigation. In: Barratt, T.M., Avner, E.D., Harmon, W.E. (eds) *Pediatric Nephrology*, 4th edn, pp 343–364. Baltimore: Lippincott, Williams & Wilkins.

Fogo, A. (1999) Renal pathology. In Barratt, T.M., Avner, E.D., Harmon, W.E. (eds) *Pediatric Nephrology*, 4th edn, pp 391–413. Baltimore: Lippincott, Williams & Wilkins.

Gordon, I., de Bruyn, R. (1999) Diagnostic imaging. In: Barratt, T.M., Avner, E.D., Harmon, W.E. (eds) *Pediatric Nephrology*, 4th edn, pp 377–390. Baltimore: Lippincott, Williams & Wilkins.

Peters, A.M., Gordon, I. (1999) Quantitative assessment of the urinary tract with radionuclides. In: Barratt, T.M., Avner, E.D., Harmon, W.E. (eds) *Pediatric Nephrology*, 4th edn, pp 365–375. Baltimore: Lippincott, Williams & Wilkins.

Update on the 1987 task force report on high blood pressure in children and adolescents (October 1996). *Pediatrics* 98: 4,1: 649–658.

Valtin, H., Schafer, J.A. (1995) *Renal Function*, 3rd edn. Boston: Little, Brown.

6

Rheumatology

G Kingsley and A Calogeras

Introduction

The most important step in making any diagnosis is to take a careful history and perform a detailed examination. This is particularly important in rheumatology because most tests provide supportive rather than definitive evidence for particular diagnoses. Many hospital doctors have little rheumatology training or experience as serious rheumatic disorders are unusual in childhood and more minor conditions are often treated in general practice. If in difficulty, it is often better to seek expert advice rather than continue with a long series of investigations.

List of tests

BLOOD

Haematology
Biochemistry
Microbiology
Immunology
Acute phase response
Autoantibodies
  Rheumatoid factor
  Antinuclear antibodies
  Anti-double stranded DNA antibody
  Antibodies in scleroderma and idiopathic inflammatory myopathies
  Anticardiolipin antibodies and lupus anticoagulant
  ANCAs
Tests of immune function
HLA-B27 typing

IMAGING

Radiology
Ultrasound
Nuclear medicine
CT
MRI
Bone densitometry

BIOPSY

Synovial fluid (joint aspiration)
Synovial biopsy
Other biopsies

NEUROPHYSIOLOGICAL STUDIES

OTHER CLINICAL TESTS

Nail fold capillaroscopy
Schirmer's test
Urinalysis and urine microscopy

ABBREVIATIONS USED IN THIS CHAPTER

ANAs — anti-nuclear antibodies
ANCA — antineutrophil cytoplasmic antibody
APS — antiphospholipid syndrome
ASO — antistreptolysin-O
CK — creatine kinase
CREST — syndrome of calcinosis, Raynaud's phenomenon, oesophageal involvement, sclerodactyly, telangiectasia
CRP — C-reactive protein
ENA — extractable nuclear antigen

FMF — familial Mediterranean fever
HRCT — high-resolution computerised tomography
JCA — juvenile chronic arthritis
JIA — juvenile idiopathic arthritis
LAC — lupus anticoagulant
NAI — non-accidental injury
PAN — polyarteritis nodosa
PCR — polymerase chain reaction
RNP — ribonuclear proteins
SLE — systemic lupus erythematosus
WG — Wegener's granulomatosis

1. Tests, their underlying principles and practical details

BLOOD TESTS

Haematology

The full blood count is used, not only to help in the diagnosis of rheumatic diseases, but also to assess disease activity, monitor treatment or detect complications. Other relevant haematological tests include bone marrow aspiration (leukaemia, chronic infection) and clotting screen (SLE, clotting disorders). The acute phase response is discussed below in the section on immunology.

Conversely, primary haematological disorders must be excluded in the differential diagnosis of children with certain musculoskeletal symptoms. Leukaemia is of

Table 6.1 **Some common abnormalities of the full blood count in rheumatic diseases**

Cell type	Abnormality	Examples
Red cells	Anaemia of chronic disease	Any chronic inflammatory arthritis
	Iron deficiency anaemia	Non-steroidal anti-inflammatory
	Autoimmune haemolytic anaemia	drugs, SLE; drugs
Platelets	Thrombocytosis	Acute inflammatory states
	Thrombocytopenia	Drugs; SLE
White cells	Neutrophilia	Septic arthritis, osteomyelitis
		Systemic juvenile idiopathic arthritis
	Neutropenia	Drugs, SLE
	Lymphopenia	SLE and other connective tissue diseases

Table 6.2   Blood disorders presenting with musculoskeletal symptoms

Disease	Musculoskeletal symptoms
Acute leukaemia	40% of children with leukaemia have joint pain May mimic systemic onset juvenile idiopathic arthritis Gout can occur, particularly with treatment
Haemophilia, von Willebrand's disease	Monoarthritis due to haemarthrosis
Sickle cell disease	Synovitis during crises Increased incidence of osteomyelitis and septic arthritis Avascular necrosis (also in carriers)
Thalassaemias	Synovitis Avascular necrosis (also in carriers)

particular importance and, though usually evident from the blood film, is occasionally only apparent in the bone marrow.

Biochemistry

Biochemical tests may be used in the following main ways.

▶ *To help confirm or exclude a particular diagnosis*
   Examples: renal function tests in SLE, creatine kinase (CK) levels in dermatomyositis, bone biochemistry in rickets
▶ *To detect potential side-effects of treatment*
   Examples: liver function tests during methotrexate therapy, blood glucose during steroid therapy
▶ *To monitor disease activity*
   Examples: creatine kinase levels in dermatomyositis
▶ *To detect complications of a disease*
   Examples: 24-hour urine protein in amyloidosis complicating juvenile idiopathic arthritis.

Microbiology

There are three main types of microbiology investigation which are of use in rheumatology. They are of particular use in the diagnosis of monoarthritis, polyarthritis and the differential diagnosis of systemic juvenile idiopathic arthritis.

▶ *Isolation of the organism:* usually done by culture in association with microscopy and, where positive, an antibiotic sensitivity assay. Where tuberculosis or atypical mycobacterial infection is suspected, Ziehl–Neilsen staining for acid-fast bacilli and extended culture for typical and atypical mycobacteria should be performed.
▶ *Polymerase chain reaction:* PCR methodology is used to identify organisms which are difficult to culture (because they are fastidious in culture or present

at low levels in infected tissue). Such organisms include mycobacteria and chlamydia.

▶ *Antimicrobial serology:* recent exposure to an infection can be identified by the presence of rising titres of antibodies to the relevant bacteria in the serum. A common example in rheumatology is the use of antistreptolysin-O (ASO) or anti-streptococcal DNAase B titres to detect streptococcal infection.

Immunology

a) The acute phase response The acute phase response is the increase in many plasma proteins which occurs following injury or inflammation and is under the control of pro-inflammatory cytokines such as interleukin-6. Elevation of the acute phase response occurs in a wide variety of disease states including infection, acute and chronic inflammatory diseases, neoplasia and injury. In some patients, no cause is found despite extensive investigation. Conversely, a normal acute phase response cannot absolutely exclude the presence of serious organic disease though it is often used as a screening test.

The tests used in routine clinical practice to assess the acute phase response are the erythrocyte sedimentation rate (ESR), the plasma viscosity and the C-reactive protein. All have advantages and disadvantages but, in practice, clinicians are limited by what is readily available in their hospital.

The most widely used remains the ESR, usually recorded as the number of millimetres that red cells in a column of blood fall in one hour. It depends on the fact that an increase in the concentration of large acute phase proteins, especially fibrinogen but also serum amyloid A and alpha globulins, increases the rate of sedimentation of erythrocytes. Its main disadvantage is that it is also affected by the levels of some non-acute phase proteins such as immunoglobulins and a number of other factors including age, sex, the presence of anaemia and red cell

Table 6.3 **Some important acute phase proteins**		
Protein	**Amount of increase**	**Role in assessing acute phase response**
Caeruloplasmin	50%	Not useful in this context
C3, C4	50%	Not useful in this context
alpha-1 antitrypsin	two to fourfold	Not used in this context
haptoglobin	two to fourfold	Not used in this context
fibrinogen	two to fourfold	Major determinant of viscosity and ESR Slow to increase and subside
C-reactive protein	several hundredfold	Assay widely available Rises and falls more rapidly than ESR
Serum amyloid A protein	several hundredfold	Assay available in some centres

morphology. Its main advantage is that it is widely available and cheap. Because it primarily reflects fibrinogen levels, it rises later, and remains elevated longer, than the C-reactive protein. It is therefore mainly, and most appropriately, used to monitor chronic inflammation, though this should always be in conjunction with clinical assessment. A disproportionately elevated ESR in a patient with a known chronic disease, such as arthritis, should always raise the possibility of amyloidosis (the elevation being explained by the presence of increased levels of serum amyloid A protein) or occult intercurrent disease such as a malignancy or infection.

Plasma viscosity is dependent on the same proteins as the ESR but is not affected by red cell levels or morphology, is independent of sex and reaches adult levels by the age of three (though a further rise may be seen in the elderly). An additional advantage over the ESR is that storage for several days does not affect the result.

Measurement of C-reactive protein (CRP) is increasingly available. CRP levels rise within hours of an inflammatory event and decline rapidly with diminishing inflammatory activity. CRP is therefore particularly useful in monitoring acute inflammatory processes, but is considerably more expensive than the ESR. It has been suggested that in patients with SLE, the CRP will not rise in those with active lupus but will rise in the presence of infection; however, this remains controversial.

b) Autoantibodies

Rheumatoid factor

Rheumatoid factors are antibodies directed against the Fc fragment of IgG. The rheumatoid factor antibody can be of any immunoglobulin isotype (IgM, IgA, IgE, IgD). Classical IgM rheumatoid factor is easily detected by agglutination tests but newer tests are required for the other isotypes.

Like all IgM antibodies, IgM rheumatoid factors are pentamers and can thus cause agglutination of particles coated with the antigen which they recognise, in this case IgG. Traditional agglutination tests detect IgM rheumatoid factor by the ability to cause visible agglutination of IgG-coated particles. The particles used are either latex rubber beads coated with human IgG (Latex test) or sheep red cells coated with rabbit IgG (Rose Waaler test or SCAT). The Rose Waaler test is more specific as it does not detect anti-allotypic antibodies, but less sensitive as only a small proportion of rheumatoid factors cross-react with rabbit IgG.

These agglutination tests have now largely been superseded in routine practice by newer methods. One of the most common methods for detecting this and other autoantibodies is the ELISA (enzyme-linked immunosorbent assay). In the simplest variant of an ELISA, the specific antigen of interest (in this case human IgG) is added to each of the wells of a microtitre plate and allowed to adhere to the base of the well; unadhered antigen is then washed off. The patient's serum is then added to the wells at various dilutions and the antibody within it (in this case rheumatoid factor) allowed to bind; unbound protein is then washed off. Finally, the bound antibody (in this case rheumatoid factor) is detected using an antibody to it labelled with a suitable enzyme, an appropriate enzyme substrate and an optical densitometer able to detect the colour change resulting from the enzyme–substrate interaction. Details of more complex variants of the ELISA technique (such as sandwich or competitive inhibition ELISAs) are beyond the scope of this book. Other less commonly-used modern methods for detecting autoantibodies include nephelometry and radioimmunoassay. All these more modern methods have the advantage over traditional assays of being sensitive, quantitative and, depending on the exact assay used, capable of detecting different isotypes of rheumatoid factor.

Rheumatoid factor is not a diagnostic test for rheumatoid arthritis or connective tissue diseases, though it may provide supporting evidence for such diagnoses. In paediatric rheumatology, this is particularly true since the majority of children who have juvenile idiopathic arthritis will be rheumatoid factor negative; the only group who will be positive are a subgroup (usually older children) of those with polyarticular disease. However, the identification of rheumatoid factor in these patients is of considerable prognostic importance since they have a particularly aggressive arthritis (like adult rheumatoid arthritis) which requires intensive anti-rheumatic treatment.

Rheumatoid factor may be detected in normal people. In general, higher titres of rheumatoid factor (1:80 or greater) are likely to be of clinical significance but a proportion of the normal population, particularly but not exclusively the elderly, will have relatively high titre rheumatoid factors. Rheumatoid factor is also found in many other diseases including connective tissue diseases (especially Sjögren's syndrome and SLE), viral infections, chronic bacterial and protozoal infections (infective endocarditis, tuberculosis, malaria) and hyperglobulinaemic states (chronic liver disease). Indeed, in the tropics, the presence of rheumatoid factor is much more likely to be due to chronic infection than to arthritis, particularly in children.

In summary, rheumatoid factor should be tested in patients with clear clinical inflammatory arthritis (particularly polyarticular arthritis) and in suspected connective tissue diseases. If present, all the caveats outlined above should be considered in its interpretation. Finally, in polyarticular juvenile arthritis, the presence of rheumatoid factor should lead to early expert advice on treatment to minimise long-term disability from erosive joint damage.

Antinuclear antibodies (ANAs)

These are, as their name suggests, antibodies against components of the cell nucleus; they may be directed against almost all of the components of the nucleus including DNA (double-stranded and single-stranded), nuclear proteins (histones) and various ribonucleoproteins (RNPs). These may be useful both diagnostically (different antibodies are found in different diseases) and prognostically (certain antibodies such as those to double-stranded DNA may rise and fall with disease activity).

Antinuclear antibodies are usually detected using an indirect immunofluorescence technique. The target tissue, made permeable so that high molecular weight molecules like antibodies can penetrate, is mounted on a glass slide. The target tissue most commonly used is rat liver, but because of greater sensitivity and replicability, a smear of rapidly-dividing cells such as those from the Hep2 cell line is increasingly used in addition or instead. Next, the patient's sera, at various dilutions, are placed on the target tissue. Finally, a second fluorescent-labelled antibody, directed against human immunoglobulin, is applied. After incubation, the slide is examined microscopically for the presence, intensity and pattern of fluorescence related to the cell nuclei. The presence of fluorescence indicates a positive test since immunoglobulin from the patient's serum has adhered to the target tissue nucleus. The dilution of sera at which this occurs gives a measure of the concentration of the antibody in the serum, normally expressed as a titre. Different patterns of fluorescence are associated with antibodies directed at particular autoantigens; for example, a homogenous pattern occurs with antibodies to double-stranded DNA whereas Sm/RNP antibodies are usually associated with a speckled pattern. In practice, the various antinuclear antibodies are now usually subdivided using specific tests for double-stranded DNA antibodies and extractable nuclear antigens (ENAs) rather than on their fluorescence patterns.

In paediatric practice, a test for antinuclear antibodies is usually performed in two groups of patients, those with juvenile idiopathic arthritis or those with possible connective tissue disease. However, it is important to remember that, as with rheumatoid factor, ANA may also be found in non-rheumatological disorders including organ-specific autoimmune diseases, chronic autoimmune liver disease, viral infections and leukaemia as well as in normal individuals. The titre is again important; a weakly positive ANA is unlikely to be diagnostically relevant.

In juvenile idiopathic arthritis, a positive ANA is associated with a significantly increased risk of the sight-threatening complication of posterior uveitis. Regular slit-lamp screening for uveitis should be carried out on virtually all children with juvenile idiopathic arthritis. However, the presence of an ANA, together with certain other risk factors such as early age at onset, oligoarthritis and female sex, may indicate patients at high risk who should have a more frequent and intensive screening programme. Interestingly, the ANAs found in juvenile arthritis (with or without uveitis) are heterogenous in their reactivity and the majority are not directed against currently defined antigens. Further analysis of the ANA, using tests for currently known specific antigens, is therefore not indicated in juvenile arthritis patients.

In the context of connective tissue diseases, ANA are positive in virtually all SLE patients but are also seen in patients with other connective tissue diseases especially rheumatoid arthritis and Sjögren's syndrome. ANAs in patients with connective tissue diseases are often directed against specific known antigens and, as described in detail below, the type of antigen recognised may have diagnostic or prognostic implications. In light of this, a positive ANA in a patient with a putative connective tissue disease should be further analysed using specific tests for anti-double stranded DNA and extractable nuclear antigens (ENAs).

Anti-double stranded DNA (dsDNA) antibody

Antibodies to 'native' (double-stranded) DNA are highly specific for SLE and are particularly seen in patients with renal disease. Furthermore, they can be used to monitor disease activity in SLE since a rise in antibody titre usually precedes a clinical flare. However, clinical practice in this area remains variable since many clinicians are reluctant to treat patients with potentially toxic drugs in the absence of any clinical indication of a disease flare.

Several methods have been used to detect anti-dsDNA antibodies including the *Crithidia* immunofluorescence assay which has poor sensitivity, the Farr (ammonium sulphate precipitation) assay which detects primarily high avidity antibodies, and ELISA assays. Discrepant results from these various techniques are common and some authors recommend testing by more than one method, though this is rarely done in practice.

Antibodies to extractable nuclear antigens (ENAs)

Several autoantibodies are subsumed under this heading, which originally referred to the fact that the antigens they target can be extracted from tissue with saline. Those currently most frequently examined in service laboratories are antibodies to the RNP, Sm, Ro/SSA and La/SSB antigens; the targets for these antigens are now well-defined and often represent important nuclear functions. These antibodies are usually found in patients with SLE, mixed connective tissue disease and Sjögren's syndrome. In routine laboratories, all these are usually detected with ELISA assays using purified antigens.

The Sm and RNP proteins are complexed to uridine (U)-rich small nuclear RNAs to form snRNPs (small nuclear RNPs). The Sm protein is found on all snRNPs (U1, U2, U4–6) whilst the RNP protein is found only on U1snRNP. These snRNPs form part of the spliceosome, a molecular complex which splices the introns out of pre-messenger RNA. Anti-Sm positive sera, which are highly specific for SLE, usually contain anti-RNP antibodies; the reverse is not true and patients with high titres of anti-RNP alone usually have mixed connective tissue disease, an overlap syndrome of SLE, rheumatoid arthritis, polymyositis and scleroderma.

La is a nuclear phosphoprotein which binds to RNA polymerase III transcripts (notably transfer RNAs but also other small RNAs). RNA polymerase III is one of three RNA polymerases which transcribe RNA from DNA. It synthesises most small nuclear and cytoplasmic RNAs (whereas RNA polymerase I synthesises ribosomal RNA, and RNA polymerase II synthesises messenger RNA). The target proteins for Ro antibodies have also been clearly identified though their functions and intracellular locations have not been characterised. Anti-La and Ro antibodies are seen in patients with Sjögren's syndrome and those with subacute cutaneous lupus, a form of lupus photodermatitis. Anti-Ro is also more common in the mothers of children with transient neonatal lupus and, more importantly, the presence of anti-Ro antibody in a mother is related to a high incidence of congenital heart block in her infant.

Titres of these antigens do not, by and large, parallel disease activity and they cannot therefore be used for monitoring. However, as already mentioned, the presence of particular antibodies is associated with specific clinical features; this is further discussed in the Clinical Problems section.

Antibodies found in scleroderma and idiopathic inflammatory myopathies

Antibodies found in scleroderma and inflammatory myopathies are often analysed alongside the extractable nuclear antigens, again using ELISA and appropriate purified antigens.

One antibody characteristic of the scleroderma group of diseases is the Scl-70 antibody. This recognises topoisomerase-1, an enzyme which is involved in the unwinding of DNA strands which occurs during DNA replication and translation. Anti-Scl-70 antibody is found in 20–40% of patients with diffuse scleroderma and is even more common in those scleroderma patients with intersititial lung disease. The presence of Scl-70 antibody in patients with Raynaud's phenomenon predicts the subsequent development of scleroderma. Though Scl-70 antibodies may occasionally be found in patients with limited scleroderma (CREST syndrome), these patients more characteristically have antibodies to the centromere, the specialised domain at the constriction of a eukaryotic chromosome. Anti-centromere antibodies are also found in a small proportion of patients with primary biliary cirrhosis, a disease which can be associated with limited scleroderma.

The only myositis-related autoantibody currently routinely examined is anti-Jo-1 (anti-histidyl t-RNA synthetase). Antibodies to other aminoacyl synthetases (e.g. threonyl, alanyl and isoleucyl) can also be found in myositis sera but are much rarer. All of these anti-synthetase antibodies, including Jo-1, are found in patients with a relatively acute-onset myositis especially associated with interstitial lung disease. These Jo-1 positive patients are in general steroid-responsive. Another set of myositis-specific autoantibodies which are directed against signal recognition particles are not currently routinely analysed; these appear to occur in patients with a poorer prognosis whose disease is less steroid-responsive. Further examination of this area may allow more accurate classification and thus prognosis in patients with inflammatory muscle diseases.

Anticardiolipin antibodies and the lupus anticoagulant

Over the last twenty years, a clinical subset of SLE patients has been identified with an increased risk of thrombosis, recurrent abortion, thrombocytopenia and neurological features (especially strokes and transient ischaemic attacks). Although the syndrome was initially described as a subset of SLE, it is now recognised that patients may have this syndrome in the absence of classical SLE. Because of the laboratory abnormalities these patients have (see below), the condition is characterised as the anti-phospholipid syndrome (APS); in those without other features of SLE, it is referred to as primary APS.

The first laboratory abnormality seen in APS patients is the 'false positive test for syphilis' (among the earliest immunological abnormalities known in SLE); this phenomenon transpires to be due to the presence of anti-phospholipid antibodies in the serum. In APS, these phospholipids are not recognised in isolation but in conjunction with a coagulation factor, β_2-glycoprotein I (β_2GPI), perhaps explaining the tendency of these patients to thrombosis. Most APS patients have a second laboratory abnormality, an isolated prolongation of partial thromboplastin time without obvious derangement in other clotting factors and with no clinical bleeding diathesis. This prolongation does not correct with the addition of normal serum, suggesting the presence of an anti-thrombin activity, termed the lupus anticoagulant (LAC). In APS patients, LAC and antiphospholipid antibodies are strongly but not universally associated. In parenthesis, it is important to recognise that the anti-phospholipid antibodies seen in acute viral and bacterial infections are not identical to those seen in antiphospholipid syndrome. In particular, they do not recognise the phospholipid complexed to the coagulation factor β_2GPI which may explain why antiphospholipid antibodies found in infections are not associated with thrombosis.

The best-characterised antiphospholipid antibody, and the only one available in routine laboratories, is the anticardiolipin antibody. It is important to look for the lupus anticoagulant and anticardiolipin antibodies in any child with known SLE or with features suggestive of primary APS such as unexplained recurrent thromboembolism. In these patients, prophylactic treatment with aspirin, and in certain cases formal anticoagulation, may prevent disabling thromboembolic or neurological disease.

Antineutrophil cytoplasmic antibodies (ANCAs)
These antibodies, associated with some forms of systemic vasculitis, are directed against enzymes found in the cytoplasm of neutrophils and detected by indirect immunofluorescence using normal human neutrophils fixed in ethanol. Two types of ANCA have been identified according to different staining patterns seen on immunofluorescence and corresponding to different specific target antigens. The cANCA (diffuse cytoplasmic staining) predominantly targets an enzyme called proteinase C whereas the pANCA (perinuclear pattern) is usually directed against myeloperoxidase but also elastase and occasionally other cytoplasmic antigens.

The cANCA is fairly specific for Wegener's granulomatosis (WG; rare in children) and is found in 90% of patients with the disease. The titre of cANCA is useful in monitoring disease activity in WG in those patients who are cANCA positive. The pANCA is seen in a broad spectrum of vasculitides, particularly when there is prominent renal involvement, and also in other rheumatic and non-rheumatic inflammatory conditions. Because of this, when ordered indiscriminately, the ANCA test can be misleading and it should only be requested where there is a reasonable clinical probability of systemic vasculitis.

c) Tests of immune function Full details of the tests available and indications for their use will be found elsewhere in this volume. However, it is important to be aware of their relevance to rheumatology. Arthritis is a possible presentation of many immune deficiency states seen in paediatric practice, including the rare congenital immunodeficiencies (for example C1-esterase inhibitor deficiency), common variable immunodeficiencies and acquired diseases such as HIV infection.

Immunological tests are also of use in rheumatic diseases, especially SLE. For example the measurement of complement, particularly the C3 and C4 components, may be helpful in the diagnosis and monitoring of SLE. Circulating immune complexes are implicated in the pathogenesis of this and can also be measured. Immunoglobulin levels are elevated in many rheumatological conditions, though this is not of significant practical diagnostic use.

d) HLA-B27 typing HLA-B27 is a class I Major Histocompatibility Antigen which is found in more than 90% of patients with ankylosing spondylitis and about 60% of patients with other spondyloarthropathies. In children, it is associated with the enthesitis-related arthritis subgroup of juvenile idiopathic arthritis (previously within the late-onset oligoarticular juvenile chronic arthritis group). Despite this high sensitivity, testing for HLA-B27 is of limited value in routine clinical practice because of its lack of specificity (10–15% of normal Northern

Europeans are HLA-B27 positive); the test is also expensive. Its only relevance in paediatric practice is to help establish that a child belongs to the enthesitis-related arthritis subgroup of juvenile idiopathic arthritis, or to provide additional support for a diagnosis of spondyloarthropathy in the rare cases where these diagnoses cannot be established clinically. Its use should be reserved for the specialist.

IMAGING

Radiology

In a specialty in which the musculoskeletal system is involved, it is tempting to overestimate the value of X-rays in diagnosis and management. In addition, parents of children with musculoskeletal problems often apply considerable pressure on the doctor to arrange an X-ray. In fact, many diagnoses can be made on clinical grounds alone and radiology is often not indicated, particularly in paediatric practice when the exposure of children to ionising radiation must be kept to an absolute minimum. If used appropriately, however, radiographs can provide very useful information. The essential question therefore is 'what should we X-ray and when?' It is clearly not possible to list all the situations in which an X-ray should or should not be performed, but the following may help as a guide.

X-rays should **always** be performed in a child with persistent localised pain in whom no diagnosis can be reached. Failure to do so may lead to local malignancy, leukaemia, osteomyelitis or another serious diagnosis being missed.

There are also certain specific circumstances in which radiographs are indicated to assess diagnosis or prognosis. Examples include the following:

▶ **Hip X-ray** should be performed in a child with hip pain at a relatively low index of suspicion. Hip joints are difficult to examine clinically and X-ray may be the only way to detect serious conditions such as Perthe's disease (avascular necrosis of the hip) or slipped capital femoral epiphysis. If plain X-ray is unhelpful, ultrasound, MRI and other imaging should be strongly considered.

▶ In **Juvenile idiopathic arthritis**, X-rays of the hands and feet should be taken to look for erosive changes. If present, they generally indicate a poor prognosis and the need for intensive treatment.

▶ In **Juvenile idiopathic arthritis**, cervical spine X-rays are essential pre-operatively

▶ In **Juvenile idiopathic arthritis**, periostitis may be a feature of X-rays of affected joints and help to confirm the diagnosis.

▶ In any **chronic arthritis**, a persistently painful joint should be re-X-rayed to exclude superimposed infection (if inflamed) or to assess the extent of degeneration and suitability for surgery if not inflamed

▶ **Chest X-ray** is indicated in children with scleroderma, SLE and other connective tissue diseases to exclude respiratory system involvement.

There are also some noteworthy examples of situations in which X-rays are of little use and if wrongly relied upon may lead to misdiagnosis. These include:

▶ **Diagnosis of sacroiliitis associated with spondyloarthropathy**. X-rays of the sacroiliac joints are unhelpful in children and teenagers because the joints are poorly corticated and even when normal appear wide and ill-defined on X-ray. Alternative imaging, such as MRI, CT or bone scanning needs to be considered if it is felt essential to establish the presence of sacroiliitis.

▶ **In septic arthritis, osteomyelitis and avascular necrosis**, X-rays are often entirely normal until late in the course of disease. Alternative imaging, such as bone scanning, CT scan or MRI scan, should be used in the early stages but plain X-ray may be helpful in patients who present late.

Ultrasound

The major advantage of ultrasound is that it avoids irradiation, and sedation is not usually required even in young children. The most common use of this imaging modality in paediatric rheumatology is in assessing abnormalities of the hip joint. It is particularly useful in detecting effusions of the joint which are impossible to identify by clinical means, and may be used to guide needle aspiration. It is also used to screen for instability and congenital dislocation of the hip in neonates felt to be at high risk, and in those in whom there is clinical suspicion. It is helpful also in the follow-up of these babies as the technique is sensitive and can be useful up to the age of about 1 year even after ossification has begun to take place.

Ultrasound examination of other structures, particularly the abdomen, may be indicated in children with organ involvement from juvenile idiopathic arthritis and other connective tissue disorders and in those whose pain may arise from intra-abdominal rather than skeletal lesions.

Nuclear medicine

The most widely-used nuclear medicine technique in rheumatology remains the radioisotope bone scan using Technetium-99 tracer. Technetium is preferentially taken up in areas of increased blood flow (the early blood phase) and of increased bone turnover (the late bone phase). It is useful therefore in identifying malignancy, both primary bone tumours and metastatic deposits. A bone scan is warranted in any child with unexplained bone pain, particularly when plain X-rays are normal, to exclude malignant disease. A bone scan can also detect areas of active inflammation such as a joint involved in an inflammatory or septic arthritis and may also be helpful early on in recognising avascular necrosis, such as in Perthe's disease of the hip, when plain X-rays may still be normal. As an extension of this procedure, an indium-labelled white cell scan may sometimes help to localise soft tissue or intra-abdominal pathology.

Interestingly, whereas a bone scan may help in the diagnosis of reflex sympathetic dystrophy (Sudeck's atrophy) in adults, showing characteristic increased tracer uptake in the affected area, it is of little use in children in whom the scan uptake may be normal, increased or decreased.

Computed tomography (CT)

CT scanning has had several uses in paediatric rheumatology, although many of these indications are gradually being superseded by MRI where there is no exposure to ionising radiation and where the soft tissue images are much better. The main use of CT in paediatric rheumatology is in imaging the spine, particularly looking for evidence of infection or spinal stenosis. The sacroiliac joints are also better visualised than on plain X-ray, and assessment of pathological change in these joints may be possible in children using this image modality. CT of the abdomen and thorax is occasionally necessary in children with connective tissue disorders. High resolution CT (HRCT) of the lungs must be performed if early or mild interstitial pulmonary disease is suspected. If in doubt, as with all complex radiological tests, the choice of test should be discussed with a paediatric radiologist. In the very young, CT scanning usually requires sedation.

Magnetic resonance imaging (MRI)

MRI is set to revolutionise imaging in the rheumatic diseases, and has the potential in the future to replace more invasive techniques currently in routine use. It is especially useful in diffuse abnormalities when CT scan of the entire area would require an unacceptably high radiation exposure. It also provides a particularly clear view of soft tissue structures and medullary bone. Tumours and areas of infection are especially well visualised.

Some particular uses of MRI are shown below:

▶ **Spinal disease**, particularly when the level of involvement cannot clearly be delineated on clinical examination.
▶ **Sacroiliac disease**: this is probably the most sensitive technique for demonstrating sacroiliitis.
▶ **Hip disease** if plain X-ray is normal, for example to detect early avascular necrosis.
▶ **Soft tissue disease** including pigmented villonodular synovitis, meniscal and tendon lesions.
▶ **Muscle disease**. Characteristic changes have been described in muscle affected by inflammatory myopathy. As this is a patchy disease the benefits of MRI over the more invasive 'blind' muscle biopsy are obvious. However, the technique is not routinely available and has yet to replace this and the other standard investigation, electromyography (EMG), in the diagnosis of myositis.
▶ **Arthritis.** There is potential for its use in peripheral joint problems, including inflammatory arthritis, since synovial pathology can be visualised and erosions are evident before they can be detected by plain X-rays. Again, this is currently not available in routine practice.
▶ **Cerebral disease.** MRI brain scans may be helpful in cerebral lupus and neurological disease associated with antiphospholipid syndrome, especially in children where other causes of microvascular pathology (presenting as non-specific bright spots on MRI) are less likely than in adults. However, even in children, MRI abnormalities are not specific for SLE and expert clinical as well as radiological advice is needed on their interpretation.

MRI avoids exposure to ionising radiation, but as with CT, sedation may be required in young children. Again, if in doubt about the usefulness of a test, the situation should be discussed with a paediatric radiologist.

Bone densitometry

Dual energy X-ray absorptiometry is the most accurate and validated way to assess bone density in children at the present time. Accurate assessment of bone density may be required in children who are at increased risk of osteoporosis either because of long-standing chronic inflammatory disease or because of the use of drugs which affect bone density, most commonly corticosteroids. It is likely that children and adolescents with osteoporosis should be detected and treated to avoid the long-term consequences of reduced bone density, although at present there is some uncertainty as to exact treatment regimes.

BIOPSY

Synovial fluid (joint aspiration)

This investigation is mandatory in patients with a monoarthritis unless septic arthritis can be excluded with certainty. Joint aspiration must be performed by a trained individual using an aseptic technique. Risks of the procedure include the introduction of infection and failure to enter the joint space. A general anaesthetic with its attendant risks is usually required in small children, although the procedure can be done as a day case, older children and adolescents may tolerate the procedure or may require sedation.

The fluid obtained should be sent for microscopy (including Gram staining, Ziehl–Neelsen staining and culture. Polarised light microscopy should also be performed to exclude the rare possibility that the child has an abnormality of purine metabolism resulting in gout or a secondary cause of gout such as leukaemia; in these cases, strongly negatively birefringent needle-shaped crystals will be seen. The white cell count may give an indication of the likely cause of the effusion since a high white count is more likely to be associated with an inflammatory cause. A causative organism may be isolated on microscopy and/or culture (see Table 6.4).

Table 6.4   **Likely causative organisms in septic arthritis**

Age	Likely organisms
Neonate	Staphylococcus aureus, Streptococcal species, Candida albicans
Infant less than 2 years	H. influenzae type b (decreased since vaccination programme)
2 years to adolescence	Staphylococcus aureus, Streptococcal species
Adolescent	N. gonorrhoeae, Staph. aureus

Synovial biopsy

The main indication for synovial biopsy in clinical practice is to look for occult infection in a peripheral joint or to look for a rare orthopaedic condition, pigmented villonodular synovitis. In most paediatric cases, biopsy is usually done arthroscopically since a general anaesthetic will be necessary. The tissue specimen should be sent for microbiological analysis as well as for histology.

Other biopsies

In certain specific circumstances biopsy of other tissues may be needed.

▶ **Muscle biopsy** is needed to confirm dermatomyositis. Where possible this should be by needle rather than open biopsy. The specimen must be obtained from clinically involved but not severely weakened muscle.

▶ **Skin biopsy** or **nerve biopsy** may be indicated in suspected vasculitis.

▶ **Rectal biopsy** may aid the diagnosis of secondary amyloidosis.

▶ **Renal biopsy** may be needed in a child with possible lupus nephritis or vasculitis.

▶ **Minor salivary gland biopsy** can confirm a diagnosis of Sjögren's syndrome.

In paediatric practice these procedures should be performed after expert advice, due to their invasive nature and the frequent need for general anaesthesia particularly in younger children.

NEUROPHYSIOLOGICAL STUDIES

These specialised tests should only be performed and interpreted by a trained neurophysiologist.

Electromyography (EMG) is helpful in distinguishing myositis from non-inflammatory myopathy. A characteristic pattern of spontaneous fibrillation, short polyphasic action potentials and bizarre high-frequency repetitive discharges is virtually diagnostic of inflammatory myositis.

Nerve conduction studies are indicated in inflammatory neuropathies (as may be seen for example in SLE) and in nerve entrapment syndromes such as carpal tunnel syndrome.

OTHER CLINICAL TESTS

Nail fold capillaroscopy

This test may be used to look for dilated nail fold capillaries, as seen in dermatomyositis, scleroderma and SLE, when no abnormalities are visible by the naked eye. A small drop of lubricating gel (such as KY Jelly) is placed on the nail fold. This acts as a lens and an ophthalmoscope can then be used to view the nail fold capillaries.

Schirmer's test

This simple test is used to assess tear production looking for objective evidence of xerophthalmia as seen in Sjögren's syndrome. Standardised test papers are available which are hooked over the lower eyelid and left for 5 minutes; the result is measured as the length of the paper which becomes wet. Wetting of more than 10 millimetres is normal whilst less than 5 millimetres is clearly abnormal; results that lie between these need retesting. If tear production is abnormally low the child should be referred to an ophthalmologist for more detailed assessment to confirm the diagnosis. As there is a degree of discomfort involved, it is difficult to undertake in children who are too young to understand the procedure.

Urinalysis and urine microscopy

These tests are of great importance in screening and follow-up of children with connective tissue diseases for renal involvement. They may also be necessary in monitoring anti-rheumatic therapy in patients who are on treatment with potentially nephrotoxic drugs such as gold and cyclosporin.

2. Clinical problems and how to investigate them

Rheumatological problems in children usually present in four main ways:

▶ **joint pain with swelling** (monoarthritis, polyarthritis)
▶ **suspected connective tissue disease** (SLE, other connective tissue diseases, vasculitis)
▶ **generalised pain without swelling** (fibromyalgia, blood disorders, bone disease)
▶ **regional pain** (pain in the hip, knee, spine).

These problems are discussed in further detail below.

Two additional presentations need to be remembered. First, conditions which would present as pain in older children may present as gait disorders in children too young to localise pain clearly. Examination of the joints is, therefore, essential in any child with difficulty in walking or using their limbs. Second, rheumatological conditions must be included in the differential diagnosis of children with generalised symptoms such as pyrexia of unknown origin, malaise and weight loss; relevant diagnoses include systemic-onset juvenile idiopathic arthritis, connective tissue diseases and vasculitis. Once again, the need for expert advice early on cannot be overemphasised.

JOINT PAIN WITH SWELLING

Monoarthritis

Monoarthritis, swelling of a single joint, can be caused by a number of different conditions in children ranging from the innocuous to the very serious (see Table 6.5). Many children develop transient synovitis affecting the hip or knee following a non-specific upper respiratory infective, and this is often presumed to be viral in origin. However, diagnoses of this nature should not be made until the more serious causes of monoarthritis, especially infection and malignancy, have been ruled out. One important clue to the nature of the monoarthritis is the timescale. Very acute arthritides are likely to be infective or traumatic, whilst in long-standing disease malignancy and bacterial sepsis are unlikely and JIA (juvenile idiopathic arthritis) more likely. Additional clinical features, including preceding infection, eye disease and skin disease, may also be helpful in identifying specific pathology.

Investigation of infective arthritis The most serious cause of a monoarthritis is an acute septic arthritis (replicating bacteria within the joint). Early detection is critical because, left unchecked, infection can damage the joint irrevocably within a day or two. The organisms which cause septic arthritis vary with the age of the child (see Table 6.4) but staphylococci and streptoccocci remain common throughout childhood. In adolescents, gonococcal arthritis must be considered, particularly if the arthritis is oligoarticular (rather than monoarticular) and asso-

Table 6.5	Some causes of monoarthritis in children	
Cause	**Disease**	**Examples**
Infection	Bacterial arthritis	Acute septic arthritis, gonococcal arthritis, tuberculous arthritis, brucellosis
	Other infective agents	Transient synovitis, mumps, varicella, fungal arthritis
	Bone infection	Osteomyelitis with associated sympathetic effusion or bone abscess
	Post-infectious arthritis	Reactive arthritis, Lyme disease, streptococcal arthritis, rheumatic fever, cystic fibrosis
Unknown	Juvenile idiopathic arthritis	Oligoarthritis (persistent or extended), enthesitis arthritis, psoriatic arthritis
	Spondyloarthropathy	(Overlaps with enthesitis and psoriatic subsets of JIA)
	Sarcoidosis	
Other	Malignancy	Leukaemia, neuroblastoma, sarcoma
	Benign tumour	Pigmented villonodular synovitis
	Haemarthrosis	Haemophilias (especially after minor trauma)
	Metabolic	Familial Mediterranean fever, gout (very rare)
	Mechanical	Trauma, osteochondritis dissecans

ciated with tendinitis or a blistering, painful rash. In immunocompromised patients, the newborn and those with prosthetic joints, infections with other rarer agents such as fungi also need to be remembered. Mycobacterial infection can also cause a monoarthritis but this is likely to be subacute rather than acute. Viruses usually cause arthralgia or polyarthritis but some viruses such as mumps and varicella more commonly affect one or two large joints; the syndrome of transient synovitis (irritable hip) is also presumed to be virally-mediated. Osteomyelitis, infection in the bone near the joint, may also be confused with septic arthritis.

The most essential investigation in an acute or subacute monoarthritis is joint aspiration. Synovial fluid should be sent urgently for microscopy and culture including mycobacteria (and for polarised light microscopy to exclude gout). Whilst this will lead to a bacteriological diagnosis in many cases, patients who have been partially treated or who have low-level infections with fastidious organisms may require other procedures to identify the causative organism such as polymerase chain reaction (PCR) of synovial fluid or microscopy, culture and PCR of synovial biopsy. In some patients, despite obvious clinical septic arthritis, no organisms are ever isolated. Because of this, patients with clinical septic arthritis should be treated empirically with intravenous antibiotics as soon as joint aspiration has been completed. Such treatment should be continued, tailored by the results of any positive microbiological investigations, until the course is complete or an alternative diagnosis becomes clinically apparent. It is important to note that viruses are rarely isolated from the joint even in clear-cut infection.

Additional investigations in septic arthritis, whatever the causative bacteria suspected, should include full blood count, erythrocyte sedimentation rate, blood culture and culture of other clinically infected sites. For suspected gonococcal infection, culture of genitourinary tract swabs, fluid from skin rashes and serology (gonococcal–complement fixation test) should be performed. X-rays are unlikely to be abnormal in acute septic arthritis but may be helpful after 10–14 days in subacute diseases and osteomyelitis. ANA should be checked in all children with inflammatory arthritis unless the cause is obvious but rheumatoid factor is only relevant in those with polyarthritis; both should be negative in those with septic arthritis.

Post-infective arthritis Certain forms of arthritis in children have an established association with a preceding infective episode. These include classical reactive arthritis (due to chlamydia or enteric pathogens), streptococcal arthritis (though this is more commonly a polyarthritis), rheumatic fever (classically a flitting arthritis and associated with other systemic features such as carditis) and Lyme disease (associated with characteristic skin lesions, neurological and cardiac disease). In some of these post-infectious arthritides reliable tests exist for evidence of recent infection. These should be performed in any child presenting with monoarthritis, oligoarthritis or polyarthritis, particularly if there is a history suggesting recent infection. Table 6.6 suggests the relevant investigations, which

Table 6.6 **Investigations for a post-infective arthritis**	
Preceding illness	**Investigations**
Diarrhoea	Stool cultures ×3 for *Salmonella*, *Shigella* and *Yersinia* *Yersinia* IgM antibodies (reliable serological tests do not exist for salmonella and shigella) Hepatitis serology if liver function deranged
Possible sexually-transmitted disease	Genitourinary tract swabs for *Chlamydia* culture PCR *Chlamydia* antibodies
Rash ± upper respiratory tract infection	Paired sera 2–4 weeks apart for IgM antibodies to rubella, mumps, parvovirus, enterovirus (including Coxsackie B) and adenovirus If sore throat, ASOT + throat swab for strep culture
Rash ± neurological features	*Borrelia* IgM

depend on the nature of the preceding infective episode. In addition, the children may be mildly anaemic with some elevation of the ESR. Their ANA should also be checked, as should rheumatoid factor if there is a polyarthritis; both should be negative.

Juvenile idiopathic arthritis and spondyloarthropathy This is discussed below.

Other causes of monoarthritis The most important diagnosis to consider in this group is malignancy, particularly leukaemia, which may present with arthritis prior to obvious leukaemic changes being seen on the peripheral blood film. The most distinctive diagnostic features are the degree of pain (which is very severe) and its location (which is metaphyseal rather than true joint pain). The acute phase response is characteristically very much higher than would be expected for an oligoarthritis and there may be haematological abnormalities such as a low white count which may give a clue to the diagnosis. Radiological appearances and bone scan changes may also be helpful but the diagnosis can only be confirmed by bone marrow aspiration and biopsy.

The other conditions in this group are either obvious from the history (trauma), part of a systemic disorder which is likely to be identified from its other clinical manifestations (sarcoidosis, haemophilia) or a rare diagnosis of exclusion. Pigmented villonodular synovitis and other soft tissue and bone tumours should be considered in children with persistent swollen joints where other causes have been excluded; if plain X-rays are unhelpful, MRI scans are usually the investigation of choice. Familial Mediterranean fever (FMF), an autosomal recessive condition, should be considered in children with acute self-limiting episodes of arthritis associated with fever, peritonitis, pleurisy and erythema. It is important to make the diagnosis because of the long-term risk of amyloidosis and hence renal failure. Classical FMF sufferers are of Mediterranean or Middle Eastern origin, but other, rarer periodic syndromes have been reported in other ethnic groups such as the Irish. Until recently there has not been a routinely-available specific diagnostic test for FMF, but, as with other acutely inflammatory arthritides, patients have elevated acute phase reactants and juxta-articular osteoporosis on X-ray. However, the gene associated with FMF has now been found and genes for other periodic syndromes are gradually being identified, leading to a new era of molecular diagnosis.

Polyarthritis

The differential diagnosis of polyarthritis in children is shown in Table 6.7. The majority of children with transient polyarthritis will have viral arthritides; where relevant, these can be confirmed by the demonstration of rising titres of antibodies to relevant viruses. Common global viruses which can induce polyarthritis are shown in Table 6.7; alphaviruses other than rubella are common causes of arthritis in their geographic areas of origin, for example Ross River virus in Australia. A vast range of other viruses can more rarely induce polyarthralgia or polyarthritis. Therefore the choice of serology will depend on where the illness was contracted as well as the nature of any additional clinical features. Local microbiological advice should be sought where appropriate.

Table 6.7   **Some causes of polyarthritis in children**

Cause	Disease	Examples
Unknown	Juvenile idiopathic arthritis	Systemic JIA, polyarticular JIA (rheumatoid factor positive and rheumatoid factor negative), extended oligoarthritis, enthesitis arthritis, psoriatic arthritis
	Spondyloarthritis	(Overlaps with enthesitis and psoriatic subsets of JIA)
	Connective tissue diseases	SLE, Sjögrens syndrome, vasculitis
Infection	Post-infectious arthritis	Reactive arthritis, Lyme disease, Streptococcal arthritis, rheumatic fever, cystic fibrosis
	Viral arthritis	Rubella, parvovirus, hepatitis and many other viruses
Other	Mucopolysaccharidoses Immunodeficiencies Familial Mediterranean fever	

Post-infectious arthritides also cause a short-term arthritis; their investigation is discussed above, as is the diagnosis of FMF. Persistent arthritis in children is likely to be due to juvenile idiopathic arthritis/spondyloarthropathy or connective tissue diseases. Their investigation is discussed below. The discussion of immunodeficiences and their potential rheumatic manifestations appears elsewhere in this volume.

More persistent cases of polyarthritis most commonly fall into the category of JIA or connective tissue diseases (both are discussed below). However, some congenital diseases, such as storage disorders and dysplasias, may present with skeletal changes (including short stature and thickening with stiffness of the small joints) and thus be confused with JIA. Such children usually have typical radiological appearances and do not display true inflammatory synovitis.

Routine investigations of all children with polyarthritis should include a full blood count, an ESR and assessment of the ANA and rheumatoid factor. Most will have anaemia and an elevated ESR; the presence of autoantibodies should lead to the consideration of JIA or connective tissue diseases as discussed below.

Juvenile idiopathic arthritis and spondyloarthropathy

The classification of juvenile-onset arthritis (a heterogeneous group of idiopathic arthritides occurring in children under the age of 16) has recently undergone a substantial modification (see Table 6.8). The traditional European classification subdivided juvenile-onset arthritis, then known as juvenile chronic arthritis (JCA), into three main subgroups, systemic-onset JCA, pauci-articular JCA (further subdivided into early and late onset forms) and polyarticular JCA (again

Table 6.8 Classification of juvenile idiopathic arthritis	
Subgroup	**Major identifying features**
Systemic arthritis	Spiking fever, evanescent rash, later onset of arthritis; liver, spleen, lymph nodes and other organs may be involved
Oligoarthritis (persistent)	Arthritis of 1–4 joints in first 6 months and thereafter; posterior uveitis, ANA may be positive
Oligoarthritis (extended)	Arthritis of 1–4 joints in first 6 months, arthritis ≥ 5 joints thereafter; posterior uveitis, ANA may be positive
Polyarticular arthritis (rheumatoid factor positive)	Arthritis of ≥ 5 joints in first 6 months; posterior uveitis, ANA may be positive but RF negative
Polyarticular arthritis (rheumatoid factor negative)	Arthritis of ≥ 5 joints in first 6 months; no association with uveitis, RF negative, ANA may be positive
Enthesitis arthritis	Arthritis and enthesitis or, in the absence of enthesitis, arthritis and at least two of the following: sacroiliitis, inflammatory spinal pain, HLA-B27, anterior uveitis or relevant family history
Psoriatic arthritis	Arthritis and psoriasis, or in the absence of psoriasis, arthritis and a family history of psoriasis and either dactylitis or nail abnormalities
Unclassified	Arthritides which do not fit into the above categories

subdivided into rheumatoid factor positive and rheumatoid factor negative forms). This classification excluded other inflammatory arthropathies such as psoriatic arthritis, juvenile ankylosing spondylitis, arthritis of inflammatory bowel disease and reactive arthritis which, as in adults, were grouped as spondyloarthropathies. However, it gradually became apparent that, in children, spondyloarthropathies usually presented simply with a pauciarticular peripheral arthritis, though occasionally features such as family history, skin disease or the presence of enthesitis (inflammation of a tendon or ligament insertion such as Achilles tendinitis or tennis elbow) would give a clue to the precise aetiology. There was thus significant overlap and confusion between spondyloarthropathy and late-onset pauciarticular JCA. For this reason, many spondyloarthropathies have been incorporated into the new classification of what is now known as juvenile idiopathic arthritis within the psoriatic arthritis and enthesitis arthritis subgroups (Table 6.8). Certain spondyloarthropathies, which are not truly idiopathic, such as reactive arthritis and the arthritis of inflammatory bowel disease, remain outside this classification.

At first sight such classifications can seem far removed from daily clinical practice; however, the importance of accurate classification in children with arthritis is that the complications, prognosis and treatment of these various subgroups differs. The primary features enabling classification are shown in Table 6.8, whilst a general summary of some important considerations in investigation and follow-up are shown below. However, such patients should not be managed by the non-specialist after diagnosis but should be under the joint care of a paediatrician and a specialist rheumatologist to ensure they have access to the best advice, including the provision of physiotherapy and occupational therapy.

Systemic juvenile idiopathic arthritis is usually suspected in children with a pyrexia of unknown origin and a rash; the arthritis which may help to narrow down the diagnosis is often absent initially. The differential diagnosis is vast, including all types of infection, malignant disease (especially leukaemia and neuroblastoma), vasculitis, SLE and immune-inflammatory diseases such as inflammatory bowel disease. Many of these conditions have specific, even curative, therapies, rendering it doubly important not to confuse them with systemic JIA. Making the diagnosis of systemic JIA requires not only the exclusion of these mimicking conditions by appropriate specific investigation, but also the finding of positive clinical evidence in favour of the diagnosis. To make a definite diagnosis of systemic JIA, the classical clinical triad of daily spiking fever, evanescent erythematous rash and arthritis should be present; in the absence of arthritis, a probable diagnosis of systemic JIA can be entertained if the child has the classical fever and skin rash in the presence of two of three other features, generalised lymphadenopathy, hepatomegaly/splenomegaly or serositis. There is no specific laboratory test to identify systemic juvenile idiopathic arthritis, although the diagnosis should not be made unless a very high acute phase response, neutrophilia and thrombocytosis are present and autoantibodies are absent. Posterior uveitis is very rare in these children but screening, at least initially, may be considered since the diagnosis can be confused with that of fulminant onset seronegative polyarthritis where the children are at risk. Untreated systemic JIA can progress to the macrophage-activation syndrome (also known as the haemophagocytic syndrome) which has a high mortality rate even with expert intensive care.

Oligoarthritis is usually suspected in relatively well children who classically have problems with their wrists, knees and ankles. Because these children are very young (the peak age is around 3 years), they often deny pain and may present with less specific features such as mood changes and reluctance to walk; the detection of arthritis in this situation requires careful clinical examination. Although the outlook for the joints is good in these children, the complication of posterior uveitis, which may result in blindness unless identified early, means that, once again, accurate diagnosis is important. Investigations should include a full blood count and ESR (though the latter may be normal if only a very few joints are involved) and an ANA. The risk of uveitis is higher in ANA-positive children but cannot be excluded in those who are ANA-negative; therefore all children with oligoarthritis should be referred for urgent slit lamp examination and continuing ophthalmological follow-up. In some children, the number of joints involved in their disease increases after the first six months to more than 5; these children are now separately defined as **extended oligoarthritis**; they have more long-term joint problems than children with persistent oligoarthritis, and anti-rheumatic drug therapy with methotrexate should be considered.

Polyarthritis can occur in two varieties, distinguished by the presence or absence of rheumatoid factor; this is the only indication for the assessment of rheumatoid factor in children with arthritis. The group of **rheumatoid factor negative polyarthritis** is poorly defined; investigations will reveal anaemia, a variably elevated ESR, in some cases a positive ANA and, by definition, a negative rheumatoid factor. These children are at risk of posterior uveitis, and therefore ophthalmological screening and follow-up is required. **Rheumatoid factor positive polyarthritis** is much rarer, usually occurs in teenage girls and is the juvenile equivalent of adult rheumatoid arthritis. These children are likely to be moderately anaemic and their ESR is likely to be significantly raised. They will, by definition, have a positive rheumatoid factor but may also have, as do adults with rheumatoid arthritis, a low level positive ANA. X-rays may well be normal initially but will later develop the classical erosive changes associated with rheumatoid arthritis. They are not at risk of posterior uveitis and do not require eye-screening if the diagnosis is established with certainty. However, they have an extremely poor prognosis with regard to their joints, necessitating early intensive anti-rheumatic therapy. They may also develop, at onset or later, the systemic manifestations associated with adult rheumatoid arthritis including lung disease, neuropathy and vasculitis, and these should be specifically looked at.

Enthesitis-related arthritis and **psoriatic arthritis** are primarily defined clinically as described in Table 6.8. Initial investigation will include a full blood count and ESR, though these may well be normal. Such children will also be negative for autoantibodies. As discussed in the Imaging section above, plain X-rays will be unreliable in establishing a possible diagnosis of sacroiliitis and MRI or CT scan will be required. HLA-B27 testing is rarely required and interpretation can be confusing, so is best left for the use of specialists (see HLA-B27 typing, above).

SUSPECTED CONNECTIVE TISSUE DISEASE AND VASCULITIS

With the exception of systemic lupus erythematosus (SLE) in certain ethnic groups and some vasculitides (Kawasaki disease and Henoch–Schönlein purpura), these diseases are rarely seen in paediatric practice. For this reason, and because of their considerable morbidity and mortality, such patients should not be managed by the non-specialist. They should be under the joint care of a paediatrician and a specialist rheumatologist and, in difficult cases, early referral to a tertiary centre should be considered. However, all doctors looking after children need to have a strategy for initial investigation since they may present acutely or in a non-specific fashion and, unlike many other rheumatic conditions, appropriate investigations may be rapidly diagnostic.

One very important issue for the non-specialist is to recognise the clinical situations in which a connective tissue disease or vasculitis should be considered. These children may present in outpatients with chronic progressive symptoms or as an emergency with an acute illness (especially SLE and some forms of vasculitis). The diagnosis is particularly likely to be missed in those who present acutely because emergency teams are attuned to standard acute childhood illnesses such as infection and because the doctors may have little clinical experience of acute connective tissue disease. The following features should raise suspicion of these diagnoses:

▶ children with unexplained general symptoms such as malaise, fever and weight loss
▶ children with abnormalities involving more than one body system (multisystem disorders)
▶ children with abnormalities in the most commonly-affected body systems, especially skin lesions (rashes and/or apparent bruising), renal/urinary abnormalities and joint pain/swelling
▶ children who have one of the above plus abnormalities in other body systems including blood, nervous system, respiratory system, muscle and gastrointestinal tract.

There are two major groups of conditions which are considered under the heading of connective tissue diseases, **autoimmune connective tissue diseases** (SLE, dermatomyositis, scleroderma, Sjögren's) and **vasculitis**. Brief descriptions outlining the major clinical features and investigations are shown, disease by disease, below. It must be borne in mind that some children defy exact classification, presenting with overlap syndromes which include features of more than one condition. One example of this is mixed connective tissue disease (overlap between SLE, scleroderma, rheumatoid arthritis and myositis) defined by the presence of anti-RNP antibodies.

Systemic lupus erythematosus (SLE)
Typical clinical features:

▶ general — fever, malaise, lymphadenopathy
▶ skin lesions — butterfly rash, photosensitivity, mouth ulcers, alopecia, Raynaud's syndrome
▶ other systems — arthritis, serositis, renal disease, haematological disorders, neurological disorders
▶ equal sex incidence before puberty; more common in girls thereafter.

Investigation of SLE Investigations are performed in SLE (Table 6.9) to make the diagnosis (ANA, anti-dsDNA antibodies, occasionally skin and renal biopsies), to assess disease activity (acute phase response, blood film, complement), to assess organ involvement (especially renal but also liver, pulmonary and cardiac tests) and to look for complications requiring specific treatment (autoimmune thrombocytopenic purpura or coagulation abnormalities suggestive of anti-phospholipid syndrome).

Dermatomyositis (DM)/polymyositis (PM)
Typical clinical features:

▶ Both DM and PM — proximal muscle pain/weakness, respiratory muscle weakness, cardiac involvement, fever
▶ DM only — heliotrope rash, other skin rashes, calcinosis, arthritis, vasculitis, Raynaud's, pulmonary fibrosis.

Table 6.9 Investigation of systemic lupus erythematosus		
Investigation	**Result**	**Interpretation**
Haematology		
Full blood count	Anaemia	Usually normochromic normocytic but can be haemolytic; exclude with film/Coombs test
	Leucopenia/lymphopenia	Usual in active SLE
	Neutropenia	Requires specific investigation and treatment
	Thrombocytopenia	Requires specific investigation and treatment
Acute phase response	Elevated ESR, CRP	Acute disease or complication such as infection
Immunology		
Antinuclear antibodies	ANA positive	Positive in almost all patients but not specific for SLE; if negative, virtually excludes SLE
	anti-DNA, anti-Sm positive	Virtually specific for SLE; positive in most SLE patients, especially those with or likely to develop renal disease; DNA antibody titre varies with disease activity
	anti-Ro, anti-La positive	Positive in substantial minority with SLE, especially with Sjögrens; also associated with neonatal lupus syndromes
Coagulation abnormalities	Lupus anticoagulant and anticardiolipin antibodies	Suggest anti-phospholipid syndrome which may require aspirin or anticoagulant treatment
Complement	Reduced C3 and C4	Active disease especially nephritis
Renal		
Urinalysis and urine microscopy	Proteinuria, haematuria, abnormal urinary sediment, evidence of infection	Proteinuria in active or previous renal disease; haematuria/red cell casts in active nephritis; other cell casts in severe renal disease
Urea, creatinine, electrolytes (U&E)	Elevated urea, creatinine Abnormal electrolytes	Impaired renal function
Further testing		If U&E or urinalysis abnormal, arrange 24-hour urine protein, renal ultrasound and radionuclide glomerular filtration rate. Obtain renal advice with regard to renal biopsy

Table 6.9 (continued)		
Investigation	**Result**	**Interpretation**
Other organs		
Respiratory	Chest X-ray, lung function	These tests are used to assess
Cardiac	ECG, echocardiogram	involvement of major organ
Nervous system	Lumbar puncture, MRI scan, nerve conduction studies, psychometrics	systems. Simple tests (chest X-ray and ECG) should be performed routinely. Other tests should be ordered and interpreted with expert advice
Skin	Skin biopsy	
Muscle biopsy	Creatine kinase, EMG, muscle biopsy	

Appropriate investigation of dermatomyositis/polymyositis (Table 6.10):

▶ Diagnosis — acute phase response (to differentiate from non-inflammatory muscle disease), creatine kinase, EMG and muscle biopsy; muscle MRI helpful where expertise is available
▶ Monitoring — ESR and creatine kinase, in conjunction with clinical examination, are normally used in outpatients; in inpatients with possible respiratory impairment, spirometry should be monitored frequently in children who can cooperate, to assess the need for ventilatory support.

Scleroderma
Typical clinical features:

▶ spectrum of disease from localised forms (morphoea, linear scleroderma), through limited scleroderma (CREST syndrome), to true systemic sclerosis
▶ skin lesions (tethering, telangiectasia, calcinosis), Raynaud's phenomenon, musculoskeletal symptoms (including true muscle inflammation), dysphagia, malabsorption, cardiac disease, renal disease, pulmonary disease (pulmonary hypertension and fibrosis).

Investigation of scleroderma (Table 6.11):

▶ Diagnosis — primarily clinical diagnosis; if Raynaud's phenomenon and/or ANF absent, rarer fibrosing diseases should be considered
▶ Monitoring — no test accurately assesses disease status overall; monitoring comprises clinical examination (with appropriate further investigation of any problems detected) and routine assessment of systems which are associated with significant morbidity and mortality, especially renal, cardiac and pulmonary disease.

Table 6.10 **Investigation of dermatomyositis (DM)/polymyositis (PM)**

Investigation	Result	Interpretation
Haematology		
Full blood count	Leucocytosis and anaemia	May occur though uncommon at onset.
	Eosinophilia	Trichinosis should be considered.
Acute phase response	Raised ESR usual in active disease	Used to differentiate from non-inflammatory muscle disorders (muscular dystrophy, myotonia) and to monitor disease.
Muscle		
Muscle enzymes	Raised creatine kinase usual in active disease (but may rarely be normal)	Used in diagnosis and to monitor disease activity. Other muscle enzymes (aldolase, LDH) no better than creatine kinase; transaminase elevation not specific for DM/PM.
EMG	Characteristic pattern of polyphasic spikes and fibrillation	Problematic in young children since may require sedation; not mandatory unless diagnosis in doubt.
Muscle biopsy	Muscle fibre degeneration, necrosis, inflammatory cell infiltrates, vascular lesions	Samples must be prepared with expert advice; false negatives may occur since muscle involvement patchy; not mandatory unless diagnosis in doubt.
MRI of muscle	Extent of inflammation in muscle	May be used to select involved muscle for biopsy or to monitor disease.
Other organs		
Respiratory	Spirometry, other lung function, chest X-ray	Spirometry to monitor ventilation (decrease in vital capacity first sign of deterioration).
Cardiac	ECG, echocardiogram	If cardiac involvement suspected.
Skin	Skin biopsy	No features specific for DM/PM.
Autoantibodies	Positive antinuclear factors in minority of patients	Not routinely clinically useful in children (see text for specific antibodies).
Infection		
Microbial serology and other appropriate tests for infection	May be positive (relevance and interpretation depend on clinical features and geographical location)	Acute myositis can be due to viruses (especially influenza A and B, Coxsackievirus B) and other agents (trichinosis, toxoplasma, schistosomiasis, trypanosomiasis, staphylococcal pyomyositis).

Table 6.11   **Investigation of scleroderma**

Investigation	Result	Interpretation
Haematology Full blood count and acute phase response	Anaemia	Chronic disease (need to exclude vitamin B_{12} or folate deficiency from malabsorption).
	Leucocytosis	Leucocytosis may occur in advanced disease.
	Eosinophilia	May occur in minority of patients.
	Raised ESR	Not a reliable overall indicator of disease status.
Autoantibodies	Positive antinuclear factor (speckled) frequent; target Scl-70 or centromere	Useful in diagnosis and classification — anti Scl-70 occurs in true systemic sclerosis and anti-centromere antibody in limited scleroderma
Renal Urinalysis, urea, creatinine and electrolytes	Proteinuria Elevated urea, creatinine abnormal electrolytes	Proteinuria and hypertension most common signs of renal impairment but elevated urea or creatinine may also be first indicator.
Further investigation		Renal disease has a poor prognosis and may worsen rapidly. Arrange renal ultrasound and radionuclide glomerular filtration rate, control blood pressure as priority and seek expert advice.
Other organs Respiratory	Echocardiogram	Assessment of pulmonary hypertension.
	Chest X-ray, lung function tests, high resolution CT	Detection and assessment of pulmonary fibrosis.
Cardiac disease	ECG, echocardiogram	Assessment of cardiac involvement.
Gastrointestinal tract	Barium studies, oesophageal manometry, tests for malabsorption	Appropriate in patients with significant symptomatic involvement.

Table 6.12	Investigation of Sjögren's syndrome	
Investigation	**Result**	**Interpretation**
Haematology		
Full blood count and acute phase response	Anaemia	Anaemia of chronic disease.
	Leucopenia	Lymphopenia and neutropenia occur in active disease.
	Raised ESR	Common, indicating active disease.
Immunology		
Immunoglobulins	Polyclonal hypergammaglo-bulinaemia	Consistent though non-specific feature.
Autoantibodies	Rheumatoid factor	Most common autoantibody (seen in >75%).
	Antinuclear factor	Present in 40–70% patients.
	Anti-Ro and anti-La	Present in many patients (higher specificity for Sjögren's than ANF or rheumatoid factor).
Eye disease	Schirmer's test	Reduced tear production.
	Ophthalmology assessment	Superficial erosions by Rose–Bengal or fluorescein staining; filamentous keratitis characteristic on slit-lamp examination.
Salivary glands	Minor salivary gland (labial) biopsy	Diagnostic test showing lymphoid aggregates and plasma cell infiltrate.
	Sialogram and salivary flow	Reduced salivary flow with ectasia of ducts.
Other organs		
Respiratory	Chest X-ray, lung function tests, high resolution CT	Detection and assessment of pulmonary fibrosis.
Renal	Abnormalities in urinalysis, urea, creatinine, electrolytes	Detection and assessment of interstitial nephritis and renal tubular acidosis

Sjögren's syndrome

Typical clinical features:

▶ may be primary (rare) or secondary to other connective tissue diseases (commoner in children)

▶ essential features are dry eyes (keratoconjunctivitis sicca) and dry mouth (xerostomia) sometimes associated with salivary gland enlargement, especially of the parotid

▶ additional systemic features in primary Sjögren's include arthralgia/arthritis, myositis, lung disease and renal abnormalities including renal tubular acidosis
▶ in adults with primary Sjögren's, increased incidence of lymphoma requiring long-term follow up.

Investigation of Sjögren's syndrome (Table 6.12):

▶ diagnostic tests — demonstration of dry eyes (Schirmer's test and further ophthalmological examination), characteristic changes on minor salivary gland biopsy, autoantibodies
▶ monitoring should include regular ophthalmological assessment, assessment of salivary gland flow and monitoring for complications.

Vasculitis

This heterogeneous group of diseases is characterised by inflammatory cell infiltration and necrosis of blood vessels. Any organ of the body may be affected by the process and the clinical consequences depend upon the size, site and number of vessels involved. It can be localised, for example to the skin, when it may be clinically less significant, but often it is generalised and potentially life-threatening. It is important for the non-specialist to have a clear idea of when to suspect these serious disorders, and a series of pointers is outlined in the introduction to this section (pp. 180–181).

Classification of vasculitis in adults and children has proved controversial in view of the considerable overlap between the various syndromes described. One classification commonly used for childhood vasculitis is given in Table 6.13.

Brief notes on the presentation and investigation of the more common or important forms of childhood vasculitis are given below.

Kawasaki disease A relatively common childhood systemic necrotising vasculitis, Kawasaki disease affects small and medium-sized arteries including coronary

Table 6.13 Classification of Childhood Vasculitides

Subgroup	Disease
Polyarteritis	Polyarteritis nodosa
	Microscopic polyarteritis
Kawasaki's disease	
Granulomatous vasculitis	Wegener's granulomatosis
	Churg–Strauss syndrome
Leucocytoclastic vasculitis	Henoch–Schönlein purpura
	Hypersensitivity vasculitis
	Mixed cryoglobulinaemia
Giant cell arteritis	Takayashu's arteritis
Other	Vasculitis secondary to connective tissue disease; Behcet's disease

vessels. It most often affects infants and young children, particularly boys, with a particularly high incidence among those of Oriental and Afro-Caribbean origin. There is some seasonal variation in incidence, and the disease occasionally occurs in epidemics, suggesting an infective cause.

Clinical features

There are six diagnostic criteria, of which five must be present to make the diagnosis: fever, polymorphous rash, conjunctival injection, cervical lymphadenopathy, erythema and oedema of mucous membranes and of the palms and soles with subsequent desquamation.

Other features which may be seen are pneumonitis, arthritis, diarrhoea and vomiting, cardiac involvement (including carditis and coronary artery aneurysms causing acute myocardial infarction), renal and neurological manifestations, including irritability.

Investigations in Kawasaki disease

▶ *Full blood count and acute phase response*
Mild anaemia common; elevated ESR, platelet count and white cell count are usual (though early neutropenia or thrombocytopenia may occur and thrombocytosis occurs during the third week of fever)
▶ *Immunology*
Positive ANCA in some patients; increased circulating immune complexes and immunoglobulins (these tests are not performed routinely)
▶ *Biochemistry and urinalysis*
Moderate elevation in liver enzymes common; if renal involvement, sterile pyuria and abnormal urea and electrolytes
▶ *Cardiac studies*
ECG, echocardiography (occasionally coronary angiography) to assess initial and subsequent cardiac status including presence of aneurysms and coronary artery disease.

Henoch–Schönlein purpura This common small vessel vasculitis affects particularly 5–15-year-olds. It usually occurs in the winter, often with a preceding history of upper respiratory tract infection. There is no specific diagnostic test.

Clinical features

▶ Fever
▶ Palpable purpura in dependent pressure-bearing areas such as the buttocks and lower limbs
▶ Arthritis/arthralgia, usually transient and may slightly precede the rash
▶ Abdominal pain and gastrointestinal haemorrhage, rarely precedes the rash
▶ Glomerulonephritis, rarely precedes the rash, severity variable but extent of renal disease over first few months determines ultimate renal outcome.

Investigations in Henoch–Schönlein purpura

▶ *Full blood count and acute phase response*
Anaemia is common (in part related to gastrointestinal blood loss); modest leukocytosis may be seen and the ESR is elevated.
▶ *Coagulation studies*
Studies of the coagulation pathway including platelet levels and function are normal.
▶ *Immunology*
This is not routinely helpful; autoantibodies are negative but there may be elevated IgA, elevated IgM, immune complexes and alternative (not classical) complement pathway activation.
▶ *Renal function*
Impaired renal function may be suggested by haematuria, proteinuria (occasionally inducing hypoalbuminaemia) or abnormal urea and electrolytes.
If renal disease persistent, severe or recurrent, further investigation including renal biopsy may be warranted and expert advice should be sought.
▶ *Skin biopsy*
May be helpful diagnostically in difficult cases, shows characteristic leucocytoclastic vasculitis with IgA and C3 deposition.

Polyarteritis nodosa (PAN) PAN is characterised by a necrotising vasculitis associated with aneurysmal nodules along the walls of medium-sized muscular arteries. It is rare but does occur in childhood.

Clinical features

▶ Malaise, fever, weight loss
▶ Skin rash, classically livedo reticularis
▶ Abdominal and testicular pain
▶ Myalgia, arthritis, neuropathy
▶ Hypertension, coronary disease and renal involvement.

Investigations in PAN

▶ *Full blood count and acute phase response*
Anaemia, elevated ESR and neutrophilia.
▶ *Hepatitis serology*
The association of PAN with hepatitis B is rare in children.
▶ *Immunology*
Classical cANCA (anti-proteinase 3) are negative but pANCA (anti-myeloperoxidase) may be found (non-specific finding in many forms of vasculitis); immunoglobulins and immune complex levels are elevated.
▶ *Renal function*
Haematuria, proteinuria and abnormal urea and electrolytes suggest renal disease.
▶ *Diagnostic imaging*
Angiographic demonstration of small aneurysms involving the renal, hepatic, coeliac or coronary arteries is pathognomonic; magnetic resonance angiography may gradually replace contrast studies.

▶ *Biopsy*
Biopsy of involved tissue (especially sural nerve, kidney or skin) may support the diagnosis by showing vasculitis with granulocytes ± monocytes in the vessel wall; also helpful in detecting degree of renal involvement.

Wegener's granulomatosis (WG) and other granulomatous vasculitides WG is a necrotising granulomatous vasculitis of the upper and lower respiratory tract. Limited forms may be confined to the upper respiratory tract, but generalised WG is associated with glomerulonephritis and small vessel vasculitis affecting other organs. It is rarely seen in children.

Clinical features of WG

▶ Malaise, fever and weight loss
▶ Upper airway lesions (sinusitis, otitis media, epistaxis/lesions of nasal septum and subglottic stenosis)
▶ Lower airway lesions (pulmonary infiltrates common on X-ray but clinical disease rarer)
▶ Skin, joint, ocular, renal, neurological and cardiac involvement.

Investigations for WG

▶ *Full blood count and acute phase response*
Anaemia, elevated ESR and neutrophilia
▶ *Immunology*
cANCA (anti-proteinase 3) antibodies are strongly associated with, and relatively specific for, WG (but may be absent in WG limited to the upper respiratory tract and in inactive disease).
▶ *Renal function*
Haematuria, proteinuria and abnormal urea and electrolytes suggest renal disease; if severe, further tests including renal biopsy may be warranted and expert advice should be sought.
▶ *Imaging*
CXR classically shows multiple nodular pulmonary infiltrates, but reticulonodular shadowing and other less specific abnormalities may be present.
▶ *Biopsy*
Biopsy of skin, nasal or sinus submucosa shows necrotising granulomata with little arteritis. Renal biopsy shows a focal necrotising proliferative glomerulonephritis with crescent formation.
▶ *Organ involvement*
Further investigation of other potentially involved organs may be required to enable accurate assessment and treatment, for example eyes for uveitis and ulceration.

Churg–Strauss syndrome, the other main granulomatous vasculitis in adults, is excessively rare in children. It should be suspected in patients with asthma, fever and eosinophilia. Mononeuritis multiplex is common but renal disease is rare. The diagnosis is made by biopsy showing a necrotising vasculitis with an eosinophilic infiltrate and extravascular necrotising granulomata.

NON-ARTHRITIC MUSCULOSKELETAL PROBLEMS

Widespread pain without swelling

Non-inflammatory musculoskeletal pain is very common in childhood. In most cases, no serious cause is identified. However, it is important to make as accurate a diagnosis as possible as rapidly as possible, to ensure serious medical conditions are not missed and to avoid unnecessary or prolonged investigation. Since the potential causes of musculoskeletal pain are numerous, the mainstay of diagnosis

Table 6.14   **Some causes of non-inflammatory musculoskeletal pain in children**

Cause	Examples
Mechanical disorders	Accidental and non-accidental trauma Regional pain syndromes
Idiopathic pain syndromes	Fibromyalgia Chronic fatigue syndrome Reflex sympathetic dystrophy Benign nocturnal limb pains (incorrectly termed 'growing pains')
Neoplasia	Bone and soft tissue tumours Hypertrophic osteoarthropathy (usually but not always associated with malignant disease) Acute leukaemia and lymphoma
Infection	Osteomyelitis and soft tissue infections usually associated with clinical inflammation but chronic disease may not be
Haematological disorder	Sickle cell disease (pain due to microinfarcts in older children) Sickle cell disease (dactylitis or hand–foot syndrome in infants) Thalassaemia Haemophilia (acutely, bleeds into joint or soft tissue; later degenerative changes)
Metabolic/endocrine disease	Rickets Osteoporosis Thyroid disorders Hypervitaminosis A Scurvy
Genetic disorders	Hypermobility (Benign, Marfans, Ehlers–Danlos) Storage disorders Skeletal dysplasias

remains a careful history and clinical examination. A formal functional assessment, usually by a physiotherapist, can also be very revealing where the child or his/her parents allude to substantial problems with daily living yet examination is relatively normal.

As shown in Table 6.14, the list of potential diagnoses for a child with musculoskeletal pain is long. However, after consideration of clinical features (for example, malignancy is unlikely as a cause of long-standing disease), only a relatively few simple investigations are initially required to rule out serious organic pathology in the absence of clinical evidence.

First-line investigations in musculoskeletal pain without inflammation:

▶ Full blood count
▶ Acute phase response including ESR and/or CRP
▶ Biochemistry including urea and electrolytes, bone biochemistry and creatine kinase
▶ Anti-nuclear factor
▶ Thyroid function tests
▶ Haemoglobin electrophoresis, sickle test and coagulation screen
▶ Imaging of one or more involved areas (especially if localised or severe pain or deformity); plain X-ray usually sufficient but other tests such as bone scan may be required.

If initial tests are abnormal, further or repeat investigations should be performed.

Where the diagnosis is initially unclear, review over time may be necessary since symptoms and signs often evolve. A second opinion should be sought if the doctor feels uncertain for two reasons. First, it minimises the chance of missing serious or treatable pathology. Second, if the ultimate diagnosis is an idiopathic pain syndrome, a psychological and rehabilitative approach rather than the traditional curative therapy will be needed; this is not likely to be accepted if the child and his parents do not perceive the doctor to be confident in his/her diagnosis.

Localised pain: the regional pain syndromes

An important and common group of rheumatological disorders are the regional pain syndromes. They usually present with pain localised to one limb or joint; diagnosis is generally reached by careful history-taking and clinical examination. Investigations may occasionally be used to make a firm diagnosis or, more often, to exclude serious disease such as non-accidental injury, malignancy, infection or monoarticular onset juvenile idiopathic arthritis. Although it is important not to miss serious pathology in such children, it is equally critical to avoid erroneously labelling them as suffering from serious disease which may lead to inappropriate treatment or lifestyle changes. Table 6.15 sets out some common causes of regional pain.

Investigations are rarely helpful in the diagnosis of local soft tissue problems or many other regional conditions such as patellar disease, Osgood–Schlatter's disease and reflex sympathetic dystrophy. A child with reflex sympathetic dystrophy presents with a characteristic clinical picture of severe burning pain in the distal portion of a limb, sometimes following trauma. The limb, usually the leg,

Table 6.15 Some common causes of regional pain	
Hip disorders	Secondary avascular necrosis
	Perthe's disease (idiopathic avascular necrosis)
	Slipped capital femoral epiphysis
	'Transient synovitis' ('irritable hip')
	Congenital dislocation of the hip
Knee disorders	Chondromalacia patellae
	Patellar dislocation
	Osgood–Schlatter's disease
	Osteochondritis dissecans
Spine disorders	Discitis/osteomyelitis
	Spondylolisthesis
	Mechanical back pain
	Scheuermann's disease (osteochondritis)
Other local lesions	Achilles tendinitis, plantar fasciitis, pes planus.
	Lateral epicondylitis ('tennis elbow')
	Rotator cuff tendinitis
	Stress fractures (especially feet and tibia)
	Osteochondroses (described at most sites)
Reflex sympathetic dystrophy. Serious disease masquerading as regional pain	Bone tumours (benign and malignant)
	Osteomyelitis
	Trauma including non-accidental injury
	Monoarticular arthritis

may be diffusely swollen, cold, discoloured or hyperaesthesic. Laboratory investigations are normal. Unlike in adults, the bone scan is unhelpful but X-ray should be performed to exclude other conditions and, late in disease, may show patchy osteoporosis.

There are, however, a variety of circumstances where investigations are appropriate and some of these are outlined below:

▶ A **full blood count and ESR** should be undertaken in any child where the diagnosis is not clinically clear.

▶ Screening for **haemoglobinopathies** should be performed where indicated by the child's ethnic origin or family history.

▶ **Plain radiographs** are required in any child who has significant localised or persistent pain, local tenderness or another reason to suspect significant pathology (infection, benign tumour, malignancy). Further investigation with a radioisotope bone scan, CT or MRI may be required if the XR is normal yet clinical suspicion persists; expert advice should be sought.

▶ **Bone tumours** are often demonstrated on plain radiographs (though a CT or bone scan may be needed); in some cases further assessment by biopsy of the abnormal area is necessary.

- ▶ If **leukaemia** is suspected, a bone marrow is essential.
- ▶ A skeletal survey or bone scan should confirm the suspicion of **non-accidental injury**.
- ▶ **Back pain** in children (particularly those under 10) warrants a high index of suspicion; all children should have a full blood count, ESR and plain X-ray. Further imaging with isotope bone scan, CT scan or MRI may be required to exclude infection or benign or malignant tumours.
- ▶ **Hip pain** is difficult to diagnose clinically with certainty because the joint is deep below the surface; a low index of suspicion for investigation is needed. Plain XRs may diagnose late-stage avascular necrosis, congenital dislocation of the hip, Perthe's disease and slipped capital femoral epiphysis but CT or MRI scan will be needed to identify early disease. Bone scan can also identify early avascular necrosis. Ultrasound or MRI is useful in demonstrating synovitis (irritable hip and other causes) with aspiration if an effusion is present.
- ▶ In a child with **knee pain**, aspiration of the joint is mandatory if there is any swelling (to exclude septic arthritis); if there is local bone pain or inflammation, X-ray should be requested to exclude osteomyelitis or malignancy.

FURTHER READING

Athreya, B.H. (ed) (1997) Rheumatic Disease Clinics of North America. *Paediatric Rheumatology* Vol. 23, no. 3. Philadelphia: W.B. Saunders.

Cassidy, J.T., Petty, R. (1995) *Textbook of Paediatric Rheumatology*, 3rd edn. Philadelphia: W.B. Saunders.

Davidson, J. (2000) Juvenile idiopathic arthritis: a clinical overview. *European Journal of Radiology*. 33: 128–134.

Malleson, P.N. (1997) Management of childhood arthritis. Part 1: Acute arthritis. *Arch Dis Child* 76: 460–462.

Malleson, P.N. (1997) Management of childhood arthritis. Part 2: Chronic arthritis. *Arch Dis Child* 76: 541–544.

Woo, P., Wedderburn, L.R. (1998) Juvenile chronic arthritis. *Lancet* 351: 969–973.

7

Metabolic Disease

J Collins

Introduction

Although primary metabolic disorders are individually rare, their number and range mean they make an important contribution to childhood disease and disability (see Scriver et al. 1995). Most are inherited and many are treatable. Any organ of the body can be affected, and as the symptoms and signs are often non-specific, diagnosis depends on clinicians having a high index of suspicion. Metabolic disorders can be broadly divided into defects in intermediary metabolism and defects of peroxisome and lysosome metabolism. It is beyond the scope of this chapter to include every disorder.

ABBREVIATIONS USED IN THIS CHAPTER

CDG — carbohydrate-deficient glycoprotein syndrome

MCAD — medium chain acyl-CoA dehydrogenase deficiency

MELAS — mitochondrial encephalomyopathy, lactic acidosis and stroke-like episodes

OTC — ornithine transcarbamylase deficiency

PKU — phenylketonuria

VLCFAs — very long chain fatty acids

BACKGROUND

The enzyme defect may or may not have been defined. Clinical features arise due to excess substrate or its metabolites or due to deficiency of products.

The same enzyme defect may present at different ages, for example the neonatal onset and late onset group of urea cycle defects. The phenotype and genotype are likely to be very different.

Some disorders are sporadic but most are inherited. Inheritance can be:

▲ autosomal recessive — most common
▲ X-linked — e.g. OTC deficiency, adrenoleukodystrophy, Menkes syndrome
▲ autosomal dominant — e.g. respiratory chain defects, some forms of porphyria
▲ maternal inheritance — e.g. respiratory chain defects.

RANGE OF DISORDERS

Metabolic diseases can affect:

Protein metabolism — organic acidaemias

amino acidopathies

urea cycle

Carbohydrate metabolism — glycogen synthesis and breakdown

gluconeogenesis

pyruvate metabolism

galactosaemia

Respiratory chain function

Fat metabolism — oxidation

ketone body formation

Purine and pyrimidine metabolism

Lysosomal function — glycosaminoglycans (mucopolysaccharides)

— glycoproteins

— lipid storage

Peroxisomal function — peroxisome biogenesis

— peroxisome beta oxidation

The diagnosis may be made because of screening tests, or suggestive or diagnostic clinical features.

CLUES TO DIAGNOSIS

Family history

Clues within the family history include:

▲ Consanguinity

▲ Neonatal death

▲ Sudden infant death

▲ Death in siblings at any age

▲ Illness in siblings

▲ Familial illnesses

Time of onset of symptoms

This is particularly important in disorders of intermediary metabolism.

▲ Relationship to introduction of milk feeds

▲ Relationship to other protein loads

▲ Relationship to intercurrent illness

▲ Relationship to fasting, including for surgical procedures.

Loss of developmental skills (regression)

In the early years when acquisition of new skills is so rapid, it can be very difficult to be sure whether the pathological process is a degenerative disease. Rather than loss of skills, there may be slowing of the rate of development, at least to start with.

DYSMORPHIC/OTHER DIAGNOSTIC FEATURES

Most children with metabolic disorders do not have any diagnostic signs, but the following list may help:

▲ Microcephaly
 — Seen in, for example, pyruvate dehydrogenase deficiency, peroxisomal disorders
▲ Agenesis of the corpus callosum
 — Seen in, for example, non-ketotic hyperglycinaemia, respiratory chain defects, peroxisomal disorders, Menkes' syndrome.
▲ Hair abnormalities
 — Pili torti seen in Menkes' syndrome, arginosuccinase deficiency
 — Alopecia seen in biotinidase deficiency
▲ Skin abnormalities
 — Ichthyosis in steroid sulphatase deficiency
 — Eczema seen in untreated PKU, biotinidase deficiency
▲ Eye abnormalities
 — Cherry red spot seen in infantile or type I GM1 gangliosidoses, all types of GM2 gangliosidoses, Niemann–Pick disease type IA, type I sialidosis
 — Cataracts seen in galactosaemia, Wilson's disease, peroxisomal disorders
▲ Smell
 — Characteristic of some of the organic acidaemias, e.g. maple syrup urine disease (maple syrup), isovaleric acidaemia (sweaty feet)

Tests

Depending on the main clinical features, the following may be useful. Blood and urine will obviously be the commonest samples collected. Single samples can be helpful but sometimes a profile may be more useful, e.g. blood sugar profile with concurrent blood lactate measurements in the hepatic glycogenoses.
Samples may include:

▲ blood — plasma and whole blood, including ECTA sample for storage for DNA
▲ urine
▲ cerebrospinal fluid
▲ tissue samples for histology, EM, enzymology:

 — skin for fibroblast culture
 — muscle
 — liver
 — bone marrow
 — heart
 — brain

Dynamic tests, e.g. fasting studies and glucagon stimulation tests, etc. (see Chapter 4), may be very useful but are potentially dangerous and should only be carried out in specialist tertiary centres.

Clinical problems and how to investigate them

Unfortunately clinical problems often overlap, but the broad range listed below should alert the paediatrician to the possibility of a primary metabolic disorder. It is assumed baseline investigations will have been done.

METABOLIC ACIDOSIS

Exclude renal and cardiac causes and consider septicaemia. The metabolic acidosis is likely to be severe, recurrent, and to coincide either with the introduction of protein feeds or intercurrent illness.

INVESTIGATIONS IN METABOLIC ACIDOSIS

Blood
▲ Sugar
▲ Ammonia
▲ Anion gap
▲ Lactate

Urine
▲ Ketone bodies
▲ Organic acids
▲ Dicarboxylic acids
▲ Lactate

This is a common way for the organic acidaemias and congenital lactic acidoses to present, particularly in the neonatal period (see Collins 1990).

The blood sugar may be low and there will be a large anion gap. Lactate will be markedly elevated in the lactic acidoses and mildly so in the organic acidaemias. Ammonia will be elevated in the organic acidaemias, especially propionic acidaemia. In the organic acidaemias the urine will test positive for ketone bodies. Urine organic and dicarboxylic acids should be diagnostic during the acute phase in most organic acidaemias and fat oxidation defects.

HYPERAMMONAEMIA

The infant or child with neonatal-onset disease is likely to be encephalopathic with signs of raised intracranial pressure and liver dysfunction. Poor feeding and vomiting are early signs, as is hyperventilation which often leads to a respiratory alkalosis. In the late-onset group intermittent vomiting and altered mental status, seizures and developmental delay are common.

INVESTIGATIONS IN HYPERAMMONAEMIA

Blood
▲ Glucose
▲ Arterial gas
▲ Clotting
▲ Ammonia
▲ Amino acids
▲ Acylcarnitine profile on blood spots

Urine
▲ Orotic acid
▲ Organic acids

In the urea cycle disorders the ammonia will be very high, particularly in those presenting neonatally, but may be an intermittent finding in late presenters. Hyperammonaemia may be a feature of the organic acidaemias and severe liver disease.

LIVER DYSFUNCTION

Acute:

Galactosaemia
Tyrosinaemia
Alpha-1-antitrypsin deficiency
Urea cycle disorders
Fat oxidation defects
Organic acidaemias
Niemann–Pick type C disease

INVESTIGATIONS IN ACUTE LIVER DYSFUNCTION

Blood	**Urine**	**Other**
▲ Liver function tests including clotting	▲ Reducing sugars	▲ Bone marrow
▲ Amino acids	▲ Succinyl acetone	▲ Skin biopsy
▲ Galactose-I-phosphate uridyltransferase	▲ Orotic acid	
▲ Alpha-1-antitrypsin phenotype	▲ Organic acids	
▲ Ammonia	▲ Dicarboxylic acids	
▲ Glucose		
▲ DNA for MCAD mutation (negative result does not exclude diagnosis)		
▲ Acylcarnitine profile on blood spots		

Chronic:

Hepatic glycogenoses
Tyrosinaemia
Galactosaemia
Alpha-1-antitrypsin deficiency
Respiratory chain defects
Peroxisomal disorders*
Lysosomal disorders*
Niemann–Pick Type C disease

*Liver dysfunction unlikely to be the only sign.

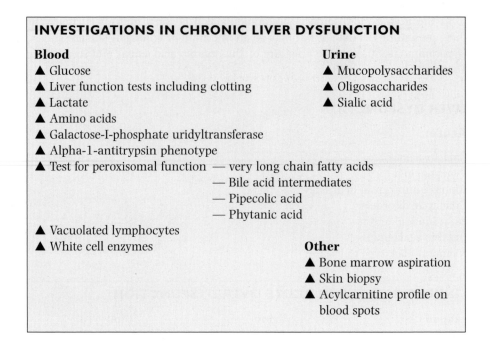

INVESTIGATIONS IN CHRONIC LIVER DYSFUNCTION

Blood
▲ Glucose
▲ Liver function tests including clotting
▲ Lactate
▲ Amino acids
▲ Galactose-I-phosphate uridyltransferase
▲ Alpha-1-antitrypsin phenotype
▲ Test for peroxisomal function — very long chain fatty acids
— Bile acid intermediates
— Pipecolic acid
— Phytanic acid

▲ Vacuolated lymphocytes
▲ White cell enzymes

Urine
▲ Mucopolysaccharides
▲ Oligosaccharides
▲ Sialic acid

Other
▲ Bone marrow aspiration
▲ Skin biopsy
▲ Acylcarnitine profile on blood spots

HEPATOMEGALY/HEPATOSPLENOMEGALY

This is characteristic of storage disorders. In hepatic glycogenoses there is only hepatomegaly unless portal hypertension supervenes. Hepatosplenomegaly is characteristic of the lysosomal disorders.

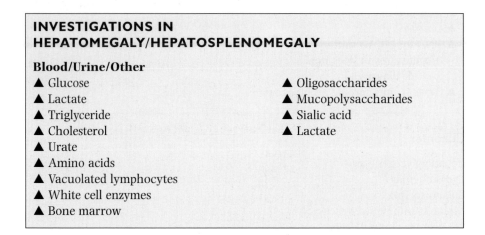

INVESTIGATIONS IN HEPATOMEGALY/HEPATOSPLENOMEGALY

Blood/Urine/Other
▲ Glucose
▲ Lactate
▲ Triglyceride
▲ Cholesterol
▲ Urate
▲ Amino acids
▲ Vacuolated lymphocytes
▲ White cell enzymes
▲ Bone marrow

▲ Oligosaccharides
▲ Mucopolysaccharides
▲ Sialic acid
▲ Lactate

HYPOGLYCAEMIA

See also chapter 4.

Symptoms can be subtle or more florid and precipitated by fasting, often when the feed interval is increased, e.g. the night-time feed is cut out in a baby.

Hypoglycaemia is seen in:

▲ Hepatic glycogenoses
▲ Disorders of gluconeogenesis
▲ Hyperinsulinism (transient and persistent)
▲ Organic acidaemias
▲ Fat oxidation defects
▲ Abnormalities of ketone body formation
▲ Any severe liver dysfunction (see above).

INVESTIGATIONS IN HYPOGLYCAEMIA

Blood
▲ Glucose (a profile may be helpful)
▲ Liver function tests
▲ Lactate
▲ Triglycerides and cholesterol
▲ Urate
▲ Ammonia
▲ Amino acids
▲ Ketone bodies
▲ DNA for MCAD screening (if dicarboxylic aciduria)
▲ Blood spots for acylcarnitine profile

Urine
▲ Organic acids
▲ Dicarboxylic acids
▲ Ketone bodies
▲ Lactate

NEUROLOGICAL DYSFUNCTION

Features which may be included are set out in Table 7.1, together with relevant conditions.

Investigations in neurological dysfunction

The precise investigations will depend on the clinical problem (see Aicardi 1992). Reasonable baseline investigations should include those set out in the information box.

INVESTIGATIONS IN NEUROLOGICAL DYSFUNCTION

Blood
▲ FBC and film
▲ Acanthocytes
▲ VLCFAs
▲ Urate
▲ Ammonia
▲ Amino acids
▲ Lactate
▲ Isoelectrofocusing of transferrin
▲ White cell enzymes
▲ Cooper/Caeruloplasmin

Urine
▲ Organic acids
▲ Amino acids
▲ Orotic acid
▲ Oligosaccharides
▲ Mucopolysaccharides
▲ Sialic acid

CSF
▲ Lactate
▲ Glycine

Table 7.1 **Neurological dysfunction: possible features and relevant conditions**

Feature	Relevant condition
Microcephaly	Pyruvate dehydrogenase deficiency Peroxisomal disorders
Macrocephaly	Glutaric aciduria type I Canavan's disease Alexander's disease
Mental retardation	May be associated with almost any metabolic disease causing acute or progressive neurological symptoms
Eye movement disorders: Nystagmus	Abetalipoproteinaemia Any disorders with ataxia
Ophthalmoplegia	Gaucher's disease Niemann–Pick Type C disease Carbohydrate-deficient glycoprotein (CDG) syndrome
Retinal abnormalities	Retinitis pigmentosa Respiratory chain defects Abetalipoproteinaemia Peroxisomal disorders Ceroid lipofuscinosis CDG syndrome
Macular abnormalities	Cherry red spot (see above in Dysmorphic features section) Optic atrophy, grey discolouration — metachromatic leukodystrophy
Sensorineural deafness	Peroxisomal disorders Lysosomal disorders Respiratory chain defects Purine disorders Organic acidaemias (biotinidase deficiency)
Encephalopathy	Organic acidaemias Hyperammonaemia syndromes Fat oxidation defects Any disorder with acute liver dysfunction
Seizures — Early (soon after birth)	Non-ketotic hyperglycinaemia Pyridoxine dependency Peroxisomal disorders

Table 7.1   (continued)

Feature	Relevant condition
Seizures–Later	Amino acid disorders Organic acidaemias Metal defects (Menkes' disease, molybdenum cofactor deficiency) Peroxisomal disorders Lysosomal disorders Pyrimidine defects
Hypotonia	Commonly associated with encephalopathy Respiratory chain defects Peroxisomal disorders
Movement disorders	
Pyramidal tract	Seen in amino acid disorders, urea cycle disorders, metachromatic leukodystrophy, arginase deficiency
Extrapyramidal	Inborn errors of biopterins, Lesch–Nyhan, Pelizaeus–Merzbacher Glutaric aciduria type I, other organic acidaemias
Ataxia	Lysosomal disorders (metachromatic leukodystrophy, Tay–Sachs, Krabbe's, Niemann–Pick type C, Gaucher's, GM1 and GM2 gangliosidosis) CDG syndrome Respiratory chain defects and Leigh's syndrome Purine disorders Urea cycle disorders Organic acid disorders (late onset propionic acidaemia, glutaric aciduria type I, biotinidase deficiency, maple syrup urine disease) Others (abetalipoproteinaemia, Batten's disease, Refsum's disease)
Myopathy	Respiratory chain defects Hepatic glycogenoses, particularly GSD type III Fat oxidation defects
Regression/dementia	Lysosomal disorders, e.g. mucopolysaccharidoses, mucolipidoses, gangliosidoses, Niemann–Pick type C,

Table 7.1 (continued)	
Feature	**Relevant condition**
Regression/dementia	metachromatic leukodystrophy Amino acid disorders, e.g. type I tyrosinaemia, homocystinuria Acute intermittent porphyria OTC deficiency Respiratory chain defects Peroxisomal disorders, e.g. X-linked adrenoleukodystrophy Purine defects, e.g. adenylosuccinase deficiency Others, e.g. Wilson's disease
Stroke	Respiratory chain defects, homocystinuria, Fabry's disease, CDG syndrome, organic acidaemias, molybdenum cofactor deficiency, Menkes' disease

BONY DISORDERS

Bony abnormalities are seen in the mucopolysaccharidoses and mucolipidoses, where they consist of dysostosis multiplex. Rickets are a feature of the Fanconi syndrome, which is seen in association with a number of metabolic disorders (see Renal Disease below and Chapter 5).

SKIN AND HAIR ABNORMALITIES

Alopecia is seen in biotinidase deficiency and pili torti in the conditions described above. Eczematous skin reactions are also seen in biotinidase deficiency and in untreated phenylketonuria, and ichthyosis in steroid sulphatase deficiency.

INVESTIGATIONS IN SKIN AND HAIR ABNORMALITIES

Blood
▲ Plasma biotinidase
▲ Lactate
▲ Copper and caeruloplasmin
▲ Ammonia
▲ Amino acids
▲ DNA testing for steroid sulphatase deficiency

Urine
▲ Organic acids
▲ Orotic acid

RENAL DISEASE

In the hepatic glycogenoses there is enlargement of the kidneys due to deposition of glycogen. This can also occur in other storage disorders. A Fanconi syndrome is common. It is seen in the following conditions:

- ▲ Cystinosis
- ▲ Galactosaemia
- ▲ Tyrosinaemia
- ▲ Glycogen storage disease
- ▲ Respiratory chain defects.

HEART

The heart is affected in the following conditions:

- ▲ Pompe's disease
- ▲ Glycogen storage disease type III
- ▲ Respiratory chain defects
- ▲ Fat oxidation defects
- ▲ CDG syndrome.

MULTI-ORGAN DISEASE

In many conditions more than one organ is involved. This is a particular feature of the respiratory chain defects, where apparently diverse organ systems can be affected. For example, in Pearson's syndrome there is involvement of the bone marrow and if the child survives, affected individuals will go on to develop a neurological condition (MELAS or Kearns–Sayre syndrome). Peroxisomal disorders and CDG syndrome are also multi-organ disorders.

What needs to be done

Initial investigations can be carried out at the district general hospital but when dynamic tests or tissue samples are required, referral to a tertiary centre is recommended. Where there is evidence of a neurodegenerative process or some other progressive condition, early referral to a paediatric neurologist is advised so that appropriate investigations can be coordinated (see Chapter 12). Neuroimaging, particularly MRI scans, may be helpful to show and define the position of a leukodystrophy. Neurophysiological studies, including electroretinograms, visual evoked responses, nerve conduction studies, EMG and of course EEG, all play a part in the work-up of these conditions. Diagnostic features may be present, for example the ERG in ceroid lipofuscinosis.

Practical details of tests

TIMING

Timing of the samples is very important. In disorders of intermediary metabolism it is most important to take the samples when the child is ill (decompensated). For example, in the organic acidurias and fat oxidation defects there may be few, if any, distinctive metabolities in the urine when the child is well. It is essential to label the samples with their time of collection so that changes in different metabolites can be examined together. In non-ketotic hyperglycinaemia, where the diagnosis rests on the plasma/CSF glycine ratio, the blood and CSF samples must be taken at the same time.

Causes of error

▲ Reliance on BM Stix or other dipsticks — these are merely a screening technique and are unsuitable on their own for accurate blood glucose estimation.

▲ Difficulties obtaining blood samples, including squeezing to get the blood to flow, will cause errors. Blood lactate is particularly sensitive to this. It will also rise with prolonged fitting, and care needs to be taken interpreting results.

▲ Fits/encephalitis — frequent fits and/or encephalitis appear to affect the CSF lactate concentration and the results should be interpreted carefully. This causes difficulties because such symptoms may be a feature of respiratory chain defects, and therefore the CSF lactate may be truly raised.

▲ Blood contamination of CSF — this will affect measurements of CSF glycine and lactate and make interpretation impossible.

▲ Ammonia estimation — the sample must be taken to the laboratory immediately or the concentration will rise.

▲ Instability of pyruvate and acetoacetate — both these metabolities are notoriously unstable and relatively difficult to measure. Care needs to be taken in interpreting results even in specialist centres.

▲ Interference of drugs — urine organic acids and dicarboxylic acids are analysed using gas chromatography — mass spectrometry. This is a very sensitive technique but the results can be confused by interference with drugs. Full details of drugs taken by the child should be on the request form.

▲ Analytical techniques — some of the results are qualitative and therefore dependent on the experience of the operator and the analytical technique used. For example, urine organic acids should be measured using gas chromatography — mass spectrometry to be reliable, and although techniques such as high pressure liquid chromatography have their place they usually cannot be used for the final diagnosis. A clinician needs to be aware of the techniques used.

Sample collection

Blood	Standard venepuncture techniques, with care over stasis
Urine	The sample should be collected in a bottle without preservative.
Cerebrospinal fluid	This should be collected for routine studies as well as for CSF glycine and lactate if clinically indicated. A plasma sample should be taken for glycine at the same time if non-ketotic hyperglycinaemia is suspected. Other CSF amino acids and neurotransmitters may be analysed in specialist centres
Skin biopsy	This is for fibroblast culture, fibroblasts providing a very useful source of tissue for enzymology. In an emergency the skin can be cleaned and a small sample removed

from the palmar surface of the lower arm using a scalpel. The sample need be no bigger than a few mm across and should be deep enough to cause a small amount of bleeding. A local anaesthetic spray can be used if necessary. The sample can then be stored in sterile N-saline, and kept in a refrigerator overnight until culture medium becomes available. If many biopsies are being performed then curved forceps make the procedure easier. After the biopsy a dressing should be applied and the arm kept dry for 24 hours.

Liver biopsy   This procedure should be performed in specialist centres unless in an emergency, when a Trucut biopsy needle should be used in the standard way. Fresh samples should be sent for histology, electron microscopy and histochemistry. The sample for enzymology should be immediately snap-frozen by wrapping it in a small piece of silver foil, and placing it either on dry ice or in liquid nitrogen. The sample should be stored at $-70°C$ until it can be sent for enzymology.

Muscle biopsy   Again this should be done in a specialist centre unless in an emergency, when a Trucut needle open biopsy could be performed. Again a fresh sample is required for histology, electron microscopy and histochemistry, but a frozen sample, as detailed above, for enzymology.

Dynamic tests

These basically consist of fasting studies and stimulation tests.

They should only be performed in specialist centres as they are not without risk and interpretation of results can be difficult. They are particularly useful in the diagnosis of the carbohydrate disorders and fat oxidation defects. The allopurinol loading test is used to diagnose carriers of OTC deficiency.

Interpretation of test results

Many results will give a clear-cut answer, e.g. this child has propionic acidaemia. However, sometimes interpretation is much more difficult, particularly if the child is extremely ill or near to death. There will be excretion of large amounts of metabolites such as lactate, and it is difficult to distinguish primary and secondary metabolic defects. Advice should be sought from the tertiary centre.

Checklist

History — onset of symptoms
        — death of siblings
        — other family history.

Take samples when decompensation has occurred.
Store blood for DNA

Urine is one of the most important sample to collect in disorders of intermediary metabolism.

Always discuss handling of samples with relevant laboratories before they are taken. Correct handling for enzymology is essential.

Prenatal testing — not usually possible unless a firm, i.e. enzymatically or DNA mutation proven, diagnosis has been made.

Getting the correct samples is therefore essential.

REFERENCES

Aicardi, J. (1992) *Diseases of the Nervous System in Childhood*. Oxford: Blackwell Scientific.
Collins, J.E. (1990) A practical approach to the diagnosis of metabolic disease in the neonate. *Developmental Medicine and Child Neurology* 32: 90–97.
Scriver, C.R., Beaudet, A.L., Sly, W.D., Valle, D. (1995) *The Metabolic and Molecular Bases of Inherited Disease*. New York: McGraw Hill.

8

Hepatology

C S Ball

Introduction

Paediatric hepatology impinges on every other area of paediatric medicine. A good understanding of clinical medicine combined with an attempt to understand pathobiological processes provides the basis for good clinical practice. Inevitably, clinical presentations seldom provide the complete answer and all hepatology relies on investigation for the whole picture. It is impossible to conceive a comprehensive investigation sequence which will provide all the answers, but a sensible progression is outlined in this chapter. The real skill relies heavily on expert interpretation. Use the information in this chapter as a guide. In general, blood and urine investigations provide many diagnoses without liver biopsy. These investigations are highly portable and may be sent to relevant centres from a distance with relative ease. Invasive investigations such as liver biopsy should not be performed without thorough training and resident paediatric surgical back-up — COMPLICATIONS CAN BE FATAL. Consultant Paediatric Hepatologists are always pleased to offer telephone advice, and this should be sought at an early stage even by those reading this chapter! Commonly occurring clinical problems are discussed. Decision-making points are emphasised.

1. List of tests

BLOOD

Biochemical liver function tests
Prothrombin time/INR
Full blood count/Film
Direct Coombs test
Procoagulation studies (Protein C, S, AT3, etc.)
Ham's test
Fat-soluble vitamins A, D, E
Cholesterol
Triglycerides
Quantitative amino acids
Ammonia
Alpha-fetoprotein
Transcobalamins
Copper/caeruloplasmin
Immunoglobulins
Complement
Autoantibodies
T-lymphocyte subsets
Alpha-1-antitrypsin phenotype
Galactose-1-phosphate uridyl transferase

WBC storage enzymes screen for Gaucher's, Niemann–Pick, A, B, Wolman's GM1 gangliosidosis, alpha mannosidosis, beta mannosidosis, fucosidosis

WBC GSD assay
Bile acid studies
Lactate
Pyruvate
Blood glucose
CPK
Cortisol (stressed)
T4, TSH
Hepatitis serology
Virology
Amylase
Very long chain fatty acids (VLCFA)

URINE

Culture
Amino acids
Organic acids
Orotic acid
Succinyl-acetone
Dicarboxylic acids
Bile acids

IMAGING

Ultrasound/Doppler
X-ray
Contrast studies (small bowel meal, etc.)
CT
MRI/MRA/MRCP (Magnetic resonance cholangiopancreatography)
Digital subtraction angiography/arteriography
Aortoportogram

Right heart cardiac catheter
Percutaneous transhepatic cholangiography (PTC)
Endoscopic retrograde cholangiopancreatography (ERCP)
Methyl bromida scanning (biliary scintigraphy)
Technetium colloid scan
Lymphangiogram
Echocardiogram

TISSUE

Percutaneous liver biopsy
Transjugular liver biopsy
Bone marrow
Skin fibroblast culture
Muscle biopsy
Colonic biopsy
Laparoscopic/open biopsy
Skin biopsy
Lymph node biopsy

ENDOSCOPY

Oesophagogastroduodenoscopy (OGD)
Colonoscopy
ERCP

OTHERS

Sweat test/IRT/CF genotype
Detailed ophthalmic examination/Slit lamp examination
Sigmoidoscopy
Saturation/macroaggregated albumin scan
Procoagulation studies (factor C, S, AT3, etc.)

ABBREVIATIONS USED IN THIS CHAPTER

ANA/ANF — antinuclear antibodies
AVM — arteriovenous malformation
CPK — creatine phosphokinase
DCT — direct Coombs test
G6PD —glucose 6 phosphate dehydrogenase deficiency
ERCP — endoscopic retrograde cholangiopancreatography
FFP — fresh frozen plasma
GGT — gamma-glutamyl transpeptidase
GSD — glycogen storage disease
HLH — haemophagocytic lymphohistiocytosis
ICP — intracranial pressure
KF — Kayser-Fleischer rings

LCH — Langerhans cell histiocytosis
LKM — liver/kidney microsomal
MBIDA scan — methyl bromide imino-diacetic acid
OGD — oesophagogastroduodenoscopy
PTC — percutaneous transhepatic cholangiopancreatography
PV — portal venous
SMA — smooth muscle antibodies
TBB — transbronchial biopsy
TORCH — toxoplasmosis, rubella, cytomegalovirus, herpes screen
TPN — total parenteral nutrition
VLCFA — very long chain fatty acids

2. Clinical problems and how to investigate them

The information box sets out the many manifestations of liver disease in children.

MANIFESTATIONS OF LIVER DISEASE IN CHILDREN

- Increased cardiac output
- Vasodilation
- Varices
- Warm skin
- Hepatorenal syndrome
- Poor digestion, especially fats
- Malabsorption fat-soluble vitamins
- Aldosteronism
- Decreased body fat stores
- Hepato/splenomegaly
- Jaundice
- Clubbing
- Cutaneous shunts
- Intrapulmonary shunts
- Rickets and osteopenia
- Arthritis
- Purpura
- Bruising
- Ascites
- Increased body water
- Muscle wasting
- Itching
- Spider naevii
- Palmer erytheme
- Pale stools
- Diarrhoea
- Gastrointestinal bleeding

ACUTE LIVER FAILURE

Acute liver failure can be divided into three clinical entities:

1. Commonly referred to as fulminant hepatic failure, which is the clinical syndrome of severe hepatic dysfunction with encephalopathy within 8 weeks of the onset of the illness. Overall mortality 70%.
2. 'Late onset', hepatic failure starting 8–24 weeks after the onset of the illness. Overall mortality 90%.

3. 'Severe', with prolongation of INR > 5 but WITHOUT encephalopathy as occurs particularly in infants. Overall mortality 95%.

NB: All suspected cases of acute liver failure should be discussed with a paediatric hepatologist as soon as possible. Children with an INR of > 4.0 should be listed for liver transplant.

Clinical features of acute liver failure

◆ Jaundice with a small/shrinking liver
◆ Encephalopathy
◆ Prolonged INR unresponsive to IV Vitamin K
◆ Hypoglycaemia
◆ Hyperammonaemia
◆ Raised intracranial pressure

The encephalopathy may be due to accumulation of toxic substances, and may be clinically graded at several levels.

Grade I

Irritable and inappropriate behaviour. Lethargy. Flap/tremor of outstretched hands. Recognises parents. Often sleepy. Can still draw picture with difficulty.

Grade II

Irritable, inappropriate behaviour. Mood swings. Flap/tremor of outstretched hands. Photophobia. NOT recognising parents.

Grade II Agitated

Aggressive outbursts and bad language. May thrash around in bed and be very difficult to control. Unable to stay still. Pulls at drips, etc.

Grade III

Rousable but mostly sleeping. Incoherent. Pupils sluggish and dilated. Flap/tremor. Hypertonia/clonus and episodes of extensor spasm.

Grade IV

Areflexic. Irregular gasps. Respiratory failure imminent. Bradycardia. Unresponsive to painful stimuli.

80% of cases of fulminant hepatic failure above grade II have increased intracranial pressure (ICP). The end result is brain death with fixed dilated pupils, bradycardia, hypertension and papilloedema. Papilloedema is often only apparent as a late sign.

Causes of acute liver failure

Some chronic liver disorders may only declare themselves when liver function deteriorates considerably, and may therefore present as acute liver failure. In all cases the processes listed in the information box should be considered.

> ## PATHOGENIC MECHANISMS FOR CONSIDERATION IN ACUTE LIVER FAILURE
>
> ◆ Infection, e.g. Hepatitis A, B, C, D, E, *Herpes simplex*, CMV, adenovirus, EBV, measles, leptospirosis, salmonella, malaria
> ◆ Drugs, e.g. Carbamazepine, sodium valproate, paracetamol, halothane, anti-tuberculous therapy, cytotoxic agents
> ◆ Toxins, e.g. *Amanita phalloides*, carbon tetrachloride
> ◆ Metabolic, e.g. galactosaemia, fructosaemia, tyrosinaemia, Wilson's disease, alpha-1-Antitrypsin deficiency, Niemann–Pick type C, neonatal haemo-chromatosis
> ◆ Ischaemic, e.g. septicaemic shock, Budd–Chiari syndrome, circulatory failure, heatstroke
> ◆ Infiltrative, e.g. leukaemia, lymphoma, haemophagocytic lymphohistio-cytosis (HLH).
> ◆ Autoimmune, e.g. autoimmune hepatitis, giant cell hepatitis with Coombs-positive haemolytic anaemia in infancy.

Investigations in acute liver failure

Figure 8.1 gives a flow diagram outlining action to be taken following diagnosis of acute liver failure.

Blood FBC, INR, LFTs, serum copper and caeruloplasmin and ophthalmoscopy for KF rings, Hepatitis serology (hepatitis A IgM, hepatitis B IgM anticore), Hepatitis C antibody, Hepatitis E antibody, *Herpes simplex*, CMV, VZV, Adenovirus, EBV, HIV, Alpha-1-antitrypsin phenotype, Serum iron and ferritin. Arterial blood gases. Bank serum and plasma for any later analyses. Triglycerides, fibrinogen. Immuno-globulins, complement, autoantibodies, T lymphocyte subsets. Alpha-fetoprotein.

Urine Culture, urinary organic acid screening (esp. succinyl acetone-tyrosi-naemia), toxicology screen and banked serum and plasma for drug level or later tests. Pre and post penicillamine copper excretion.

Imaging/others Chest X-ray, USS of liver and spleen with visualisation of portal and hepatic veins, echocardiography, CT scanning for tumours, angiography/MRI if in doubt of vascular details. ECG. Bone marrow examination to exclude infiltrative disorders.

HEPATOMEGALY

Hepatomegaly may even be obvious on inspection if the organ is massive or has an irregular margin. It is not unusual to feel a soft smooth liver edge in a slim child, especially in the infant where the liver may be up to 2 cm palpable below the costal margin under physiological circumstances. The differential diagnosis of hepatomegaly is considerable and not exclusive to liver disease alone. Occasionally no specific cause may be found.

Acute liver failure flow diagram

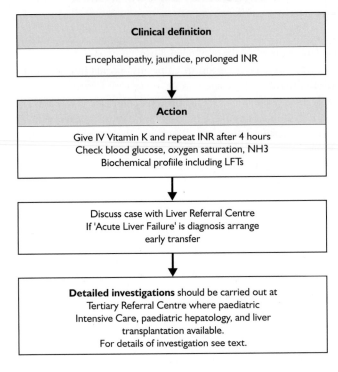

Clinical definition
Encephalopathy, jaundice, prolonged INR

Action
Give IV Vitamin K and repeat INR after 4 hours Check blood glucose, oxygen saturation, NH3 Biochemical profiile including LFTs

Discuss case with Liver Referral Centre If 'Acute Liver Failure' is diagnosis arrange early transfer

Detailed investigations should be carried out at Tertiary Referral Centre where paediatric Intensive Care, paediatric hepatology, and liver transplantation available. For details of investigation see text.

Caution
DO NOT SEDATE
DO NOT PERFORM LIVER BIOPSY (see text for details on liver biopsies)
DO NOT KEEP PATIENT IF COMA STAGE 1 AS **DETERIORATION CAN BE RAPID AND WITHOUT WARNING**
DO NOT TRANSFER PATIENTS WITHOUT MEDICAL ESCORT (see text for details on transfer)

Points
INR >4.0 AFTER IV VITAMIN K = LIST FOR TRANSPLANTATION
INFANTS MAY HAVE PROLONGED INR
WITHOUT ENCEPHALOPATHY

Fig. 8.1 **Acute liver failure: flow diagram.**

Causes of hepatomegaly

Alpha-1-antitrypsin deficiency
Autoimmune hepatitis
Arteriovenous malformations
Bile acid metabolism disease
Biliary atresia
Budd–Chiari syndrome
Caroli's disease
Cholesterol ester storage disorder
Choledochal cyst
Congenital hepatic fibrosis
Cystic fibrosis
Cytomegalovirus infection
Dengue haemorrhagic fever
Diabetes mellitus
Extramedullary erythropoiesis
Fat infiltration
Fatty acid oxidation defects
Fructosaemia
Gaucher's disease
Glycogen storage diseases
Granuloma
Heart failure
Hepatic cholesterol storage disease
Hepatic fibrosis
Hepatitis of infancy

Hepatitis
HIV
Haemochromatosis
Haemosiderosis
Haemophagocytic lymphohistiocytosis
Hypopituitarism
Langerhans cell histiocytosis
Inborn errors of metabolism
Liver tumours
Liver abscess
Niemann–Pick disease
Parenteral nutrition
Pericarditis
Polycystic disease
Progressive intrahepatic cholestasis
Reye's syndrome
Schistosomiasis
Sclerosing cholangitis
Sickle cell disease
Storage disorders
Urea cycle disorders
Veno-occlusive disease
Viral infections
Worm infestation
Zellweger's syndrome

Clinical findings

Although the differential diagnosis of hepatomegaly is vast, clinical features and presentation will often assist considerably in suggesting the likely aetiology. This is significantly age-related.

Preterm infants The preterm infant in the neonatal nursery is most likely to have multifactorial neonatal hepatitis. This is commonly associated with intravenous feeding, hypoxia, necrotising enterocolitis, and patent ductus arteriosus. These infants can also have any of the diseases seen in OLDER infants.

Infants Idiopathic neonatal hepatitis is the most likely cause BUT other causes must be excluded (see section on neonatal jaundice). Tumours, cysts and malformations are to be particularly excluded in infancy.

Children Virtually the entire differential diagnosis applies. If child is jaundiced, see section on jaundice. If all the biochemical liver function tests are normal, congenital hepatic fibrosis is the most likely cause.

Investigations in hepatomegaly

The flow diagram of clinical definition and sequence of investigations is given in Figure 8.2.

Which of these tests are performed at a referring local paediatric department shoud be agreed with a liver unit in advance.

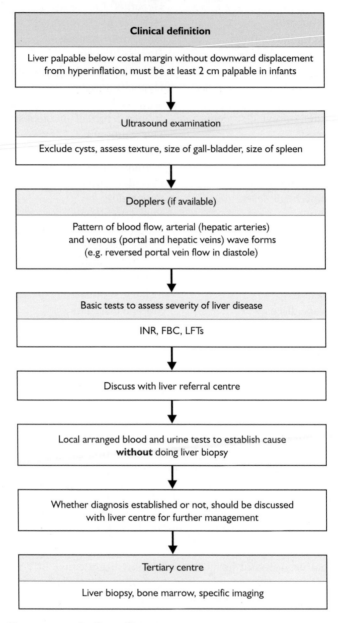

Hepatomegaly flow diagram

Fig. 8.2 **Hepatomegaly: flow diagram.**

Blood tests FBC and film, reticulocytes, DCT and G6PD status, Hb electrophoresis, INR, LFTs, biochemical profile, alpha-1-antitrypsin phenotype, CF gene probes (in conjunction with a sweat test), copper and caeruloplasmin, immunoglobulins, complement levels, autoantibodies, hepatitis A, B, C, D, E serology, virology for CMV, EBV, adenovirus, *Herpes simplex*, parvovirus, measles, VZV,

HIV, cholesterol, triglycerides, lactate, pyruvate, CPK, alpha-fetoprotein, transcobalamins, urate, fibrinogen, blood cultures, lymphocyte subsets, procoagulation screen (AT3, factor S and C), Ham's test, serum bile acids, malaria thick and thin blood film, ammonia, quantitative amino acids.

Urine tests Urine culture, organic acid screening for urinary succinyl acetone; orotic acid; dicarboxylic acids. Bile acid screening, amino acid screening, reducing sugars, pH, osmolality, electrolytes, urea and creatinine, bilirubin (look at colour first), stix analysis, 24-hour urine copper excretion pre and post penicillamine.

Imaging

Ultrasound scan
Technetium colloid scan
CXR
Echocardiogram
CT scan
MRI
MRA
Angiography

ERCP
PTC
Laparoscopy
Operative cholangiography
Right heart catheter
Endoscopy upper and lower Gl
Sigmoidoscopy
Spinal X-rays

Tissue

Bone marrow aspirate and trephine
Liver biopsy
Skin fibroblast culture
Muscle biopsy

Rectal biopsy
Lymph node biopsy
CT/US guided liver biopsy
Skin biopsy

JAUNDICE

Jaundice is the most easily and widely recognised symptom of liver disease and is particularly useful at disclosing the possibility of liver disease which may otherwise go unnoticed. The primary cause, however, may not be hepatological. Of key importance is the colour of urine and stool which determines whether cholestasis is part of the clinical picture. In all circumstances, the physician should himself/herself examine stools and urine, as the history given by parents may be misleading. If there is NO evidence of cholestasis, then haematological causes must be considered first. Hyperbilirubinaemia is said to be conjugated when this is greater than 20% of the total bilirubin.

THE JAUNDICED INFANT

Examine infant for signs of hypothyroidism, poor feeding, dysmorphism, sepsis (check cord), observe feeding, check genitalia and muscle tone.

Causes

Same as for hepatomegaly except for most glycogen storage diseases and Reye's syndrome, which are not associated with jaundice.

Investigations

Stools yellow/green/brown (older child) and urine colourless. Check:

Split bilirubin
Total bilirubin
Urine for reducing sugars
Urine for culture
Thyroid function tests
FBC, film, reticulocytes
G6PD status
DCT
Blood group of mother and child

If mostly unconjugated hyperbilirubinaemia, need to consider risk to developing CNS and phototherapy/exchange transfusion may be indicated. Remember, phototherapy will produce bilirubin in the urine due to water solubilising effect. If jaundice is prolonged beyond 10 days postnatally, repeat evaluation and above investigations to ensure that conjugated hyperbilirubinaemia is not developing. If stools fully pigmented and urine clear, breast-feeding is the most likely explanation, and the infant should thrive and behave normally. If there are episodes of hypoglycaemia or the infant is male and has small genitalia, exclude hypopituitarism. Galactosaemia, hypothyroidism, hypopituitarism, and UTI can all produce jaundice in the infant with a mixed conjugated/unconjugated presentation. A urine test positive for reducing sugars suggests galactosuria, which can occur in ANY cause of neonatal hepatitis. Galactose should then be excluded from the diet until definitive proof of galactosaemia as the possible diagnosis is obtained by assay of RBC galactose-1-phosphate uridyl transferase.

Conjugated hyperbilirubinaemia

Pale stools and dark urine. Remember, the normal breast fed infant has bright yellow stools which are almost fluorescent and the urine is almost completely colourless. Bottle fed babies may produce green/brown stools. If the parents can see that the child has passed urine without feeling the nappy, the urine is probably pigmented. ALWAYS see the urine and stool for yourself, parents often do not appreciate when stools are paler than normal. All of these infants are abnormal and must be investigated as a matter of urgency. Contrary to popular medical mythology, infants with cholestatic liver disease usually THRIVE, and failure to observe FTT should NOT be taken as reassuring, and is a common cause of false reassurance and late referral of children with biliary atresia.

Clinical examination in the infant with prolonged jaundice

Figure 8.3 sets out clinical definition and sequence of investigations in the infant with prolonged jaundice.

Examine colour of stool and urine. Examine infant for birth weight (often <10th centile if Alagille or intrauterine infection), craniotabes, strawberry naevi (may have liver AVM), micropenis and hypotonia (hypopituitarism/septo–optic dysplasia may also have a midline facial defect such as cleft lip), features of Down syndrome (neonatal hepatitis), dysmorphism with hypotonia and possible visual impairment (Zellweger's), purpura (thrombocytopenia of intrauterine

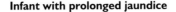

Infant with prolonged jaundice

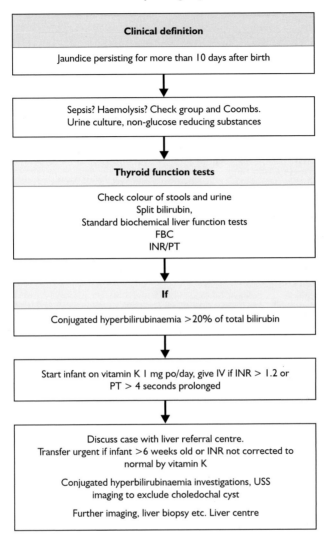

Clinical definition
Jaundice persisting for more than 10 days after birth

Sepsis? Haemolysis? Check group and Coombs.
Urine culture, non-glucose reducing substances

Thyroid function tests
Check colour of stools and urine
Split bilirubin,
Standard biochemical liver function tests
FBC
INR/PT

If
Conjugated hyperbilirubinaemia >20% of total bilirubin

Start infant on vitamin K 1 mg po/day, give IV if INR > 1.2 or
PT > 4 seconds prolonged

Discuss case with liver referral centre.
Transfer urgent if infant >6 weeks old or INR not corrected to
normal by vitamin K

Conjugated hyperbilirubinaemia investigations, USS
imaging to exclude choledochal cyst

Further imaging, liver biopsy etc. Liver centre

Fig. 8.3 **Infant with prolonged jaundice: flow diagram.**

infection or HLH), cardiac murmur (Alagille's or biliary atresia — especially with polysplenia/asplenia), asymmetry (Beckwith syndrome associated with hepatoblastoma), ascites (advanced liver disease, often metabolic or storage), splenomegaly (storage disorders/intrauterine infection), cataract (galactosaemia), choroidoretinitis (congenital infection), small optic disc/does not fix, follow (septo–optic dysplasia), odd smell (tyrosinaemia — like cabbage water). If Alagille's suspected, look at the family for facial features, and ask about heart murmurs. Listen for liver and cranial bruit and look for signs of cardiac failure if AVM suspected. Thrush, diarrhoea or delayed psychomotor development: HIV. Situs inversus abdominis (almost pathognomonic of biliary atresia). Umbilical hernia (hypothyroid or hypopituitarism as well).

Investigations

Blood tests

FBC and reticulocytes
Group and Save
PT/INR
Alpha-1-antitrypsin phenotype
Complete biochmical profile
RBC Galactose-1-phosphate uridyl transferase
Free T4 + TSH
Random cortisol
Amino acids
Cholesterol and triglycerides

Hepatitis B, C serology
HIV antibody
Blood cultures
Syphilis serology
TORCH screen
Vitamins A, D, E
Immunoglobulins
Fibrinogen
Serum for toxicology

Urine

Culture for bacteria
Culture for CMV
Amino acids
Electrolytes

Imaging

USS liver and spleen (and kidneys)
Methyl bromida biliary excretion scan
Wrist X-ray

Ophthalmology

Choroidoretinitis
Posterior embryotoxon
Cataracts

Bone marrow aspirate

Consider, if no one cause identified so far, to exclude storage disorders.

THE OLDER CHILD WITH JAUNDICE

The priority here is to differentiate between acute and chronic liver disorders, and especially conditions such as Wilson's disease and autoimmune liver disease where the onset of jaundice may represent the beginnings of imminent decompensation. A history of previous episodes of jaundice should be sought specifically, as this may be reported in chronic liver disease. The majority of cases of acute hepatitis are anicteric. It is of paramount importance to prove the diagnosis at an early stage and particularly to exclude Hepatitis A. It is NOT possible to make a 100% confident clinical diagnosis even during epidemics of known viral infections. A misinterpretation of jaundice presenting and clinically diagnosed as Hepatitis A could have fatal consequences for the child with Wilson's disease.

Investigations in the older child with jaundice

Blood tests

FBC
INR
Vitamins A, D, E
Biochemical profile including LFTs and split bilirubin
Quantitative amino acids
Ammonia
Cholesterol
Triglycerides
Lactate
Alpha-1-antitrypsin phenotype
Viral serology for CMV, EBV, HSV, toxoplasmosis, measles, HIV, HBV IgM anticore, HCV antibody (PCR if relevant), hepatitis E if travel to endemic area

Immunoglobulins incl. IgE if drug reaction suspected
Complement levels C3, C4
Autoantibodies
Blood culture
Leptospira antibodies
Malarial parasites if relevant
Copper and caeruloplasmin
Bile acids
VLCFA
Fibrinogen
Save serum and plasma for later analyses

Urine

24-hour urinary copper excretion pre and post penicillamine
Urine culture
Urine culture for CMV

Urine bile acids
Urine organic acids
Toxicology screen

Other

Sweat test
Stool culture for salmonella, etc.
Skin fibroblast culture for metabolic disorders
Bone marrow if infiltration or storage disorder a possibility

Ophthalmic examination for KF rings, cataract, choroidoretinitis, posterior embryotoxon
Bile assay for conjugates if Crigler–Najaar suspected

Imaging

USS liver and spleen to rule out choledochal cyst, stone duct dilatation
CXR
DISIDA
CT/MRI

ERCP/MRCP
PTC
Angiogram
Operative cholangiogram
Endoscopy upper and lower GI
Sigmoidoscopy

Tissue

Liver biopsy only if INR and platelet
count permit this
Rectal biopsy if colitis suspected or
Niemann–Pick disease

Skin biopsy if LCH suspected
Skin fibroblast culture

Management of the older child with jaundice

The sequence of investigations and management is set out in Figure 8.4.

◆ Look at colour of stools and urine
◆ Previous history of jaundice/illness
◆ Pain?
◆ Diarrhoea?
◆ Weight loss
◆ Abdominal swelling

Jaundice in the older child

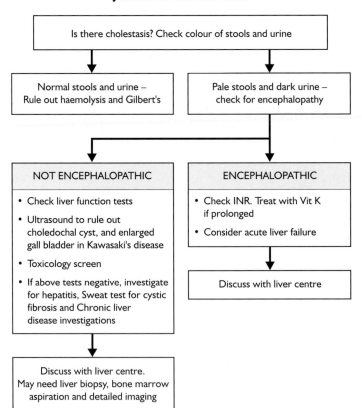

Fig. 8.4   Jaundice in the older child: flow diagram.

◆ Check LFTs, FBC, INR split bilirubin and test urine stix and culture. If NOT cholestasis, check DCT, retics, film, Hb electrophoresis, G6PD if relevant. In teenagers, Gilbert's very common and associated with fatigue and lethargy and abdominal pain.
◆ If cholestasis, rule out HepA IgM
◆ Send all virology, and toxicology tests
◆ Urgent USS to identify ducts, gall bladder, vessels. rule out choledochal cyst
◆ Small gall bladder suggests cholestasis
◆ Large gall bladder suggests stone or Kawasaki's
◆ Immunology (see Chapter 1)
◆ Copper levels (blood and excretion)
◆ Slit lamp eye examination
◆ Bone marrow examination
◆ Alagille investigations
◆ Alpha-1 — autotripsin screen
◆ Sweat test
◆ Liver biopsy if possible
◆ Alpha-fetoprotein imaging as determined by likelihood of tumour, sclerosing cholangitis or biliary anomaly (discuss with hepatobiliary surgeon)

HAEMATEMESIS

Haematemesis/melaena is a very frightening event. The majority of children presenting in this way have known liver disease. Occasionally, the Gl haemorrhage is the first presenting problem. The differential diagnosis includes all possible causes of cirrhosis, jaundice, and hepatomegaly. Investigations should be targeted in a logical manner to ensure that the patient has portal hypertension, and then to see if this is due to chronic liver disease.

Investigations in haematemesis
The sequence of investigations and management is given in Figure 8.5.

◆ FBC, INR, biochemical profile including LFTs
◆ USS liver and spleen
◆ Chronic liver disease workup if CLD suspected
◆ Upper Gl endoscopy to examine for bleeding, ulcers, varices
◆ Angiography if PV sclerosis suspected or shunt planned

CIRRHOSIS

Cirrhosis of the liver is defined by a diffuse process affecting the whole liver in which normal architecture is replaced by structurally abnormal nodules encircled by fibrous tissue.

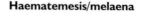

Haematemesis/melaena

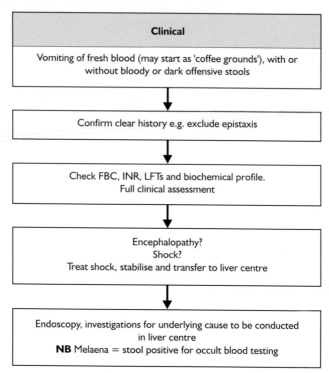

Fig. 8.5 **Haematemesis/melaena: flow diagram.**

Clinical features of cirrhosis

Chronic hepatocellular failure and portal hypertension cause the symptoms seen in cirrhosis. Patients have a firm nodular liver, occasionally a small right lobe or splenomegaly. Sometimes the liver is so small as to be impalpable, but is typically large in biliary cirrhosis.

Causes of cirrhosis

Extrahepatic biliary atresia
Intrahepatic biliary hypoplasia
Choledochal cyst
Cystic fibrosis
Progressive intrahepatic cholestasis
Bile duct stenosis or obstruction
Choledocholithiasis
Pancreatic fibrosis
Pancreatic tumours
Sclerosing cholangitis
Familial intrahepatic cholestasis
Bacterial ascending cholangitis

Cholangitis due to *Fasciola, Ascaris,* etc.
CMV cholangitis
Langerhans cell histiocytosis
Post hepatitic — any cause
Venous congestion, e.g. constrictive pericarditis
Veno-occlusive disease
Indian childhood cirrhosis
Other copper-associated liver disease
Ulcerative colitis

Wilson's disease
Gaucher's disease
Galactosaemia
Wolman's disease
Fructosaemia
Fatty acid oxidation defects
GSD types III, IV
Abetalipoproteinaemia
Sickle cell disease
Hurler's syndrome
Thalassaemia
Porphyria

Alpha-1-antitrypsin deficiency
Haemochromatosis/haemosiderosis
Tyronaemia
OCT deficiency
Zellweger's syndrome
Cystinosis
Byler's disease
Niemann–Pick disease type C
Coprostanic acidaemia
Cholesterol ester storage disease
Shwachmann's syndrome
Hereditary hypofibrinogenaemia

Investigations in cirrhosis

All cases

Full biochemical profile including liver function tests
FBC
Cholesterol and triglycerides
Alpha-fetoprotein
USS
Arterial blood gases
Barium meal/endoscopy

Selected patients

Alpha-1-antitrypsin phenotype
Copper and caeruloplasmin
Fasting blood sugar, pyruvate, and lactate
RBC glycogen content
RBC galactose-1-phosphate uridyl transferase
Hb electrophoresis
Serum iron and TIBC
Serum quantitative amino acids
Lipoprotein profile
Serum bile acids
Hepatitis B, C, D serology
TORCH
Immunoglobulins
Complement
Autoantibodies

Urine tests

24-hour copper pre and post penicillamine
Urinary porphyrins

Amino acids
Non-glucose reducing substances
Mucopolysaccharides
Fatty acid degradation products

Imaging

IVU
ERCP
PTC
Inferior venacavagram
Hepatic venogram
CT scan of liver and biliary system

Miscellaneous

Sweat test
MBIDA scan
Fibroblast culture
Liver biopsy
Skin biopsy

GALLSTONES

Gallstones are amorphous or crystalline materials which have precipitated in bile. They can obstruct bile flow and lead to cholecystitis, cholangitis, biliary cirrhosis, and, rarely, cause rupture of the biliary tree. Most stones are of mixed type containing cholesterol, bile pigment, calcium, and an organic or protein matrix. These stones are usually multifaceted and radio-opaque. Pure cholesterol stones, however, are round and often single and non-radio-opaque unless infection has produced secondary calcification with a ring-like appearance round the stone. Black bile pigment stones are small, hard and amorphous and are usually associated with haemolytic conditions. They are radio-opaque because they contain calcium. Brown stones are similar but are associated with recurrent biliary system infection.

Causes of gallstones

Abnormal bile formation due to liver disease
Decreased bile salt concentration in bile
Increased biliary cholesterol concentration
Ileal disease causing reduced enterohepatic circulation
Abnormal gall bladder function
Abnormal bile constituents — excess bilirubin in haemolysis, abnormal mucoprotein in CF, bacteria, parasites, cell debris
Stasis due to bile duct obstruction
Stasis due to abnormal bile duct
Drugs causing cholestasis or change in bile chemistry

Contributory factors

Cholecystitis

Obesity

Intra-abdominal infection

Intra-abdominal surgery

Family history

TPN/frusemide

Cholestyramine treatment

Selective IgA deficiency

Investigations in gallstones

FBC, film, reticulocytes, Hb electrophoresis, G6PD assay, DCT

Biochemical profile including LFTs

INR

Investigate underlying liver disease if this is apparent

Blood culture if patient febrile

Imaging

USS very sensitive and useful for serial monitoring. Detects 95% of gallstones

Oral cholecystography rarely necessary

Plain abdo X-ray

ERCP/PTC sometimes necessary for biliary tree details.

3. Practical details of tests

Most investigations in paediatric hepatology are based on blood and urine analyses and require no particular skill in their execution. Interpretation can be difficult, but a synopsis of interpretations is presented.

IMAGING

Ultrasound

Ultrasound has become an indispensable tool of the trade. Ultrasound will sometimes allow dilated biliary structures (e.g. choledochal cyst) to be diagnosed antenatally. Tumours may also be detected early on, even antenatally. The size of gallbladder is easily assessed and stones detected. The presence of duct dilatation, and AV malformation, or significant ascites, contraindicates liver biopsy. A suitable liver biopsy site may be planned. No liver biopsy should be performed without ultrasound findings being known first. Situs inversus abdominis can also be completely missed clinically, but easily detected on ultrasound.

Endoscopic techniques

Older children may be capable of cooperation with sedation only, but most children require general anaesthetic for endoscopic procedures. The quality of information and images obtained (e.g. ERCP) is very operator-dependent, and except for emergencies should probably be performed only in large centres with paediatric endoscopy experience.

LIVER BIOPSY

Always check ultrasound findings, FBC, and INR/PT before starting. In infants under the age of 1 year, may be performed with only and sedation if required. In the older cooperative child, apply local anathestic cream locally over site after percussing liver in the anterior axillary line 1 hour before procedure to check that this is at least one intercostal space below the point of dullness (e.g. 7th–8th intercostal space on right mid axillary line). Sedate with imidazolan 0.1 mg/kg iv in a suitable environment for controlled anaesthesia, immediately prior to injecting 1% lignocaine into the skin overlying biopsy site, which is normally in the right mid-axillary line. Wait 2 minutes — check anaesthesia, incise to create opening of 2 mm.

Whilst waiting for local anaesthetic to work, take 1.4 mm Menghini disposable needle biopsy pack. Use sterile technique at all times. Aspirate at least 2 ml of N-saline into syringe of biopsy pack, attach needle and tighten on Luer. Once sealed, check air-tightness by placing gloved finger over end of needle and pulling back on barrel of syringe — there should be NO leak of air into barrel of syringe. With the bevel pointing cephalically, the needle is advanced through the incision as far as the intercostal ligament when a resistance is felt. Flush a few drops of saline under slight resistance to clear tip. The barrel of the syringe is then pulled back to the click stop position (10 ml vacuum) and the needle advanced rapidly in and out of the liver 2–5 cm in depth following an imaginary line at right angles to the liver surface. The biopsy is best taken during expiration. Expel the needle contents carefully to retrieve the biopsy.

For routine histology, the biopsy should be preserved in formal saline. For culture, place small 1–2 mm of tissue in N-saline in sterile universal container. For later biochemical analyses, it is useful to store some in liquid nitrogen wrapped in aluminium foil. If specific (e.g. glycogen storage) assays are required, this may require fresh tissue and should be carefully arranged BEFORE taking biopsy material.

After the biopsy, the patient should have a small dressing placed over the incision site, and rest in bed lying on the right-hand side for 4 hours. This is often very difficult, especially with young children. Observation of pulse, respiration and blood pressure should be recorded every 15 minutes for 2 hours, every 1/2 hour for 2 hours and hourly thereafter for a minimum of 2 hours in LOW RISK cases. Observations should be more frequent or for longer in cirrhotic patients who are more at risk of haemorrhage after liver biopsy.

Complications of liver biopsy

Kept to a minimum by using experienced operators ONLY. Complication rate may be as low as 1/1000. Local pain and haematoma are the commonest. Sometimes the haematoma is subcapsular or intrahepatic. Haemorrhage can be serious, especially if either an hepatic arterial vessel or intercostal artery is damaged by the needle. Bleeding may then occur into the thorax, lung or biliary system which may continue uncontrolled. Pain, signs of shock, and respiratory difficulty are signs to watch for. If this is seen, a CXR should be ordered immediately, IV FFP, blood and if indicated platelets obtained, and emergency ultrasound exam to look for haematobilia, etc. Inform surgical colleagues! Taking the biopsy too low will allow the needle to traverse the thinnest part of the right lobe and may hit the gall-bladder or structures at the portahepatis. A viscus may be perforated, and even a renal biopsy unwittingly performed.

Advice on liver biopsy

Liver biopsy in children is potentially hazardous. It is not advisable to perform the procedure without adequate previous experience, and preparation is crucial in reducing the known risks. Surgical cover should always be available to deal with post-operative emergencies. Post-mortem biopsy, taken as soon as possible after death with the largest available Menghini needle, allows liver tissue WITHOUT autolysis to be studied and is invaluable in assessing the cause of death in liver disease. This may also increase the opportunity for experience in using the Menghini technique.

SKIN FIBROBLAST CULTURE

A small full-thickness skin biopsy may be taken from the skin of the forearm or even at the site of liver biopsy. A piece no more than 2 mm in diameter is sufficient, taken under sterile technique and transferred to transport medium. Sterility is important, as bacterial contamination prejudices the chance of successful fibroblast culture. If transport medium is not available, then sterile N-saline will suffice especially if refrigerated and transported rapidly to the relevant laboratory. This specimen may be collected post mortem. Studies on fibroblasts have been used to accurately diagnose inborn errors of metabolism and thus facilitate appropriate genetic counselling and in many cases enable antenatal diagnosis.

BONE MARROW ASPIRATE

Examination of bone marrow will often reveal a diagnosis of storage or proliferative disorders which may be difficult or impossible to diagnose on liver histology alone. In order to exclude Niemann–Pick type C disease, we recom-mend that bone marrow aspirate be carefully examined in all cases of idiopathic neonatal/infantile hepatitis. The procedure is also particularly important in undiagnosed acute liver failure, especially in infants where haemophagocytic lymphohistiocytosis (HLH) is an important part of the differential diagnosis.

OPHTHALMOLOGY

Clinical examination of the eye by an experienced operator and with slit lamp where available is of considerable value. The opinion of a consultant paediatric ophthalmologist should be sought. **NB**: Children under 10 years with Wilson's disease often do not have KF rings.

SCANNING

Techniques of CT and MRI are familiar. The scans which most practitioners are not familiar with are those using nuclear medicine scintigraphy. The ^{99m}-Tc methylbromida scan ('DISIDA', similar, 'HIDA' scan) has replaced the Rose Bengal test in assessing BILIARY EXCRETION. The agent rapidly enters hepatocytes and is then excreted into bile and through the biliary system into bowel. This test is useful in demonstrating poor biliary excretion in cholestatic disorders. Adequate excretion is helpful in excluding biliary atresia, but impaired excretion may occur in any cause of conjugated hyperbilirubinaemia. If there is no excretion into bowel over 24 hours, then this describes complete cholestasis and further investigations are required to exclude biliary atresia (liver biopsy/ERCP/laparotomy). All infants should have 5 mg/kg/day of phenobarbitone for at least 72 hours before performing the test, as the choleretic effect helps to discriminate between the causes of cholestasis.

^{99m}-Tc sulphur colloid images reflect reticuloendothelial function and hepatic blood flow. The label, injected intravenously, is taken up by Kupffer cells in the liver, with most of the isotope being visible over the right lobe of liver under normal circumstances. Splenic uptake should be minimal, and there should be NO uptake in bone marrow. Liver uptake is patchy in fibrotic/cirrhotic liver disease or poor in severe parenchymal disease, especially Wilson's disease. Good uptake in only the caudate lobe is seen in Budd–Chiari syndrome. The relative uptake of spleen and bone marrow as seen in the spine can be used as an index of assessing disease progression.

CHOLANGIOGRAPHY

Percutaneous transhepatic cholangiography (PTC) and endoscopic retrograde cholangiopancreatography (ERCP) are the techniques used for imaging details of the anatomy of the biliary tree.

PTC provides particularly good images for demonstrating the site of obstruction of bile ducts within or outside the liver, and may have a therapeutic advantage of clearing biliary sludge and relieving obstruction. Balloon dilatation of strictures may also be performed. The three main complications are bacteraemia/septicaemia, bile leak or haemorrhage.

Operative cholangiography may be helpful during lapartomy performed via the gall bladder or cystic duct, and is especially useful if there are unexpected surgical findings, or poor images from ERCP or PTC taken preoperatively.

ERCP provides good imaging of the extrahepatic and intrahepatic bile ducts. The technique is particularly useful in defining extrahepatic biliary obstruction and sclerosing cholangitis. Gallstones may also be removed, sphincterotomy performed, and transbiliary prostheses inserted. Complications include cholangitis, bacteraemia, pancreatitis, raised serum amylase, biliary leak, haemobilia, damage to the ampulla, and perforation of the duodenum.

ANGIOGRAPHY

Splanchnic catheterisation of the coeliac and superior mesenteric arteries via the femoral artery is helpful in defining anomalies of the hepatic artery and space-occupying lesions within the liver. Venous phase films outline the portal venous system, including the superior mesenteric vein.

Percutaneous transplenic portal venography performed by splenic puncture helps to demonstrate patency of the portal vein, but may not identify the site of obstruction or may fail to opacify the portal vein because of retrograde flow.

Digital subtraction angiography allows images to be collected of arterial and venous systems after intravenous rather than intra-arterial injection of contrast, and thus reduces operative risks.

Transhepatic portography where a catheter is inserted through a needle in the liver, may be used if patency of the portal vein is in doubt prior to liver transplantation.

Hepatic vein catheterisation allows pressure measurement in an unobstructed major branch of hepatic vein and is related to portal vein pressure. The normal wedged pressure is 5 mmHg but pressures of 20 mmHg may be found in sinusoidal or post-sinusoidal hypertension. In extrahepatic portal vein obstruction the hepatic vein wedge pressure is normal.

Cavography, and **right heart cardiac catheter**, may be required if liver disease is thought to be due to venous outflow block.

BLOOD TESTS

Standard biochemical liver function tests

Bilirubin, aspartate transaminase, gamma glutamyl transpeptidase, alkaline phosphatase, total protein, and albumin are assayed using automated equipment in most hospital biochemistry laboratories. The main value of these tests is in monitoring progress of liver disease, and identifying those patients suspected of having a liver disorder. These tests are not diagnostic and over-interpretation of the values can cause confusion. For bilirubin and the liver enzymes it should always be remembered that the measured level relates not only to production but also clearance.

Bilirubin Produced in the reticuloendothelial system from RBC degradation and the waste product of haem, this yellow pigment is transported in blood in its fat-soluble from largely bound to albumin. Removed into the hepatocyte, bilirubin is water-solubilised by conjugation with glucuronic acid and becomes excretable, passing into bile. Thus, conjugated bilirubin adds colour to the bowel contents and is responsible for normal stool pigmentation. Under normal circumstances, very little bilirubin in the circulation is conjugated. When the total value is 100 micromoles/l or more, the conjugated fraction should be less than 20%. If conjugated hyperbilirubinaemia exists, it is usual for the majority of the bilirubin to be conjugated. The conjugation process is commonly impaired in physiological jaundice of the newborn, Gilbert's disease in the older child/adolescent, and extremely rarely due to absence of the enzyme conjugating process in Crigler–Najaar syndrome. All conjugated hyperbilirubinaemia is pathological and requires further investigation.

Aminotransferases Found in nearly every tissue, these intracellular enzymes leak from damaged cells. A high AST (or ALT) is associated with hepatitis of liver cell necrosis. In liver transplant, AST is the most widely-available sensitive indicator of rejection.

Gamma-glutamyl transpeptidase An elevated GGT is associated with biliary processes, particularly biliary obstruction. Interpretation of GGT can be difficult, however, as infants with successful Kasai portoenterostomies typically have an elevated GGT, and some intrahepatic cholestatic conditions seem to be associated with normal GGT levels. Newborn infants commonly have GGTs three times the normal adult reference level without obvious explanation.

Albumin Albumin is synthesised in the liver. Low albumin concentrations are found in advanced chronic liver disease, or after alimentary bleeding. Children with chronic liver disease may also have proteinuria or protein-losing enteropathy (due to increased portal pressure) so that increased loss may be part of the cause rather than reduced synthesis. As albumin has a half-life of 20 days, acute liver diseases do not usually present with hypoalbuminaemia.

Immunoglobulins Elevated immunoglobulins formed in the reticuloendothelial system may be found in chronic liver disease. IgM may be raised in viral hepatitis, total immunoglobulins may be raised in any chronic liver disease (including Wilson's disease), and elevated IgG is typically found in autoimmune liver disease. Low levels of IgA and C4 complement are sometimes found in autoimmune chronic active hepatitis.

Autoantibodies Although non-organ specific, these tests are very useful in detecting autoimmune liver diseases. Smooth muscle (SMA) and/or antinuclear (ANA/ANF) antibodies may be seen in autoimmune chronic active hepatitis, autoimmune sclerosing cholangitis, and Wilson's disease. Liver kidney microsomal (LKM) antibodies may be found in some cases of autoimmune chronic active hepatitis.

Prothrombin time/international normalised ratio (INR) This is the single most useful liver function test. The prothrombin time or INR reflects liver-dependent coagulation synthesis. If corrected within 4 hours of vitamin K given intravenously, then prolongation of PT/INR is due to impaired vitamin K absorption. If resistant to vitamin K, then significant liver disease or disseminated intravascular coagulation is present. Patients with portal vein obstruction often have mildly prolonged PT/INR without obvious explanation.

Serum cholesterol Synthesised in liver and in the gut wall, cholesterol values less than 2 micromol/l are associated with poor prognosis in chronic liver disease. Very high levels may be found in cholestatic liver disorders, particularly bile duct paucity (e.g. Alagille's syndrome).

Ammonia Produced in the colon by bacterial urease or synthesised in liver, kidney or small bowel, the blood concentration of ammonia is regulated by the liver. Elevated ammonia levels are found in most chronic liver disorders, but the main purpose of measurement is to establish a link between the liver and unexplained neurological dysfunction.

Serum bile salts Bile salts are synthesised, conjugated, and secreted from the liver into the biliary system. They are reabsorbed from the intestine (ileum), extracted from portal venous blood and recirculated through hepatocytes. Impaired liver extraction leads to a rising level which is specific for liver disease. Normal bile salt levels are higher in young children until at least 8 years. If specific bile salts are abnormal, then the test may be diagnostic for bile salt metabolism defects.

URINE TEST

Urine bile salts A useful screening test for bile acid metabolism defects and should be measured before serum bile salts.

SPECIFIC INVESTIGATIONS

Copper and caeruloplasmin Caeruloplasmin, the liver-synthesised copper binding protein, is low in up to 95% of cases of Wilson's disease. Unfortunately, the specificity of the test may be poor because other chronic liver diseases are associated with poor caeruloplasmin synthesis. The copper level tends to follow the caeruloplasmin concentration, but a low caeruloplasmin and relatively normal copper level would suggest Wilson's disease.

Urinary copper excretion This is a more specific test for Wilson's disease using 24-hour urine collections before and after Penicillamine 500 mg given at 0 and 12 hours, into acid-washed containers. A value in the second 24-hour collection rising to over 25 micromoles/24 hours is highly specific for Wilson's disease.

Alpha-1-antitrypsin deficiency Isoelectric phenotyping is the investigation of choice. As Alpha-1-antitrypsin is an acute phase protein, serum levels may even be normal in individuals with an abnormal genotype. New DNA techniques are also helpful. Normal phenotype is PiMM, classical deficiency is PiZZ.

Alpha-fetoprotein Synthesised in fetal life and by poorly differentiated liver cells, AFP is typically high in the newborn period, mean value 50,000 ng/ml, decaying exponentially after birth to 12.5 ng/ml by 6 months; a process which may be delayed in some cholestatic infants. Very high levels are useful markers for hepatoblastoma and hepatocellular carcinoma, and if present can be used for monitoring response to treatment.

4. Summary

Paediatric liver problems may be investigated successfully following logical sequences, commencing with full clinical history and examination. Basic investigations can all be performed at outside specialist centres and will often serve to narrow the diagnosis if not establish it. Early discussion and prompt referral to a tertiary centre helps to avoid delayed diagnosis. In principle it is often helpful to consider all jaundiced infants as having possible biliary atresia, and older children Wilson's disease. If the problems are viewed this way, then serious pathology comes to mind first and not last.

FURTHER READING

Hadzic, N., Mieli-Vergani, G., Sokal, E. (1998) *Chronic Liver Disease in Childhood. International Seminars in Paediatric Gastroenterology and Nutrition,* Vol. 7, no. 4, pp 1–15.

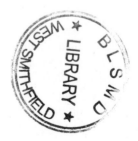

9

Gastroenterology

S Devane

Principles of physiology, anatomy and biochemistry

The gastrointestinal tract is a tubular structure that derives from the endodermal layer of the embryo. The fore-gut forms the pharynx, oesophagus, stomach and proximal small intestine, the mid-gut forms the small intestine and the proximal large intestine and the hind-gut forms the remainder of the gastrointestinal tract.

The functions of the gastrointestinal tract are divided into those related to transit, i.e. moving the luminal contents at the right pace, at the right time to the right part of the bowel, those relating to digestion, and those relating to absorption. The time, place and duration of digestion is regulated by transit. Absorption includes both absorption of nutrients and reabsorption of water secreted into the intestine as part of the digestive process. In the adult, approximately 9 litres per day of fluid is secreted into the gastrointestinal tract, of which almost all is reabsorbed.

The different parts of the gastrointestinal tract are specialised to different functions. The oesophagus is purely a conduit. The stomach is a mixing and storage organ and for the latter purpose has the capacity for receptive relaxation. It also performs some digestive functions. The small intestine is concerned with further digestion and absorption, but the orderly transit of its contents is very important. The colon is responsible for water reabsorption and for waste elimination.

Digestion occurs both in the lumen and in the brush border, a layer of microvilli that covers the luminal surface of the enterocytes that line the intestine. Absorption may be transcellular by active or passive processes, or may be paracellular, i.e. between cells across the tight junctions that seal them together. Large molecules may be absorbed by an endocytotic method. Enterocytes are produced in the depths of the crypts within the luminal wall and migrate upwards onto the luminal surface. In the case of the small intestine, the luminal surface is magnified greatly in area by the presence of villi. Enterocytes are lost from the tip of the villi and replaced from below.

Control of the functions of the gastrointestinal tract occurs at three levels. The first of these is that of the gastrointestinal cells themselves. The mucosal cells play a part in regulating absorption. The smooth muscle cells have an intrinsic regular fluctuation in their transmembrane electrical potential, that (because of coupling between adjacent cells) regulates the frequency of muscle contraction.

The second level is that of the enteric nervous system. The intestine has approximately the same number of nerve cells within it as does the spinal cord, giving an indication of its complexity. The enteric nervous system utilises the same neurotransmitter molecules as the central nervous system. The fasting intestine undergoes a cyclical fluctuation in its activity from quiescence to regular rhythmic contractions over a period of 60–90 minutes that is reminiscent of the cyclical pattern of REM and non-REM sleep in the central nervous system. The third level of control is that of the paracrine and endocrine substances that circulate in the microenvironment of the gastrointestinal wall. The substances involved in these processes inter-relate with one another and fluctuate in concentration under the influence of ingested food in a manner that is not yet fully understood. The effect of ingested food includes both a cephalic (a very rapid) phase and a later, slower phase mediated by luminal contents.

The transit functions can be investigated by adding marker substances to the luminal contents. Such markers may be radiographic contrast (Barium, gastrograffin), radiologically traceable solid markers, radioactive isotopes complexed to nutrients (labelled chicken, etc.), and non-absorbable substances (carmine red, lactulose) whose arrival in the caecum or at the anus can be detected by indirect or direct methods. These last methods are useful for detecting the first arrival of a meal (the 'head' of the meal).

The digestive functions can be measured either by urinary detection of the products of digestion (pancreolauryl test, disaccharide excretion tests), or by direct measurement of enzymes (secretin–pancreozymin test, stool chymotrypsin). The absorptive functions can be assessed by urinary detection of the products absorbed (d-xylose, lactulose, Cr-EDTA), or (rather poorly) by measuring nutrient repletion (serum iron, ferritin, calcium, etc.).

The control functions can be assessed by measuring gastrointestinal electrical activity (electrogastrography), motor activity (manometry), and circulating hormones (motilin, etc.). These methods are rather crude, and there is no method for assessing the function of the enteric nervous system.

The immunological and inflammatory problems that affect the gastrointestinal tract can be assessed by measuring acute phase reactants (ESR, CRP, platelet count, orosmomucoid), immunological function (leucocyte counts, leucocyte migration, opsonisation, immunoglobulin concentration, chemiluminescence), immunological activity (labelled leucocyte scan) and specific immunological substances (antigliaden antibodies, gut auto-antibodies).

A paediatric gastroenterology department needs the support of a modern and comprehensive haematology and biochemistry laboratory, and the support of a histopathology department with expertise in gastrointestinal histology. Additional equipment that may not be present in all hospital laboratories but that may be required include a mass spectrography system to enable C^{13} urea breath tests to be undertaken, chromatographic equipment for detecting and measuring carbohydrates in liquid stool and in urine after permeability and absorption tests, and a hydrogen detector for breath hydrogen tests.

The paediatric gastroenterology department also requires the support of a radiology department with child-friendly access to fluoroscopy systems and a Gamma camera. Ideally the fluoroscopy system should be a modern system with freeze frame facilities to minimise radiation exposure. The paediatric gastroenterology department should include or have access to a member of staff with full radiological protection training.

Additional equipment that should be available to the department includes the following:

- A jejunal biopsy capsule — Watson or Crosby type. These may be a single or double port type. They are available in paediatric and adult sizes. Metal parts need to be autoclaved and the tubing may be sterilised using ethylene oxide.
- Breath hydrogen detector. The electrochemical detector type is suitable for installing in a ward setting, and provides immediate results, obviating the need to store samples in a vacuum tube for later measurement in the laboratory.
- pH electrode digital recorder, and analysis system. The pH electrode may be of the semi-disposable antimony electrode type or of the much more expensive glass electrode type. The latter is reusable ad infinitum. The digital recorder will need an interface with a computer which will subsequently analyse the pH data recorded.
- Endoscopy system. An endoscopy suite, ideally in a child-friendly environment, may be required and this should include adequate equipment for sterilising the endoscopes in use. The endoscopy equipment may be of the traditional ocular type or the more modern video-chip variety. The latter allows narrower bore endoscopes, as a single connection wire can bring the data from the end of the endoscope to the screen. Endoscopes suitable for neonatal use are now available, though these suffer from the disadvantage of sharing a single channel for the air feed and the biopsy forceps. The endoscopy equipment will need to be accompanied by biopsy forceps for obtaining tissue samples, a diathermy snare for removing colonic polyps, and retrieval tools for grabbing polyps to be extracted.

List of tests

ANATOMY AND MACROSTRUCTURE

Radiological contrast studies
Contrast cine-swallow
Contrast meal
Contrast follow-through
Contrast and double contrast small bowel enema
Contrast and double contrast colonic enema
GI ultrasound scanning
GI computerised tomographic scanning
MRI scanning
ERCP
Endoscopy

Oesophago-gastro-duodenoscopy
Colonoscopy
Small intestinal enteroscopy

MICRO AND ULTRASTRUCTURE

Oesophageal and antral biopsy
Jejunal biopsy
Rectal biopsy

MOTILITY

Oesophageal manometry
Antroduodenal manometry
Rectal manometry

Electrogastrography
Oesophageal pH monitoring
Lactulose mouth to caecum transit time
Carmine red marker study
Solid marker study
Scintigraphy — gastric
Scintigraphy — small intestinal

LUMINAL DIGESTIVE AND MUCOSAL FUNCTION

Absorption
Permeability
Disaccharidase excretion test
Pancreolauryl test
Stool chromatography
Stool-reducing substances
Stool electrolytes
Disaccharide breath hydrogen test
Secretin–pancreozymin test
Stool chymotrypsin and elastase

MICROBIOLOGY

Glucose breath hydrogen test
C13 and C14 urea breath test
Helicobacter pylori serology
Stool culture and sensitivity
Stool microscopy
Stool electron microscopy

Yersinia antibodies
Stool immunofluorescence
Stool C. difficile toxin
Mantoux test

BLOOD TESTS

Haemoglobin and ferritin
Calcium, phosphate and alkaline phosphatase
Zinc, copper and selenium
Antigliaden, anti-reticulin, anti-endomysial and anti-tissue transglutaminase antibodies
Platelet count
ESR, CRP, orosmomucoid
Immunoglobulins, opsonisation, leucocyte migration and chemiluminescence

OTHER

Labelled leucocyte scanning
Food challenges — open
Food challenges — blind
Sweat test
Sputum microscopy and lactose
Gut auto-antibodies
Serum motilin, VIP, and other hormones
Stool alpha-1 anti-trypsin
Urine toxicology

ABBREVIATIONS USED IN THIS CHAPTER

CCK — cholecystokinin
Cr-EDTA — chromium-ethylene-diaminetetraacetic acid

EGG — electrogastrography
VIP — vasoactive intestinal peptide

Tests

I ANATOMY AND MACROSTRUCTURE

(a) Radiological contrast studies

These are probably the most readily available tests of the gastrointestinal tract, using equipment already present in most hospital services. Contrast agents may be barium or iodine based; the former should not be used where there is a risk of aspiration or of perforation. Most contrast agents are hypertonic, and where such agents are used, care must be taken with monitoring fluid balance.

- Contrast cine-swallow. This will display the quality of co-ordination of the pharyngeal swallowing system and also any pooling of contrast in the mouth as a result of poor co-ordination of the mouth and tongue. It is useful in the assessment of feeding problems, particularly in children with neuromuscular problems. The consistency of the contrast can be varied to suit the patient.
- Contrast meal. The main function is to show the anatomy of the upper gastro-intestinal tract. It will show any major delay in gastric emptying, and the con-trast can be followed into the jejunum to show malrotation. In rare cases marked oesophageal varices or peptic ulceration may be diagnosed, although endoscopy has superseded it as a test for these.
- Contrast follow-through. This will show abnormalities in small bowel calibre, major abnormalities in transit time, and mucosal thickening or irregularity. Flocculation of the contrast medium suggests malabsorption.
- Contrast and double contrast small bowel enema. A development of the follow-through examination, this requires small intestinal intubation. It provides better definition. Air can be instilled to allow increased mucosal detail by pro-viding a 'double contrast'.
- Contrast and double contrast colonic enema. To show colonic mucosal lesions or distal obstructive lesions this study is available, but is contraindicated if a toxic megacolon is suspected. It is uncomfortable and in most cases has been superseded by colonoscopy. It has a particular role in suspected intussuscep-tion, where it is often therapeutic, though pneumatic reduction is increasing in popularity.
- Gastrointestinal ultrasound scanning. Ultrasound scanning of the gastroin-testinal tract is the best method of detecting pyloric muscle hypertrophy in pyloric stenosis. It can also be used to detect malrotation of the intestine by showing an abnormal relationship of the superior mesenteric artery to the superior mesenteric vein, which is present in > 95% of children with this problem.
- Gastrointestinal computerised tomographic scanning. Providing good informa-tion on pancreatic structure, this may be used for detecting retroperitoneal and mesenteric lymph node enlargement. It requires sedation in young chil-dren and sometimes general anaesthesia.
- MRI scanning. An alternative to CT scanning in some circumstances, MRI scanning offers the advantage of avoiding ionising radiation. It provides better definition of abnormal tissues such as lymphomatous infiltration. It requires sedation in young children and sometimes general anaesthesia.
- Endoscopic retrograde cholangiopancreatography. ERCP provides an image of the pancreatic and bile duct. It requires skilled endoscopy under general anaes-thesia with a side-viewing endoscope. It carries a small risk of ascending cholangitis.

(b) Endoscopy

- Oesophago-gastro-duodenoscopy. This provides direct vision of the oeso-phageal, gastric and duodenal mucosa, and allows an opportunity to take biopsies from any of these sites. It is the best method of detecting oesophageal inflammation and sources of bleeding, and of detecting peptic ulceration. In children, general anaesthesia is almost invariably required, but heavy sedation may be sufficient in some older children.

- Colonoscopy. Providing similar information on the colonic and terminal ileal mucosa, colonoscopy requires heavy sedation, and some paediatricians prefer general anaesthesia. The use of a general anaesthetic demands even greater care during the procedure as perforation is more likely. It has superseded contrast enema in almost all situations.
- Small intestinal enteroscopy. This new technique offers the opportunity for inspection of the small intestinal mucosa in children with suspected occult bleeding. It is only suitable for older children, and requires sedation and patience (while the enteroscope, with its terminal balloon inflated, passes the length of the small intestine).

2 MICRO- AND ULTRASTRUCTURE

- Oesophageal and antral biopsy. Biopsies are obtained at endoscopy by the use of avulsion forceps and may be subjected to haematoxylin and eosin staining (for histology), to modified Giemsa staining (to show *Helicobacter pylori* relatively cheaply), to Walthin–Starey silver staining (to show *H. pylori* well) or to other special stains. The same suitability factors apply as to endoscopy.
- Jejunal biopsy. A necessary investigation in suspected enteropathy, jejunal biopsy may be obtained either by using a Crosby or Watson capsule or by using avulsion forceps at endoscopy. Both methods require sedation in young children, and the endoscopic method may require general anaesthesia. Endoscopy provides a greater number of but smaller and less well-oriented samples. Biopsies may be preserved in formalin for histological staining, in cocodylate buffer for electron microscopy, or frozen for later measurement of enzyme levels in the brush border.
- Rectal biopsy. Where Hirschsprung's disease or other colonic neuronal dysplasia is suspected, this is the investigation of choice. Rectal biopsies are obtained using a suction capsule and may be stained with haematoxylin and eosin for histology, with a silver stain to show nerve fibres, or with an acetylcholinesterase stain to show this neurologically-active enzyme. Other special stains may also be applied.

3 MOTILITY

- Oesophageal manometry. This provides pathophysiological information on oesophageal function, and its role is confined to those patients with achalasia, or with severe oesophageal dysfunction not responding to management. It may be undertaken with a single channel manometry system pulled slowly through the gastro-oesophageal area, with multiple manometry probes placed carefully and left in situ, or with a combination of manometry transducers and a 5 cm-long pressure-sensitive sleeve straddling the oesophageal–gastric junction. It requires sedation in young children if excessive movement artifacts are to be avoided.

- Antroduodenal manometry. The role of this test, available in only a few centres, is confined to the investigation of suspected pseudo-obstruction. This requires a multiple transducer probe to be placed in the antroduodenal area and left in situ. Insertion and monitoring requires sedation in young children.
- Rectal manometry. This investigation may be helpful in severe refractory constipation. It is best performed using a specially-constructed series of balloons connected to a series of transducers, and will show inco-ordination between stimulation of sensation on filling and sphincter responses.
- Electrogastrography. A new technique, electrogastrography detects gastric electrical control activity using surface electrodes. It is helpful in suspected pseudo-obstruction. It requires adequate signal processing and analysis equipment, and is therefore a specialised test available in a few centres only.
- Oesophageal pH monitoring. Using an indwelling pH-sensitive electrode, this detects acid reflux into the oesophagus. It is the gold standard for quantification of oesophageal acid reflux. It is probably most useful in patients with atypical symptoms which may be due to gastro-oesophageal reflux. It is tolerated well by young children, but supervision of toddlers is necessary to prevent interference with the probe.
- Lactulose mouth-to-caecum transit time. Providing a measure of the transit of the head of a meal from the mouth as far as the caecum, this uses the conversion of some of a non-absorbable carbohydrate to hydrogen by caecal bacteria. It requires a means of collecting expired air and a hydrogen detector. Air collection is more difficult from younger children. It is not applicable if there is small intestinal bacterial over-growth, or in the small number of children without hydrogen-producing enteral bacteria.
- Carmine red marker study. This provides a measure of the transit of the head of a meal from the mouth as far as the anus.
- Solid marker study. Combined with X-rays, this provides a measure of the transit of a meal from ingestion of shaped radio-opaque markers to the time an X-ray is taken. It is most useful for detecting transit delay in the proximal or distal colon.
- Scintigraphy — gastric. Gastric scintigraphy, using a gamma camera, provides a continous measure of the transfer of a radio-labelled meal out of the stomach. It can detect reflux of the labelled material into the oesophagus or aspiration into the lungs ('milk scan'). It requires use of ionising radiation.
- Scintigraphy — small intestinal. This can provide a continuous measure of the transfer of a radio-labelled meal out of the stomach and into the caecal area. Comparison of gastric emptying with arrival of the radio-labelled material at the caecum gives a small intestinal transit time.

4 LUMINAL DIGESTIVE AND MUCOSAL FUNCTION

- Absorption. The urinary excretion of D-xylose can be used to indicate the adequacy of absorption. A timed urine collection is required, and so it is not suitable for incontinent children. Other carbohydrates can be measured in a similar manner, for example 3-0-methyl glucose. Laboratory facilities to measure these substances are necessary.

- Permeability. In a similar manner to absorption tests, urinary excretion of substances that should not be absorbed can be detected. Substances used include lactulose and chromium EDTA (the latter involving a radioactive isotope). These tests are limited by the ability to collect a timed urine sample and are not appropriate to very young children unless in a specialist metabolic ward.
- Disaccharidase excretion test. A small proportion of inadequately-digested disaccharides is absorbed intact and may be detected in a timed urine collection. This excretion must be compared to that of absorbable and non-absorbable carbohydrates for interpretation. The test requires urinary continence, and equipment for accurate carbohydrate concentration determination.
- Pancreolauryl test. This test of pancreatic function requires two timed urine collections to measure excretion of a dye (fluorescein), successively complexed to a non-absorbable substance unless cleaved from it by pancreatic enzyme activity, and non-complexed. While validated in adults, it is still experimental in children. The standard doses are not appropriate to young children.
- Stool chromatography. Malabsorption of carbohydrates can be detected by performing chromatography on liquid stool. This is suitable for young children but is irrelevant unless the stool is watery. Watery stool can be collected by reversing a nappy to prevent liquid soaking away into it.
- Stool reducing substances. The presence of more than 1/4% reducing substances in liquid stool is usually abnormal, though 1/2% is not necessarily so in all cases. It indicates malabsorption of carbohydrates. Sucrose is not a reducing substance, so sucrose isomaltase deficiency does not produce a positive result unless the stool is pretreated with acid to cleave the sucrose molecules into fructose and glucose.
- Stool electrolytes. Measurement of stool electrolytes will differentiate a secretory diarrhoea (when the sodium concentration is high) from osmotic diarrhoea (when it is usually low). It is impractical unless the stool is watery.
- Disaccharide breath hydrogen test. Malabsorption of a carbohydrate can be detected by measuring breath hydrogen resulting from bacterial metabolism of the carbohydrate in the caecum. Breath sample collection is easiest in children who can co-ordinate blowing, but can be accomplished using a mask in younger children. Malabsorption of lactose, sucrose and fructose can be detected. The test cannot be relied upon in the presence of small intestinal bacterial over-growth, or in the small number of children (<2%) without hydrogen-producing bacteria in the caecum. A hydrogen detector is required.
- Secretin–pancreozymin test. The gold standard test for pancreatic function, this requires collection of duodenal juices for 10-minute periods after intravenous injection of pancreozymin (CCK) and later of secretin. It requires sedation and radiographic screening to place the collection tube in situ, and to keep it there. There is a small risk of anaphylactic responses to the injected hormones.
- Stool chymotrypsin and elastase. This provides an indirect measure of pancreatic enzyme production by detecting chymotrypsin activity in the stools. A positive result suggests good pancreatic activity but a negative result is not reliable.

5 MICROBIOLOGY

- Glucose breath hydrogen test. This test is identical to the disaccharide breath hydrogen test in its conduct. Unless there is glucose malabsorption, a rise in breath hydrogen following glucose administration suggests small intestinal bacterial over-growth.
- C13 and C14 urea breath test. *Helicobacter pylori* carries a urease that produces CO_2 from urea. A rise in C13 or C14 in exhaled CO_2 following administration of labelled urea suggests the presence of *H. pylori* in the stomach. The C14 urea breath test is not suitable for children, as the label is radioactive. The C13 urea breath test is suitable for children, but requires access to a mass spectrometer. This access is increasingly being made available by post by commercial companies.
- *Helicobacter pylori* serology. Serological tests for this organism, which has been called the cause of the 'world's most common infection', are now available, and can detect positive serology on finger-prick blood samples. While they will determine seropositivity with good sensitivity and specificity, this does not indicate causation except in proven peptic ulceration.
- Stool culture and sensitivity. Readily available in most medical facilities, this detects enteric pathogens. Ideally, a series of fresh stool samples is required.
- Stool microscopy. Stool microscopy detects the presence of cysts, ova and parasites, and requires a fresh stool taken immediately to the laboratory.
- Stool electron microscopy. This detects the presence of viral pathogens. In young infants, a positive result may be incidental.
- Stool immunofluorescence. Stool immunofluorescence can be used to detect selected viral pathogens. It is most often used to detect rotavirus.
- Stool *Clostridium difficile* toxin. Pseudomembranous colitis may occur in children on broad-spectrum antibiotics, and can be diagnosed by detecting the toxin produced by the responsible organism in the stool.
- *Yersinia* antibodies. *Yersinia* antibodies are raised in the presence of *Yersinia* enterocolitis, which may be mistaken for inflammatory bowel disease.

6 BLOOD TESTS

- Haemoglobin and ferritin. This indicates iron status and is a proxy index of malabsorption.
- Calcium, phosphate and alkaline phosphatase. Abnormalities may indicate malabsorption, though alkaline phosphatase concentrations will not be raised in the presence of zinc deficiency.
- Zinc, copper and selenium. Low concentrations of these may indicate prolonged failure of adequate nutrition. They must be measured in prolonged gastrointestinal failure.
- Antigliaden, anti-reticulin, anti-endomysial and anti-tissue transglutaminase antibodies. These are present in coeliac disease and are supportive evidence but not diagnostic evidence for the diagnosis. Specificity is better for IgA antibodies than for IgG antibodies, and for the latter two rather than for antigliaden antibodies. IgA antibodies may not be detected in the presence of IgA deficiency.

- Platelet count. The platelet count behaves as an acute-phase reactant and may indicate gastrointestinal inflammation. It is useful in monitoring inflammatory bowel disease.
- ESR, CRP, orosmomucoid. Acute-phase reactants, these are raised in the presence of gastrointestinal inflammation.
- Immunoglobulins, opsonisation, leucocyte migration and chemiluminescence. In the presence of an unexplained enteropathy these immunological tests may be required, as enteropathy may be the presenting feature of an immunodeficiency.

7 OTHER

- Labelled leucocyte scanning. Leucocytes taken from a patient, labelled with indium or technetium, and reinjected, may be detected using a gamma camera as they congregate in areas of inflammation. This allows the detection of active areas of inflammation in the gastrointestinal tract in inflammatory bowel disease. Indium produces too much radiation to be acceptable in young children, so technetium is preferable.
- Food challenges — open. Repeated open challenges may help establish a diagnosis of food allergy. Good record keeping is necessary. The carer must be cautioned against the over-meticulous recording of normal variations in children's moods and behaviour.
- Food challenges — blind. This is the gold standard method for proving a gastrointestinal food allergy. It is very difficult to organise in the clinical setting, as a non-identifiable placebo for a suspected substance is difficult to construct. A relevant symptom score and diary sheet is required.
- Sweat test. Measurement of sweat sodium and chloride will make a diagnosis of cystic fibrosis in a child presenting with meconium ileus or malabsorption. A sweat sodium of > 70 mM/l is positive, < 50 mM/l is negative, and values in between need a repeat sample. A positive result needs to be repeated for confirmation. Results based on a collection of < 100 mg of sweat are unreliable, and it is difficult to get this quantity of sweat under the age of 6 weeks. A sweat test should be undertaken in children with malabsorption, in children with neonatal meconium ileus, with neonatal meconium plug syndrome, and in infants with in-utero intestinal perforation.
- Sputum microscopy and lactose. These tests may be used to detect aspiration of milk in an intubated child in an intensive care unit. Fat-laden macrophages will be seen on microscopy, and lactose detected on assay.
- Gut auto-antibodies. Auto-antibodies to gut mucosa are present in a small number of children with severe protracted enteropathy. These can be detected by incubating serum with gastrointestinal tissues such as monkey oesophagus.
- Serum motilin, VIP, and other hormones. These hormone concentrations may be raised in children with a secretory diarrhoea secondary to a tumour producing gastrointestinally-active hormones. The assay is available in few centres.
- Stool alpha-1 anti-trypsin. In the presence of a protein-losing enteropathy, this protein is found in appreciable quantities in the stool.

- Urine toxicology. Occasionally this may be required to detect factitious diarrhoea due to laxative administration.
- Mantoux test. This may be required to exclude tuberculosis in the presence of gastrointestinal inflammation.

Clinical problems

I PERSISTENT VOMITING

Vomiting is the return of gastric contents to the outside world. This may be passive or active. The former is frequently called regurgitation or reflux vomiting, and the latter called true or reflex vomiting. The former is mainly driven by gravity and the dynamics of pressure differences and flow across the chest. The latter is a complex reflex co-ordinated in the brain stem and involving simultaneous activity by the pyloric muscle, gastric smooth muscle, gastro-oesophageal junction, oesophagus, diaphragm, anterior abdominal wall muscles and associated with changes in sweat gland, skin blood vessel, and eye muscle activity. It is this latter form that is preceded by and associated with the sensation of nausea. The clinician must initially try to distinguish which form of vomiting is occurring.

While regurgitation or reflux vomiting is usually passive, the vomiting described may occasionally take on some of the characteristics of reflex vomiting initiated by the irritation of the pharynx and stimulation of the gag reflex produced by the regurgitation.

A sensible approach to the investigation of vomiting must take into account the age of onset of symptoms.

Vomiting in the first 48 hours of life, particularly if bile-stained, requires investigation for gastrointestinal obstruction. A plain film of the abdomen at this stage is in effect a contrast X-ray, with swallowed air acting as the contrast medium. The plain film of the abdomen must be examined for absence of gas in the lower bowel, and for the characteristic bubbly appearance of inspissated meconium that occurs in meconium ileus. Dilated bowel may be seen and fluid levels may be seen in a lateral decubitus X-ray.

In the absence of signs of obstruction, investigations for systemic infection such as septicaemia or urinary tract infection must be undertaken. In rare circumstances, acidosis may indicate a congenital metabolic abnormality such as maple syrup urine disease. Where obstruction is uncertain, a formal contrast X-ray study may be helpful, with the contrast administered either by enema or by nasogastric tube.

True vomiting in infancy without bile-staining may be due to pyloric stenosis, and suspicion is heightened by the association of alkalosis and hypochloraemia. Ultrasound examination of the pyloric region is now the best investigation for this condition. Persistent true vomiting not due to pyloric stenosis may be due to intermittent bowel obstruction associated with malrotation, and an X-ray contrast study will indicate whether the duodeno-jejunal junction is normally placed to the left of the mid-line or abnormally placed on the right of the mid-line, the differentiating feature. Other investigations required include those for systemic infection such as urinary tract infection and in rare circumstances investigation for congenital metabolic defects.

Vomiting in infancy that is predominantly passive is due to incompetence of the gastro-oesophageal junction area. A small amount of passive regurgitation, called posseting, is a normal phenomenon. Excessive regurgitation causing parental distress, or causing medical compromise (failure to thrive, anaemia, or recurrent chest symptoms), is called gastro-oesophageal reflux. A contrast X-ray study of the oesophagus and stomach is a necessary investigation in order to demonstrate that the anatomy is normal and that malrotation is not present, but is not in itself a good test of the competence of the gastro-oesophageal sphincter

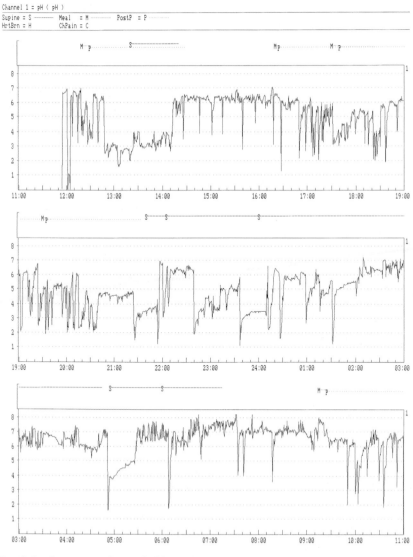

Fig. 9.1 **Intraoesophageal pH monitoring.**

area. (It may demonstrate incompetence during the short period of the study, and particularly if aggressive stress of competence is introduced by turning the child upside-down and applying external pressure to the abdomen). Intra-oesophageal pH monitoring and recording for a 24-hour period (Fig. 9.1) is the gold standard for the detection and quantification of gastro-oesophageal acid reflux. It is most useful to the clinician where the presenting symptoms are of uncertain aetiology, for example recurrent respiratory symptoms.

Where facilities are available, gastric scintigraphy may provide quantification of gastro-oesophageal reflux over a longer period than a contrast X-ray, and has the added advantage that aspiration into the lungs will show as a hot-spot in this area. This study is sometimes called a milk-scan. Oesophageal manometry will show the underlying pathophysiological basis of reflux but is not necessary in the vast majority of cases.

Oesophageal endoscopy is useful where significant oesophagitis is suspected, either because of symptoms suggesting chest pain or blood present in the vomitus. Its place is in elucidating the cause where the symptoms are of uncertain origin.

Persistent or recurrent vomiting in older children requires contrast studies to define any anatomical abnormality, and probably intra-oesophageal pH studies. These must be preceded by a thorough physical examination which must include fundoscopy. In some cases cranial MRI scanning to examine the brain stem is warranted. In addition, it may be necessary to exclude unusual metabolic abnormalities by measuring urinary and serum amino acids and organic acids, and pH, after an overnight fast. If all of these are normal, psychological assessment may be helpful as psychogenic vomiting is common at this age, but many will fall into the unexplained category of cyclical vomiting.

Table 9.1 sets out investigations into persistent vomiting.

Table 9.1   **Investigation of persistent vomiting**

Blood electrolytes, pH, full blood count

Urine electrolytes, culture

Stool culture

Other:

If passive: If an infant and responding to treatment,
  → no investigations, otherwise
  Contrast study to establish anatomy;
  pH study to quantify acid reflux

If active: Ultrasound to detect pyloric stenosis (if age appropriate)
  Contrast study
  CNS imaging
  Urine and serum metabolic studies
  Dietary exclusion and challenge

2 FAILURE TO THRIVE

The investigation of failure to thrive (the failure to gain weight at a rate appropriate for age) must rest on a foundation of a thorough examination to exclude chronic disorders of systems other than the intestinal system and assessment of caloric intake, which may be undertaken using a 3-day dietary diary. The latter is not really possible where a significant percentage of the calories taken is derived from breast feeding. In some cases, where the question of neglect has been raised, a period of observation of calorie intake and weight gain in hospital may be necessary.

The initial investigations of failure to thrive should include a full blood count to detect anaemia, ferritin measurements to detect iron deficiency, calcium, phosphate and alkaline phosphatase measurements to detect Vitamin D deficiency (a caution is that alkaline phosphatase concentration may not be raised if zinc is also deficient), albumin to detect possible protein deficiency, and renal and liver function tests. In the presence of gluten in the child's food intake, antigliadin IgA antibiotics and anti-endomysial antibodies should be included. While awaiting the results of these investigations, unless the failure to thrive is dramatic, the rate of weight gain on an adequate calorie intake should be assessed. Where gastrointestinal symptoms are present, or the results of investigations suggest malabsorption, a jejunal biopsy should be performed. This will detect a gluten enteropathy, other dietary protein enteropathy, or infestation with giardiasis, and may occasionally detect significant rarer conditions such as lymphangiectasia or Whipple's disease. Where the biopsy suggests gluten enteropathy, then a repeat biopsy following removal of gluten from the diet followed by another biopsy in later childhood following a gluten challenge is the gold standard for proving a diagnosis of coeliac disease (the Interlaken criteria of ESPGAN). This challenge is often administered as two slices of bread a day until symptoms develop or 3 months have passed. If the biopsy is normal at that stage, coeliac disease may finally be excluded in the opinion of most but not all paediatric gastroenterologists by a repeat biopsy two years after going on to a normal diet. Where the clinical story is typical, and there is confirmatory antibody evidence, the second and third biopsies are not necessary (the Budapest criteria of ESPGAN).

3 PERSISTENT DIARRHOEA FROM BIRTH

A useful distinction can be made between protracted diarrhoea of early infancy presenting in the perinatal period, shortly after, at, or even before birth, and protracted diarrhoea with a later onset. Once the fluid balance of the infant is regulated, the most important investigations centre on the stool constituents. A distinction can then be made between diarrhoea which settles on withdrawing enteral feeds, and diarrhoea which does not settle. Stool electrolytes and chromatography will determine congenital chloride-losing diarrhoea (stool chloride > 90 mM/l, and exceeding the sum of stool Na^+ and K^+ concentrations), congenital lactase deficiency (lactose in the stool, disappearing on withdrawing milk), and glucose/galactose malabsorption (glucose in the stool, not disappearing on changing to oral rehydration solution). High stool sodium losses occur in defective Na+–H+ exchange. If these are normal, a jejunal biopsy with electron microscopy is necessary to detect congenital microvillous atrophy. A PAS stain on a formalin fixed biopsy may give an indication of the absence of the brush border. Congenital hyperthyroidism, congenital infection, and autoimmune enteropathy should also be considered. Many cases of congenital diarrhoea have an unknown basis, and some of these are hereditary.

4 PERSISTENT DIARRHOEA

Investigations for protracted diarrhoea are listed in Table 9.2.

A useful distinction can be made between persistent diarrhoea associated with poor weight gain and that associated with good weight gain. The latter situation, particularly if the stools contain recognisable food such as peas and carrots, is often normal and is termed toddler diarrhoea. Another useful distinction can be made between watery diarrhoea and other forms of diarrhoea. The former may

---

Table 9.2   Investigation of protracted diarrhoea

Blood
electrolytes, pH, ZN, CU
immune function tests
full blood count
thyroxine
VIP
congenital infection screen
gut autoantibodies

Urine
electrolytes
culture

Stool
microscopy, culture
electron microscopy or immunofluorescence
chromatography
electrolytes
C. difficile toxin
chymotrypsin

Tissue
jejunal biopsy for microscopy and electronmicroscopy
rectal biopsy
colonic biopsy

Others
contrast imaging
pancreolauryl test or secretin–pancreozymin test
sweat test
carbohydrate breath hydrogen tests
dietary exclusion and challenge

be due to a carbohydrate malabsorption, and the latter to many causes (including carbohydrate malabsorption). A description of steatorrhoea (pale floating stools) suggests malabsorption, particularly of fats (the stools float because of fermentation gas and not because of their fat content).

Diagnostic clues may be obtained from the history, and particularly from the history of the influence of feed changes. The effect of withdrawing enteral feeds will help differentiate a secretory diarrhoea from an osmotic diarrhoea. Stool electrolyte analysis will also help. In secretory diarrhoea, the sodium concentration is usually > 70 mM/l. Also the osmotic gap (the difference between stool osmolality and twice the sum of the sodium and the potassium concentration) is small. Secretory diarrhoea is much rarer than an osmotic diarrhoea.

For persistent secretory diarrhoea, it is important to exclude a tumour producing vasoactive intestinal peptide or another enteric hormone. This is done by measuring gut hormone concentrations and by imaging, looking for a pancreatic tumour or a tumour in the line of the sympathetic ganglion chain.

For persistent osmotic diarrhoea, stool chromatography is useful, as is measuring stool reducing substances.

For persistent diarrhoea which may be due to malabsorption, normal stool chymotrypsin excludes pancreatic disease. Liver function tests may exclude liver dysfunction. Serum haemoglobin, ferritin, calcium, phosphate and alkaline phosphatase will confirm malabsorption, but may be normal. Antigliaden antibodies, if positive, will suggest coeliac disease. In most cases, a jejunal biopsy will be required after completion of these initial investigations and a period of observation to confirm poor weight gain. In an atopic individual, or a child where the carer relates symptoms to dairy products, a dietetically controlled exclusion diet may be necessary as a therapeutic trial. In any case that is confusing, a radiological contrast follow-through study is required to detect surgically correctable causes of diarrhoea such as blind loop syndrome associated with a congenital abnormality. A high eosinophil count suggests the rare eosinophilic enteropathy. In some cases, gut autoantibodies, *Yersinia* antibodies, and colonoscopy should be considered.

5 BLOOD IN THE STOOLS

The presence of blood in the stools in the first days of life is usually due to swallowed maternal blood. This can be confirmed with an Apt's test. Simultaneously, the child's clotting studies should be assessed, particularly if intramuscular vitamin K has not been administered at birth, and the platelet count must be measured.

Blood in the stools in later infancy and childhood must be differentiated into its clinical types. It may be a small amount of blood at the end of the passage of a stool, often hard. This suggests constipation with an anal fissure and does not require further investigations. There may be more significant amounts of blood, associated with normal stools, but possibly associated with a small amount of mucus. This suggests a polyp and requires endoscopy. Blood associated with loose stools or mixed in with loose stools, often associated with mucus, requires investigations for colitis.

Where colitis is suspected, endoscopy is required. Ancillary investigations include measurement of acute phase reactants (platelet count, ESR, CRP or osmomucoid). Where there is a family or personal history of atopy, with possibly elevated concentrations of IgE, and a biopsy report that suggests an allergic colitis, a therapeutic trial of a diet free of cow's milk protein, which must be supervised by a paediatric dietician, is required. Where inflammatory bowel disease is suggested, a contrast follow-through examination to assess small intestinal involvement is required.

Where colonoscopy shows a polyp, endoscopic snare diathermy removal is required, together with examination of the rest of the colon for further polyps. The presence of more than 5 polyps suggests that a polyposis syndrome may be present. Histological examination of the polyps removed is mandatory, to ensure that they are juvenile and not adenomatous polyps. This is true whether or not multiple polyposis is present.

6 MUCUS IN THE STOOLS

Mucus mixed with loose stool suggests colitis or irritable bowel disease. The former must be excluded, as explained above, particularly if there is poor weight gain, loss of appetite, and abnormalities of acute phase reactants.

7 RECURRENT ABDOMINAL PAIN

Recurrent abdominal pain is a common symptom in childhood, with peaks of incidence at around 5 and 9 years of age. The investigations required are generally minimal and aimed at reassurance and exclusion of significant organic pathology. An axiom of investigation should be that a decision on the extent of investigations required should be made on the first assessment as it is detrimental to the subsequent management of the problem to add an additional investigation every time the child is assessed, with the opposite effect to reassurance. This is facilitated by the development of positive policies on the appropriate referral of children with recurrent abdominal pain, as multiple sequential investigation is more likely to occur where the child is passed from adult surgical to paediatric clinics, and from clinic to clinic.

The extent of reassurance and exclusion of significant organic pathology required depends on the family circumstances, previous investigations, and how closely the symptoms fit with the classical symptoms of benign recurrent abdominal pain of childhood. Apley's criteria still apply. If the pain is periumbilical, lasts no more than a few hours, does not wake the child at night, and if the problem has been present for a considerable period of time, then no investigations are necessary, though culture of a urine sample is common. Where the pain is away from the mid-line, further investigations of the urinary tract, including an ultrasound scan of the kidneys, is suggested. Where the pain is above the umbilicus, and particularly if there is a family history of peptic ulceration, then endoscopy should be considered to exclude an ulcer.

The requirement for other investigations depends entirely on the presence of other gastrointestinal symptoms. Lower bowel symptoms suggest that investigations for inflammatory bowel disease (acute phase reactant, indium/technetium labelled leucocyte scan, endoscopy, contrast follow-through examination) should be considered. Weight loss suggests that investigations for inflammatory bowel disease should also be considered.

Measurement of *Helicobacter pylori* antibodies, or use of a C13 urea breath test to detect *H. pylori* infection, is of doubtful value as the connection between this infection and recurrent abdominal pain is not established. The question of whether detection of infection and its eradication is worthwhile for reasons not related to the abdominal pain is an entirely separate question and related to the benefit of population screening for *H. pylori* infection.

8 CONSTIPATION

The presence of constipation can be assessed by physical examination together with an adequate history. Investigations are required if the history dates to the early neonatal period, or if the constipation is unresponsive to treatment, or if the constipation is of early onset and complicated by periods of diarrhoea suggesting enterocolitis. A rectal biopsy with examination to show abnormalities of innervation and ganglion cell presence is required. In the case of severe constipation failing to respond to treatment, occasionally rectal manometry may help delineate the underlying pathophysiology.

A plain X-ray of the abdomen is sometimes useful to quantify the severity of constipation, particularly where the retained faeces are soft rather than hard. It may also be helpful in the toddler who resists physical examination because of anxiety/separation problems.

In severe refractory cases, marker studies associated with carmine red transit studies can be used to define whether the hold-up is occurring in the colon and to define whether the hold-up/slow transit is pancolonic or predominantly distal colonic. These investigations are required in the unusual cases where surgical intervention either with a colostomy or with antegrade caecal enterostomy to allow wash-outs is being considered.

9 HAEMATEMESIS

The most common cause of haematemesis is damage to the oesophagus by vigorous vomiting caused by an incidental condition such as gastroenteritis. This is characterised by the blood coming at the end of an episode of vomiting.

Haematemesis may also take the form of small amounts of blood in the vomitus of a child with persistent vomiting due to gastro-oesophageal reflux, in which case the investigations are those appropriate for that condition. Unexpected severe haematemesis or recurrent haematemesis requires upper gastrointestinal endoscopy. This should be performed as soon as the bleeding and its associated haemodynamic complications have been brought under control. Further investigations depend on the findings. If peptic ulceration is found, then investigations for *Helicobacter pylori* infection are required. If oesophageal varices are found, then further investigations related to the hepato-biliary system are necessary.

Practical details

I UPPER GASTROINTESTINAL ENDOSCOPY

The patient having an endoscopy should have had nothing to eat for 12 hours in the case of a child and 4 hours in the case of an infant. In the older child, it can be undertaken with diazepam or midazalam sedation. In the younger child, a general anaesthetic is required. A paediatric endoscope is used. For neonates, a neonatal endoscope can be used. The endoscope should have been adequately sterilised according to standard endoscopy protocols. The patient should be placed lying on the left side. A saturation monitor should be attached to the child to monitor the effects of sedation. The endoscope should be inserted through a mouth-guard, which protects it from being bitten. The first point of difficulty is the pharynx, and this can be negotiated by putting a small bend in the endoscope which is straightened once the oesophagus is entered. The endoscope should be passed into the stomach, the stomach inflated, and the entire mucosa including the fundus examined. The latter can be examined by inserting a J-loop into the endoscope. The pylorus should be passed and the first and second parts of the duodenum examined. Antral biopsies should be taken using an avulsion forceps. Duodenal biopsies can be obtained in the same manner. After withdrawal of the endoscope, the child should be allowed to awake from the sedation. A benzodiazepine antagonist should be available in case of problems. Where good quality duodenal biopsies are required, the tubing of a Watson or Crosby capsule can be passed through the biopsy channel of the endoscope and the capsule passed into the duodenum under endoscopic vision.

Biopsies should be oriented, placed on card and placed in formalin. An antral biopsy may be embedded in a commercially available jelly containing a colour reagent affected by the urease produced by *Helicobacter pylori* (Clo-Test). A change in colour to red indicates the presence of urease and hence of *H. pylori*.

The interpretation of the histological samples obtained is beyond the scope of this book, and should be undertaken by a trained gastrointestinal histopathologist.

2 SUCTION JEJUNAL BIOPSY

The patient having a suction jejunal biopsy should have had nothing to eat for 12 hours in the case of a child and 4 hours in the case of an infant. The procedure should be conducted under sedation (chloral hydrate and trimeprazine are often used), and the time taken to appropriately place the capsule is shortened by administering metoclopramide (0.1 mg/kg) with this premedication. A Watson or Crosby capsule should be assembled and spring-loaded according to the manufacturer's instructions, having been sterilised. The biopsy can be conducted by passing the capsule into the stomach and allowing peristalsis to bring it to the duodenal-jejunal junction. This can be confirmed with a plain film of the abdomen taken 2 or 4 hours after insertion which will show the radio-opaque tubing crossing the mid-line once from left to right and once from right to left. Alternatively the capsule may be passed to the appropriate point under fluoroscopic control. The advantage of this is that it takes less time, and provides positive knowledge of the point biopsied. Care must be taken to minimise the exposure to radiation, and ideally a maximum of 2 minutes exposure time on the timer on the screening machine should be allowed. Exposure can be minimised by using modern fluoroscopy equipment with freeze frame facilities, allowing leisurely examination of the picture following a brief exposure. The first point of difficulty is the stomach, where the natural orientation sends the capsule to the left; lying on the right side, and twisting the capsule tubing, may help. The next point of difficulty is the pylorus, but provided the capsule is situated at the entrance, patience is usually all that is required; an injection of metoclopramide may help. Correct positioning at the pylorus is indicated best on a lateral view, which shows the capsule in a posterior position close to the vertebral column. Successful negotiation of the pylorus is indicated best on a lateral view also, which shows the tubing passing vertically downwards parallel to the vertebral column in a posterior position.

When the capsule is appropriately positioned, the system should be flushed with 2 ml of normal saline and then with 2 ml of air. The capsule should then be fired by suction and successful firing can be detected fluoroscopically by a movement of the blade. Excessive suction is not required, and may damage the biopsies. The capsule is then withdrawn and the biopsy sample removed. This is best achieved by manipulating it with a blunt-pointed probe onto the tip of a gloved index finger. In this position, it can be gently opened out. The glistening convex side is usually the mucosal surface, the somewhat bloodied concave side is usually the submucosa. When the biopsy is flattened it can be picked up from the finger onto a piece of card and dropped into either formalin for standard histology, cocodylate buffer for electron microscopy or normal saline. A biopsy placed on some aluminium foil may be dropped into liquid nitrogen if metabolic studies or measurement of enzyme concentrations in the brush border are required. Formalin preserved biopsies can be stained with haematoxylin and eosin for standard histology, or with PAS to show up the brush border. Complex immunochemical studies can be undertaken if required. Electronmicroscopy is mandatory if microvillous atrophy is suspected. The presence of Brunner's glands in the biopsy suggests a sample taken in the first or second part of the duodenum.

3 RECTAL BIOPSY

A rectal biopsy can be obtained under sedation. A suction capsule, similar in principle to the suction jejunal biopsy, is used. The biopsies obtained can be handled as for a jejunal biopsy. They can be stained with haematoxylin and eosin to show the presence of ganglion cells and with an acetylcholinesterase stain to show over-abundance of nerve fibres if Hirschsprung's disease is suspected.

4 MANOMETRY

Sedation is normally required in younger children. The motor activity of the upper gastrointestinal tract can be measured using multichannel manometry probes placed fluoroscopically. The manometry catheter may be a multilumen tube attached to a series of pressure transducers flushed with a low flow, high-impedance flow system, or electronic in nature. The recording should be undertaken for at least 3 hours, but with electronic recorders 24-hour monitoring may be possible. The resultant manometry recordings can be analysed for the pressure amplitudes obtained and for the co-ordination between activity in one channel and its adjacent channels. Deriving parameters of intestinal motor activity is specialised and beyond the scope of this handbook.

5 pH STUDIES

The patient should be fasting for at least 4 hours if an infant or 12 hours if a child. H2 antagonists or omeprazole must be stopped 24 hours in advance. Intra-oesophageal pH recording is undertaken with a pH-sensitive probe placed in the oesophagus transnasally and connected to an electronic recorder. A reference electrode placed on the skin is required. The pH-sensitive electrode may be of the antimony type, which can be used on approximately 20 occasions, or of the glass electrode type capable of unlimited use. The pH probe should be lubricated and passed through one nostril into the oesophagus. Correct positioning may be determined by undertaking this under fluoroscopic control when the tip of the probe should be placed opposite the junction of the 9th and 10th thoracic vertebrae. In children under one meter in height, the formula, Length $= 5 + 0.252 \times$ Ht, where Ht is the child's height, can be used to determine the approximate distance from the nose to the gastro-oesophageal sphincter, and the probe can be inserted 90% of this distance. This is reliable in infants. In older children, exact placement in relation to the gastro-oesophageal sphincter may be determined by undertaking an oesophageal manometry study initially to locate the nose to gastro-oesophageal sphincter distance, and the probe may be inserted 5 cm short of this point.

Once the probe is in place, the child should undertake as normal a day's routine activities as possible. A diary of meals, significant changes in posture, and of sleep and waking state should be kept so that the subsequent print-out of the recording can be correlated with activities. When the 24-hour recording is completed, the information can be down-loaded on to a computer which can print out a profile (Fig. 9.1) of intra-oesophageal pH and calculate the percentage time for which the pH is below 4. It can also calculate the total number of reflux episodes, the duration of the longest episode, and these parameters separately for a post-prandial period, and for sleep, awake, upright and supine periods. The result can be compared with known normal values. For children and adults, the percentage time for which the pH is below 4 should not exceed 5%. For infants, the normal oesophageal acid exposure is higher, and values of up to 12% may be normal in young infants. The most widely-known series of normal values for young children has been published by Yvan Vandenplas.

An alternative to undertaking a normal day's activities is to follow a strict protocol of regular ingestion of apple juice drinks. In this case, interpretation must be undertaken in line with the American experience of this regimented approach to the study.

6 BREATH HYDROGEN TEST

Measurement of breath hydrogen can provide information on:

1. Premature conversion of carbohydrate to hydrogen by bacteria within the small intestine

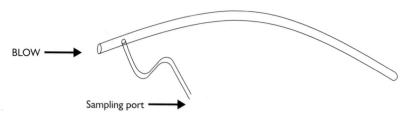

BLOW →

Sampling port →

Fig. 9.2 **Haldane–Priestley tube for collecting end-expiratory air.**

2. The arrival at the caecum of a non-absorbable carbohydrate such as lactulose
3. The arrival at the caecum of normally absorbable carbohydrates not absorbed because of a malabsorption problem.

Therefore one can undertake a glucose breath hydrogen test to look for bacterial overgrowth, a lactulose breath hydrogen test to measure mouth to caecum transit time, and a lactose, sucrose or fructose breath hydrogen test to look for evidence of malabsorption of these carbohydrates. The standard dose is 2 g/kg up to a maximum of 50 g of these carbohydrates. A side-effect is diarrhoea due to the malabsorption leading to an osmotic diarrhoea, and occasionally crampy pains due to gas production.

Expired air can be collected in older children using a Haldane–Priestley tube (Fig. 9.2). This is a long hose, with a syringe connected to a needle inserted in the proximal part, through which the patient breathes out at a steady rate. At the end of expiration, when the end-expiratory air is in the proximal part of the hose, a 20 ml sample can be aspirated. This sample can be passed through an electrochemical detector or a gas chromatography system and the hydrogen concentration obtained. Base-line samples in the fasting child must initially be obtained, and subsequent samples obtained at regular intervals after ingestion of the test carbohydrate. Where mouth to caecum transit time is being measured, samples are required every 10 minutes. Where evidence of malabsorption is required, samples can be taken at 30-minute intervals for approximately 3 hours. Where evidence of small bowel bacterial over-growth is required, samples should be taken at 10-minute intervals for the first hour. A small rise in breath hydrogen in the first 20 minutes after ingestion of carbohydrate is a normal phenomenon and due to hydrogen being produced by oral bacteria. In younger children who cannot cooperate with the Haldane–Priestley tube, mixed expiratory air can be collected via a mask and valve into a bag, or into a long tube.

In young infants, end-expiratory air may be collected in small aliquots, taken at the end of a series of normal expirations if a feeding tube is placed in the posterior nasopharynx. The operator needs to observe the breathing pattern, and as the child expires, to aspirate a few ml of air. This method is prone to blockage of the feeding tube by nasal secretions.

A rise in breath hydrogen above 10 parts per million (Fig. 9.3) is usually taken to indicate bacterial production of hydrogen. In the case of a test of malabsorption, this is a positive result. In the case of measurement of mouth to

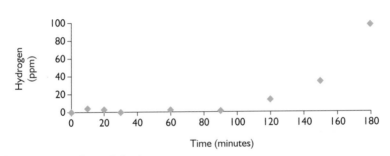

Fig. 9.3   **Lactose breath hydrogen test.**

caecum transit time, the time at which the concentration exceeds this value is taken as the transit time.

7 MARKER STUDIES

Radio-opaque markers may be followed through the gastrointestinal tract to measure transit time and to detect the sites of slow transit. Radio-opaque markers are easily obtained by cutting a radiopaque catheter into small 1-mm lengths. Fifty of these can be mixed with yoghurt and given to any child. An X-ray can be taken at 24, 48 and if necessary 72 hours, however recent European legislation has indicated that only commercially manufactured markers should be used. A more sophisticated variant of this test uses commercially available markers of different shapes. Shape A can be administered on day 1, shape B on day 2, shape C on day 3 and a single X-ray taken at 72 hours. The relative position of the different shapes can then be assessed.

The relevant information is the number of each shape in the descending colon, transverse colon and ascending colon. A significant number in the ascending colon suggests pan-colonic delay.

8 CARMINE RED TRANSIT

Carmine red is a dye which passes through the gastrointestinal tract. It can be taken orally, and the patient or parent asked to look for its first appearance in the stool. This would normally be expected 18 to 24 hours after ingestion.

9 CARBOHYDRATE PERMEABILITY AND ABSORPTION TESTS

A mixture of carbohydrates can be administered orally and a 5-hour urine collection obtained. The presence of the ingested carbohydrates in the urine gives an indication of their absorption or exclusion by the gastrointestinal tract. Ratios are more important than absolute amounts. The oldest of these tests is the d-xylose test. Modern variants use mixtures of 3-o-methyl glucose, lactulose, rhamnose, sucrose, lactose, and palatinose. These are research techniques at the present time, and no standardised doses are accepted. Disaccharides appear in the urine if they are not cleaved by disaccharidases, or if the bowel is abnormally permeable.

10 PANCREOLAURYL TEST

This is a measure of pancreatic enzyme production. Fluorescein, a dye which can be measured fluoroscopically, is administered complexed to lauric acid. The bond can be split by pancreatic enzymes. A timed urine collection is obtained. On the next day the same marker substance is administered in a non-complexed form and the same urine collection is repeated. In the presence of adequate pancreatic enzyme production the ratio of dye secreted in the urine on both days should be high. If it is less than 33% on the first day, pancreatic enzyme production is probably poor. This test has been standardised for adults and its interpretation is not fully defined for children. A side-effect is that the dye may give the skin a yellow appearance.

11 SECRETIN PANCREOZYMIN TEST

A patient having a secretin pancreozymin test should have had nothing to eat for 12 hours in the case of a child and 4 hours in the case of an infant. The procedure should be conducted under sedation (chloral hydrate and trimeprazine are often used). This test of pancreatic function requires a tube to be placed in the duodenum to collect the secretions present, and this can be placed in an identical manner to a suction jejunal biopsy capsule. It can be done in combination with a jejunal biopsy by placing a 14 French gauge adult nasogastric tube around the tubing of the jejunal biopsy capsule. A Y-tube connector can be used, with the jejunal biopsy capsule tubing emerging through one hole and jejunal juices being syphoned off through the other, with appropriate seals to prevent leakage. Two base-line 10-minute collections should be taken. An intravenous injection of CCK can then be given. Three subsequent 10-minute collections should then be taken. These should show increasing density of bile colouration. An injection of secretin is then given. Two 10-minute collections are taken and these should show a significant increase in volume produced. The collections need to be taken onto ice to preserve enzyme function. The specimens collected should be taken straight to the laboratory. Volume, bicarbonate concentration, and pancreatic enzyme concentrations can be measured (all laboratories will be able to measure amylase, but lipase and chymotrypsin can be measured in some laboratories). The normal result should be an amylase production of $28,000 \pm 16,000$ units, lipase production of $130,000 \pm 65,000$ units, trypsin production of 60 ± 30 units over 30 minutes (after CCK) and bicarbonate production in excess of 70 mM/l (after secretin).

12 C13 BREATH TEST

Labelled urea is administered. A breath sample is taken in a manner analogous to the breath hydrogen test and stored in a vacuum sample tube. Mass spectroscopy can be used to measure the C13 enrichment of the expired air. An increase in C13 suggests the presence of urease activity in the stomach.

FURTHER READING

Devane S.P., Candy D.C.A. (1992) Investigation of chronic diarrhoea. *Current Paediatrics* 2: 189–193.

Working Group of the European Society of Paediatric Gastroenterology and Nutrition (1990) Report; revised criteria for diagnosis of coeliac disease. *Archives of Disease in Childhood* 65: 909–911.

10

Respiratory Disease

A Bush

ABBREVIATIONS USED IN THIS CHAPTER

ANCA — antinutrophil cytoplasmic antibody

ARDS — adult respiratory distress syndrome

BAL — bronchoalveolar lavage

BPD — bronchopulmonary dysplasia

CMV — cytomegalovirus

DLCO — whole lung carbon monoxide transfer

DTPA — diethylnetriaminepenta-acetate

EMG — electromyelogram

FEV_1 — forced expired volume in one second

FRC — functional residual capacity

FVC — forced vital capacity

GOR — gastro-oesophageal reflux

ILD — interstitial lung disease

IRT — immunoreactive trypsin

KCO — carbon monoxide transfer per litre of accessible lung volume

LA — left atrium

LDH — lactic dehydrogenase

LV — left ventricle

M — muscarinic (receptor)

NANC — non-adrenergic, non-cholinergic (neural system)

OLB — open lung biopsy

OSA — obstructive sleep apnoea

PA — pulmonary artery

PAVM — pulmonary arteriovenous malformation

Pb — barometric pressure

PCD — primary ciliary dyskinesia (also known as Kartagener's syndrome)

PCR — polymerase chain reaction

PVR — pulmonary vascular resistance

Qp — pulmonary blood flow

RAST — specific IgE (radioallergosorbent test)

RV — residual volume

SGAW — specific airway resistance

'SPUR' — Severe, Persistent, Unusual organisms, Recurrent infections

SWVP — saturated water vapour pressure

TBB — transbronchial biopsy

TLC — total lung capacity

TV — tidal volume

VA — accessible lung volume (NOT alveolar ventilation)

VC — vital capacity

VMA — vanillylmandelic acid

Introduction

Paediatric respiratory medicine is a very clinically-based discipline. All children cough, and get upper respiratory tract infections; many children wheeze; many (particularly boys) complain that they cannot run as fast as their friends; but most are healthy. The key skill is to pick out those who are ill, on the basis of a detailed history and physical examination, and to direct investigations appropriately, rather than indulge in diagnostic trawls. Thus the diagnostic algorithms in the final section are meant as guides to possible lines of investigation of the clinical problem, rather than a recipe which must be followed in all cases in obsessive detail. Furthermore, many of the tests described should only be performed by those with special training, and who are carrying them out regularly. When evaluating a result, the physician's expectation should be compared with the observed measurements. If there is a major discrepancy, it should not automatically be assumed that the physician is wrong. All results should be evaluated critically, with the possibility of equipment error being borne in mind. The reader should not expect to perform sweat tests, ciliary studies or fibreoptic bronchoscopy just having read these pages. The final preliminary stricture to apply is that more than one condition may coexist, and the hunt for pathology should not necessarily be abandoned if one aetiological factor is found.

Principles — anatomy, physiology, development

The lung has a number of functions. The airway must conduct oxygen to the alveoli, and remove carbon dioxide, while defending against pathogens and pollutants mixed with incoming air. The circulation must feed and cleanse the alveolar–capillary unit, in addition to contributing to the defensive functions of the airway. Furthermore, the entire cardiac output must be 'arterialised' even at extremes of exercise. Blood must be filtered to prevent damaging systemic emboli and abscesses. The lungs contain as much endothelial tissue as the whole of the rest of the body put together, and this endothelial mass has important metabolic functions, which are only just becoming appreciated, but will not be discussed in detail here. The next section discusses how the lung is constructed to fulfil those functions, beginning with an account of normal development.

NORMAL DEVELOPMENT

The primitive lung bud develops as an outpouching of the foregut at the caudal end of the laryngotracheal sulcus, and is first recognisable at 4 weeks gestation. The lobar branching pattern is seen by 5 weeks gestation, and by six weeks the subsegmental pattern is visible. As the lung buds grow out they become invested with mesenchyme, and it is this primitive mesenchyme which drives the branching patterns of what will be the mature bronchial tree. The precise growth factors are as yet unknown and it is not possible to present a coherent synthesis of the genetic control and molecular basis of lung development. The intrapulmonary circulation also develops within this mesenchyme, initially as a pulmonary plexus, before making contact with the central vessels.

The main pulmonary arteries develop from the sixth branchial arches, which appear by about 32 days of gestation. Initially a series of segmental arteries supply the lung, but these regress by about seven weeks, and the plexus of the bronchopulmonary segments connects to the central pulmonary arteries. The venous drainage of the plexus is initially to the systemic circulation. At about 4 weeks gestation, the proximal pulmonary vein develops as an outgrowth of the right atrium, to connect with the intrapulmonary venous system which has developed from the primitive mesenchymal plexus. Connections persist between the systemic and pulmonary venous systems, particularly at the hila. The veins do not accompany airways and arteries, but lie in an intersegmental plane.

The bronchial arteries extend down the developing airways as a secondary system, and there are anastomoses with the pulmonary arterial tree. These subsequently regress but do not disappear, and indeed become more important in postnatal life if there is chronic airway inflammation or right ventricular outflow tract disease.

The bronchial branching pattern is laid down by 16 weeks; thereafter the bronchi increase in size, but not in numbers. Alveoli develop mainly after birth; within particularly the first 18 to 24 months of postnatal life there is a rapid increase in numbers towards the adult complement. There is evidence that there may be minor increases in numbers to age eight, but thereafter alveoli increase in size only. There is a rapid spurt in lung size in puberty particularly in boys, reflecting the rapid pubertal changes in the dimensions of the thoracic cavity.

With regard to the pulmonary circulation, the pre-acinar vessels (arteries and veins) follow the development of the airways, the intra-acinar that of the alveoli (the acinus consists of the last three generations of the bronchial tree, namely the respiratory bronchioles which by definition contain no cartilage, and the attached alveolar ducts and sacs).

The pulmonary circulation undergoes profound changes in the postnatal period. Prior to birth, the placenta is the organ of respiration, Qp is low and PVR high. Wall thickness of the muscular arteries is high, and the lumen small. At birth, PVR must fall and Qp rise dramatically if the baby is to survive. The mechanisms of this change are unknown; they may be chemically mediated, and also result from the mechanical pull on the vasculature of the first breath. Thereafter, extra-uterine adaptation takes place in three phases which may overlap. In the first, there is rapid adaptation with stretching of vessels and thinning of the muscle coat. Secondly, there is remodelling of the walls with laying down of connective tissue. Finally, growth takes place, ensuring that PVR does not rise as the baby grows and Qp rises to keep pace with peripheral oxygen requirements.

NEUROLOGICAL MECHANISMS

This is a complex field. There can be no question as to the importance of the neuromuscular mechanisms that drive the respiratory pump. The central neural control of those mechanisms is one of immense complexity. There is also a huge body of research into neural mechanisms within the lung. When assessing the clinical importance of these last, it should be remembered that the transplanted lung, which is by definition denervated, functions perfectly adequately.

Respiratory muscle disease is often not considered, and consequently not diagnosed. The main muscle of inspiration is the diaphragm, innervated by the phrenic nerves from the third through fifth cervical segments. During inspiration, descent of the diaphragm pushes down the abdominal contents onto the effectively rigid pelvic bowl as a fulcrum. The action of the ribs varies with age, babies lacking the 'buckethandle' action of older children and adults. Expiration is usually a passive process except during coughing. In clinical practice it is often inspiratory muscle disease which is most important; however, expiratory muscles are important in generating a cough pressure, and expiratory muscle failure may result in recurrent infections. Breathlessness due to diaphragmatic weakness is most obvious in the supine position, when the diaphragm has to push up the abdominal contents against gravity. The commonest causes of diaphragm palsy in paediatric practice are probably myopathy (which may predominantly or solely affect the diaphragm) and iatrogenic phrenic nerve injury, usually at the time of cardiac surgery.

A detailed description of the central control of respiration is beyond the scope of this chapter. Respiratory drive requires intact brainstem mechanisms to drive the respiratory muscles. This is unlikely to be from an anatomically discrete 'respiratory centre' but from complex interacting neural networks in the brainstem. Disorders of respiratory control are rare, and include Ondine's Curse; anatomical defects in the region of the posterior fossa and foramen magnum; and brainstem tumours. The role of peripheral mechanisms is still unclear. Central sympathetic pathways reach the lung from the hypothalamus via the upper cervical segments and synapses within the superior cervical ganglion. Parasympathetic pathways, also from the hypothalamus, reach the dorsal vagal nucleus and the nucleus ambiguus, from where the vagus conveys them to synapses within the lung; short post-synaptic fibres innervate glands and smooth muscle. Within the peripheral respiratory system, there is a rich neural and receptor network. These include the adrenergic receptor family, muscarinic receptors and the NANC system.

MECHANISMS OF VENTILATION

During spontaneous breathing, the respiratory muscles produce a negative intrapleural pressure and suck air into the lung. Contrast this with the physiology of positive pressure ventilation in the intensive care unit. Expiration is mainly a passive process, with the lung recoil pressure providing a small positive pressure to empty the lungs. In children, lung emptying stops (and FRC is reached) when lung recoil pressure balances chest wall recoil, with the airways still open. By contrast in adults, loss of elasticity in the airway walls and loss of the peripheral 'guy rope' effect of the parenchyma on the airways means that expiration is limited by airway closure.

The effects of airway malacia vary with their site and are easily determined from first principles. Extrathoracic tracheomalacia will limit inspiration, whereas intrathoracic tracheobronchomalacia will be limiting in expiration, particularly if the expiratory muscles are used in forced expiration. This has the effect of raising intrathoracic pressure above atmospheric, compressing the intrathoracic airways and limiting flow. The potential positive feedback loop (raised pressure compressing the airways resulting in an attempt to compensate by a further increase in expiratory effort to try to achieve expiration) may underlie the cyanotic spells in preterm babies with BPD and airway malacia. Ventilation exhibits a gradient in children, being distributed first and preferentially to the apices. This is in contrast to perfusion (below) which has a predominantly basal distribution. There is thus an element of ventilation: perfusion mismatch at rest, which is corrected on exercise. Furthermore, in clinical practice, if there is unilateral lung disease, it is better to have the child lying on its side with the affected side down ('down with the bad lung').

MECHANISMS OF PERFUSION

The lung has a double blood supply, the pulmonary and bronchial arterial trees. The bronchial circulation accounts for around 2% of the left ventricular output under normal circumstances. Bronchial arteries arise direct from the aorta or its branches and have important precapillary anastomoses with the pulmonary tree. They drain partly into the bronchial venous system and partly into the pulmonary veins.

The pulmonary arterial tree branches with the bronchial airway tree. Deoxygenated blood is ejected intermittently by the right ventricle. The compliance of the arterial wall ensures that flow, while remaining pulsatile, is continuous throughout the cardiac cycle. In the normal lung, perfusion can be divided into four zones. In Zone 1 at the lung apex in the upright position, pulmonary artery pressure is insufficient to oppose gravitational pressure, and there is no perfusion. The lung is saved from infarction by the bronchial circulation, which takes origin from a much higher pressure system, the aorta. In Zone 2, alveolar pressure is higher than venous pressure, and flow is determined by PA to alveolar pressure gradient. In Zone 3, left atrial pressure is greater than alveolar pressure, and PA to LA gradient determines flow. Under some circumstances there may be a fourth zone, where resistance to flow rises at the lung bases, probably due to closure of extra-alveolar vessels in areas normally kept at low lung volumes. This explanation for Zone 4 conditions is still controversial.

There are numerous pulsatile rhythms imposed on pulmonary flow. These include the intermittent nature of filling (right ventricular systole) and emptying into the left atrium. The effects of the respiratory cycle are complex. The fall in intrathoracic pressure during inspiration effectively sucks blood into the lungs. Inspiration increases lung volume; this increases the calibre and reduces the resistance of precapillary arterioles and post-capillary venules, while the expanding alveoli compress the capillary bed, increasing the resistance offered to flow at this level.

The defensive functions of the circulation are two-fold; immunologically-active cells and molecules are conducted to the site of inflammation; and secondly, access of such cells to the pulmonary parenchyma is tightly regulated by the controlled expression of families of adhesion molecules on the endothelial surface, particularly in the pulmonary venules. Also of importance are molecules such as the beta-defensins, lysozyme and lactoferrin which act as first-line airway defence mechanisms. These important and expanding fields will not be covered further in this chapter.

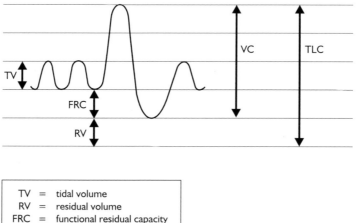

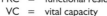

TV	=	tidal volume
RV	=	residual volume
FRC	=	functional residual capacity
VC	=	vital capacity
TLC	=	total lung capacity

Fig. 10.1 **The definition of lung volumes**

BASIC PHYSIOLOGICAL CONCEPTS

Dynamic lung volumes

The definition of lung volumes is given in Figure 10.1. Dynamic lung volumes are measured using spirometry (below) and include FEV_1 and FVC. Intrasubject reproducibility varies with disease, for example being 5% in motivated older children, but as high as 15% in CF. As with all physiological measurements, a highly-skilled operator is needed to encourage young children to perform the test well. Spirometry should also be used to record flow at low lung volumes, which is thought to be a measure of small airway obstruction, and inspiratory flow rates (below).

Static lung volumes

Available methods (discussed in detail below) include plethysmography, gas dilution, and chest radiography. Each of them is said to measure 'total lung capacity', but each of them measures something slightly different.

Plethysmography is generally taken to be the gold standard, and measures compressible gas volume. It relies on calculations using Boyle's Law, and measurements of box pressure and alveolar pressure are required. For most clinical purposes, mouth pressure is measured and at no-flow conditions assumed to be the same as alveolar pressure. In the presence of airway obstruction, alveolar pressure will be higher than mouth pressure, and lung volumes over-estimated. Furthermore, plethysmography measures intestinal gas, and gas-containing bullae as well as the volume available for gas exchange.

Gas dilution methods rely on rebreathing an inert marker gas such as helium. CO_2 is scrubbed out of the rebreathing circuit, and O_2 bled in to maintain a constant volume. The time to equilibration can also be used as a marker of the efficiency of gas mixing. This technique underestimates lung volume in the presence of airway obstruction, because gas mixing becomes so poor that the total gas volume is not accessed.

Finally, a large number of different radiological methods have been described. The most recent involves digitising posteroanterior and lateral chest radiographs using a commercially-available system of a digitising tablet linked to a personal computer. The algorithm aligns the two films in three dimensions to a given reference point (usually the arch of the aorta) and divides the digitised shape into a stack of 50 ellipses, each of a different radius. The volume of each ellipse is calculated and summed. From the total thoracic volume is deducted the volumes of the heart and mediastinum, the vertebral column, and the subdiaphragmatic structures. Allowance is made for magnification and lung tissue volume in the calculation of thoracic gas volume. Agreement with plethysmography is generally good, but occasional results differ widely, possibly due to posture or the effects of failing to take a full inspiration before the CXR is exposed.

Lung compliance

Compliance is the slope of the pressure volume curve. The curve can be measured for the lung, the chest wall, or the total respiratory system. The curve is sigmoid, and the slope is taken in the linear, mid-portion. However, compliance is a deceptively simple concept; often the phrase 'poor compliance' is used when in fact the patient has been artificially hyperventilated to the normal flat part of the compliance curve (below), or merely has severe airway obstruction. Critical thought should precede the use of this word.

A single value for lung compliance implies a one-compartment model of the lung, emptying under a single pressure. Clearly no single intrapleural pressure measurement can be representative of the complex changes within the three-dimensionally curved structure that is the pleural space. The alveoli are not one compartment but several million, and the bronchial drainage will not be uniform throughout the lungs either in airway length from alveolus to mouth, or airway calibre. This is particularly true in disease. Thus lung compliance is at best a very naïve approximation of a complex physiological concept. Strictly, there are many different compliances, particularly in what for example may be a very patchy disease like acute lung injury. In ventilated children especially, it may be better to use terms like 'stiff' and 'obstructed', or else admit that ventilation is difficult and the cause unknown.

Normal ranges

Age- and sex-matched normal ranges should be used, preferably acquired in the same laboratory with the same apparatus which is to be used for the clinical measurements. If this is not practical, then the most comparable normal equations should be taken from the literature, and compared with results obtained from a few normals in the laboratory, to ensure that the equations really are satisfactory. Results should be expressed as standard deviation (Z) scores, rather than percent predicted, because unless the variability around the mean is constant at every age, 80% predicted will mean different things at different ages. Furthermore, it gives no idea as to whether the child is within the normal range, whereas a Z score of −2.2 is obviously abnormal.

Interpretation of changes requires appreciation of the coefficient of variation of the measurement. This will vary with age, and disease state, being wider in the young and in some diseases.

TECHNICAL AND EQUIPMENT ASPECTS

Physiological equipment

It is very easy to equip a laboratory and make measurements. These will be meaningless unless the equipment is maintained and calibrated to high standards. Calibrations can be either mechanical or biological, and national standards have been set. Flow devices (e.g. pneumotachographs) are calibrated with syringes of known volume, using syringe volumes similar to those encountered during the measurements. These should be done at least daily, and preferably before and after each set of measurements. Gas analysers (whether operating in the gas or liquid phase) should have an at least daily three-point calibration, spanning the ranges encountered in clinical practice. For some measurements, e.g. plethysmography, CO transfer, a biological calibration may be all that is practical. This involves putting an experienced subject whose results are both known and tightly reproducible through the measurements. Without meticulous attention to this sort of detail, the results from the laboratory will be useless.

There are further considerations for dynamic measurements, e.g. using pressure transducers. The response time of the instruments must be known, and also the signal delay. These should be tested in the laboratory, and not taken on trust from the manufacturer's literature. Great care must be taken in ensuring that pressure transducers are accurately zeroed, particularly if relatively low pressures are being measured.

Sweat testing

Pilocarpine iontophoresis (requiring at least 100 µl sweat) or the macroduct system in which sweat is collected directly into a glass capillary (50 µl) may be used. Measurements must be carried out by someone interested, experienced, and who is performing sweat tests frequently. The occasional sweat-tester cannot be relied upon.

Skin testing

Skin prick tests can be carried out with standard lancets or (less rigorously) using an orange needle to scratch the surface of the skin. Recently, plastic lancets have been produced, which penetrate just to the correct depth. These may be less frightening for children. A positive and negative control should always be performed. Atopic status will for most purposes be detected using only six prick tests: positive and negative controls, grass pollen, house dust mite, cat and *Aspergillus fumigatus*. Other allergens may be added, but a clear idea of the value of the information should be sought *before* rather than after the investigation.

For intradermal testing, an orange needle is used, bending it to ensure an oblique entry into the skin. A successful approach is shown by a wheal being produced. Much the simplest way of performing tuberculin testing is with the disposable Heaf apparatus (below).

List of tests

PULMONARY FUNCTION TESTS

Peak flow measurement
Spirometry
Challenge testing
Lung volumes
  Plethysmography
  Gas dilution
  Radiographic
Inert gas methods
  Carbon monoxide transfer
  Pulmonary blood flow
Exercise testing
  Walking
  Free running
  Treadmill
  Bicycle
Measurement of lung compliance
Assessment of respiratory muscle function
  Using spirometry
  Pressure measurements
  Other methods

ASSESSMENT OF GAS EXCHANGE — INVASIVE METHODS

Arterial sampling
Capillary sampling
Venous sampling

ASSESSMENT OF GAS EXCHANGE — NON-INVASIVE METHODS

Oximetry
Transcutaneous gases
Capnography

IMAGING

Chest radiograph including airway imaging
Ultrasound
Nuclear medicine techniques
Computed tomography
Magnetic resonance imaging
Angiography

GENERAL BLOOD TESTS

Full blood count
Immunoglobulins and other tests of immune function
Serological studies

ALLERGY TESTING

Skin prick tests
RAST tests
Other tests
Other skin tests

EXAMINATION OF RESPIRATORY SECRETIONS

Sputum examination
  Spontaneously expectorated
  Induced sputum
Upper airway cultures
Indirect methods

SLEEP STUDIES/DETAILED PHYSIOLOGICAL MONITORING

TESTING FOR CYSTIC FIBROSIS (CF)

Sweat tests
Nasal potentials
Genotypes
Other investigations

TESTING FOR PRIMARY CILIARY DYSKINESIA (PCD)

Saccharine test
Nasal and exhaled nitric oxide
Ciliary function and structure studies

TUBERCULOSIS

Skin testing
Other tests

BRONCHOSCOPY

Neonatal fibreoptic bronchoscopy
Fibreoptic bronchoscopy in the infant
and older child
Rigid bronchoscopy

BIOPSY TECHNIQUES

Bronchoscopic biopsy

Pleural biopsy
Open lung biopsy

OTHER IMPORTANT TESTS IN OVERLAPPING FIELDS

Echocardiography
Barium studies
Immune function
pH monitoring
Neurological
Tests of malabsorption

Basic investigations

For convenience, these are described in groups, namely physiology, imaging, etc., rather than in the order they are often carried out. Most sections conclude with indications and contraindications to the performance of the test.

PULMONARY FUNCTION TESTS

Only three diagnoses can be made in a lung function laboratory: exercise-induced asthma, hyperventilation syndrome and vocal cord dysfunction. The main use of lung function tests is to demonstrate patterns, e.g. obstructive or restrictive disease, which may confirm or cast doubt on a diagnosis; and in monitoring treatment or the course of the disease. Most tests used in routine clinical practice require the subject to be cooperative, and are thus restricted to children of 4 or 5 years and over. There is a great need for easy, clinically-applicable lung function tests in children under age four years. The interrupter technique may be one such method, but requires further validation before it can be used in routine practice. Infant pulmonary function testing is a postgraduate subject in its own right, and will be considered only briefly.

Peak flow measurement

The standard peak flow meter for clinic use is likely to be reasonably accurate, but is rarely calibrated in most centres. The mini-peak flow meter used for outpatient monitoring is of low absolute accuracy and may give false positive and false negative readings. This may in part be due to the lack of linearity of the instruments over the physiological range. Despite these caveats, it is the best instrument currently available for home monitoring, and can be used by many 4-year-olds and most older children.

WHEN TO CONSIDER USING A PEAK FLOW METER

▲ Clinic routine if airway obstruction is suspected, e.g. asthma, cystic fibrosis, in a child over age 4–5 years.
▲ Clinic diagnosis of reversible airway obstruction, before and after bronchodilator administration.
▲ Out-patient monitoring, particularly for evidence of variable airway obstruction or response to treatment.

WHEN NOT TO USE A PEAK FLOW METER

▲ Monitoring restrictive lung disease; the lungs are stiff, and the problem is with inspiration, not expiration.
▲ Monitoring respiratory muscle function; the diaphragm is a muscle of inspiration, and testing it with an expiratory manoeuvre is illogical.

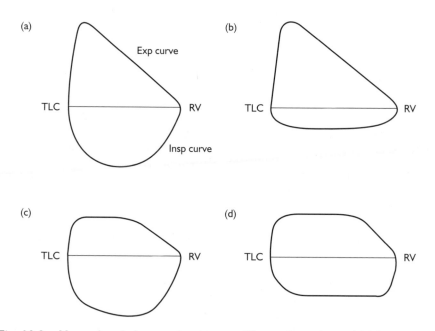

Fig. 10.2 **Normal and abnormal patterns of flow volume loop. (a) The normal pattern 'triangle on semi-circle'. (b) Extrathoracic variable obstruction — note impairment of the inspiratory curve. This pattern is also seen in stiff lungs, diaphragm weakness, and vocal cord dysfunction. (c) Intrathoracic variable obstruction, e.g. lower tracheal malacia. The expiratory curve is attenuated. (d) Fixed tracheal obstruction. Inspiratory and expiratory curves are attenuated.**

Spirometry

The most clinically useful spirometers print out the flow volume loop, and allow measurement of inspiratory and expiratory curves. The loops should be very reproducible. At least three should be recorded; the loop with the best FEV_1 and associated measurements should be recorded in the notes. The occasional child with bad airway obstruction will do progressively worse with each successive loop; the forced manoeuvre can itself cause bronchoconstriction in asthmatics; in normals, a forced manoeuvre causes mild bronchodilation. Figure 10.2 shows normal (a) and abnormal (b,c,d) patterns of flow volume loop.

Fears have been raised about the possibility of cross-infection from spirometry. The risk is fairly theoretical, but can be obviated completely by use of 'bag in a bottle' systems, in which the subject is connected to a disposable polythene bag via the mouthpiece, the bag being housed within a rigid box. The box (into which the patient does not blow) is then connected to the spirometer. An alternative is to use mouthpieces with a filter.

Portable spirometers which record only FEV_1 and FVC without displaying the loop can be bought cheaply. These are most used for monitoring lung function after lung transplantation, for the early detection of rejection.

Infant spirometry is largely confined to research laboratories. In principle, the sleeping or sedated infant is wrapped in an inflatable jacket, while breathing through a leak-proof mask connected to a pneumotachygraph. The jacket is rapidly inflated after a natural expiration to (FRC + tidal volume) or after inflating the lungs with a bag and mask to TLC. The air is thus squeezed out of the chest to record an expiratory curve. This method can be used to perform histamine challenges and determine bronchodilator responsiveness.

SOME ABNORMALITIES SEEN IN THE EXPIRATORY LIMB

▲ Impaired flow at low lung volumes — suggests small airway disease.

▲ Amputation of the top of the curve (plateau) — with normal inspiratory curve, suggests variable intrathoracic obstruction (usually bronchomalacia); with a similar amputation of the inspiratory curve, suggests rigid tracheal obstruction (e.g. tumour, complete cartilage rings).

SOME ABNORMALITIES SEEN IN THE INSPIRATORY LIMB

▲ Impaired inspiratory flow rates — typically seen in inspiratory muscle (diaphragm) weakness (see below); stiff lungs, e.g. fibrosing alveolitis; extrathoracic tracheomalacia; vocal cord dysfunction (a very useful sign).

When to perform spirometry Every clinic visit, on children old enough to make the measurements (i.e. 5 and over); especially in the asthmatic who is 'not quite right'.

When not to perform spirometry Uncooperative children; facial muscle weakness makes the measurements difficult to carry out.

Challenge testing

Most challenge testing other than exercise testing is mainly for research. Challenge testing may be carried out to determine whether a child with atypical symptoms suggestive of asthma in fact has bronchial hyperreactivity. However, there is only a weak correlation between severity of asthma and severity of bronchial hyperreactivity for an individual, although there is a better correlation for groups of asthmatics (i.e. most but not all severe asthmatics will have very reactive airways). Furthermore, there is no one challenge test that will differentiate 'asthmatic' from 'non-asthmatic' children, because they are not two separate and distinct groups but ends of a spectrum. Abnormal airway reactivity is defined as an arbitrary point on this spectrum. However, a child who has no reactivity to methacholine is not likely to have significant asthma. This may be a useful point in the child with atypical symptoms, referred as asthma.

There is considerable literature on the theoretical basis of challenge testing; for example, inhaled adenosine acts indirectly by release of mediators from mast cells, whereas methacholine may act directly on airway smooth muscle. The practical clinical importance of these distinctions is small. Before commencing any challenge test, all equipment should be calibrated and spirometry should be performed, in order to check that the child is able to perform lung function reproducibly and that it is safe to proceed. The child should have discontinued beta-2 agonists 6 hours before the test, and oral theophyllines and inhaled long-acting β-2 agonists preferably for 24 hours. Inhaled steroids, cromoglycate and nedocromil can be continued. In general, the baseline FEV_1 should be above 1 litre, and there should be no evidence of major airflow obstruction ($FEV_1 > 75\%$ predicted). If the child is obstructed, then bronchodilators can be given to document variable airflow obstruction. The simplest challenge test is free running exercise. If the child reports atypical exercise symptoms, and exhibits a significant ($> 15\%$) fall in FEV_1 after 6 minutes free running, then the diagnosis of exercise-induced asthma is established. In the pulmonary function laboratory, a treadmill in an air-conditioned room is used to maintain a level of exercise to ensure a heart rate greater than 85% predicted maximum for 6 minutes, but corridor running may be used as a screening test. As with most challenge tests, the response may vary over time. An episode of exercise bronchoconstriction causes a refractory period where further exercise will not provoke bronchoconstriction.

The next most popular challenge in clinical practice is to histamine or methacholine. After the preliminary checks above, the child puts on a noseclip and inhales normal saline for two minutes by breathing tidally from a suitable nebuliser (e.g. sidestream, flow rate 61/min). Lung function is repeated and, unless there has been a fall in FEV_1 by 20%, histamine or methacholine is inhaled in doubling concentrations for 2 minutes per dose, commencing with 0.003 mg/ml, until either a concentration of 16 mg/ml is reached or there is a fall in FEV_1 by more than 20%. FEV_1 should be measured at 30 and 90 seconds after the end of the inhalation. The hypothetical concentration causing a fall in FEV_1 of exactly 20% (PD_{20}) is found by linear interpolation. At the end of the test, unless there has been no change in lung function, beta-2 agonist is given and measurements repeated to ensure that lung function has returned to baseline.

Other challenge tests include cold air and nebulised water. These challenges are mainly research procedures. Bronchial challenge testing to specific antigens is rarely indicated in paediatric practice. Hypoxic challenge is diagnostic; is the child fit to fly in a commercial jet aeroplane? The fall in saturation while breathing 15% oxygen has been proposed as a lung function test in the uncooperative child. More practically, a fitness to fly test has been devised based on normobaric hypoxia at sea level. The required gases can be bought commercially, or mixed up in the laboratory. The child wears a noseclip and breathes 15% oxygen from a Douglas bag, via a Rudolf valve. Earlobe saturation is monitored, and if it remains above an arbitrary level which may vary with different diseases, then the child is deemed fit to fly in a commercial jet. Younger children may be studied sitting on the mother's lap in a plethysmograph filled with 15% oxygen. Note that the cabins of commercial aircraft are pressurised to the equivalent of about 6,000 feet, but light aircraft may not be pressurised at all. In such aircraft, worse hypoxia is possible at higher altitude. Within these limitations, this test predicts the need for in-flight O_2 accurately. More recently, an FEV_1 of $< 50\%$ has been suggested to be at least as good a predictor of the need for in-flight oxygen.

WHEN TO CONSIDER BRONCHIAL CHALLENGE TESTING	WHEN NOT TO DO BRONCHIAL CHALLENGE
▲ Diagnostic doubt — is this asthma? A child with asthma is unlikely to have a completely normal PD_{20}. ▲ Suppurative lung disease — is there evidence of a reversible component?	▲ Severe airway obstruction ▲ FEV_1 less than 1 litre ▲ Child unable to cope with measurements.

Lung volumes

a. Plethysmography Although equipment exists to make these measurements in the smallest infants, in clinical practice the measurements are confined to children who can cooperate. There are a number of constant-volume body plethysmographs that are commercially available. Some children may find them quite claustrophobic. In essence, all are rigid, airtight perspex boxes in which the child sits, breathing through a mouthpiece. There are two main types; constant volume, used for lung volume and resistance measurements; and constant pressure, which will not be discussed further. After thermal equilibration, the child breathes through the mouthpiece tidally, until it is occluded by a shutter at FRC. The child pants against the closed mouthpiece, supporting the cheeks with the hands. The relative changes in mouth and box pressure are used to calculate thoracic gas volume. This volume is FRC, and RV and TLC are found from a vital capacity manoeuvre.

The plethysmograph can also be used to measure specific airway conductance. Large airway calibre varies with lung volume, being highest at TLC. The ratio of pressure to flow is measured at FRC during quiet breathing or panting while seated in the plethysmograph. The measurement has the advantage of not causing bronchoconstriction, as forced manoeuvres may do; but the coefficient of intra-individual variation is high. sGAW is reduced in cases of large obstruction.

b. Gas dilution This is technically the simplest measurement, requiring least cooperation, and can thus be applied at all ages. The marker gas is usually helium, and a standard infra-red analyser is used. The child is switched into a rebreathing circuit at FRC, and breathes quietly until equilibration. Helium concentration is continuously monitored. During rebreathing, O_2 is added automatically at a rate sufficient to keep the end-expiratory volume of the circuit constant. This rate should equal the resting oxygen consumption, about 150 ml/min/m². CO_2 is scrubbed out of the circuit to prevent hyperventilation and respiratory distress. Equilibration is shown when the helium level remains constant over several breaths.

c. Radiographic The equipment required has been discussed above. If this method is to be used then it is essential to ensure that the child has had time to take a full inspiration. This limits the technique to older, cooperative children. Allowance is made for magnification by either measuring the geometry of the X-ray apparatus (tube/film and patient/film distance) or taping coins onto the side of the patient to act as scaling objects. We have used this technique to show that, in patients with CF, X-rays on which radiologists would confidently diagnose hyperinflation show lungs of normal volume!

CAUSES OF RAISED TLC AND RV	CAUSES OF LOW TLC AND RV
Any obstructive airways disease — asthma, CF, bronchiectasis.	Restrictive lung disease, whether intrinsic lung disease (fibrosing alveolitis) or chest wall problems (kyphoscoliosis). In particular, an isolated *low* RV should prompt a search for an underlying problem.

Inert gas methods

a. CO transfer This is usually measured by single breath or rebreathing manoeuvres. Single breath testing involves a vital capacity inhalation of test gas, followed by an exhalation. The rebreathing test is easier to do, and less vulnerable to disturbances of gas mixing due to airflow obstruction. To perform the manoeuvre, the child is switched into breathing from a bag of test gas at RV or FRC and then takes several deep breaths over a 10–15 second period. In each case the test gas is 0.3% CO and 10% marker inert gas such as helium in air. The final concentration of helium reflects dilution within the lung (= VA), and in normals, this is within 15% of TLC. The final CO concentration reflects both dilution and

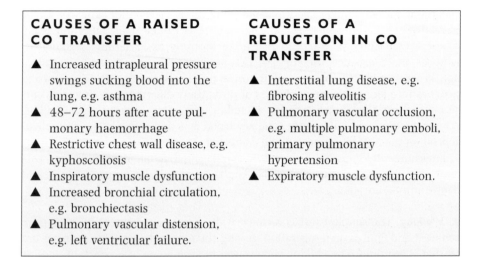

CAUSES OF A RAISED CO TRANSFER	CAUSES OF A REDUCTION IN CO TRANSFER
▲ Increased intrapleural pressure swings sucking blood into the lung, e.g. asthma	▲ Interstitial lung disease, e.g. fibrosing alveolitis
▲ 48–72 hours after acute pulmonary haemorrhage	▲ Pulmonary vascular occlusion, e.g. multiple pulmonary emboli, primary pulmonary hypertension
▲ Restrictive chest wall disease, e.g. kyphoscoliosis	▲ Expiratory muscle dysfunction.
▲ Inspiratory muscle dysfunction	
▲ Increased bronchial circulation, e.g. bronchiectasis	
▲ Pulmonary vascular distension, e.g. left ventricular failure.	

uptake (DLCO), and the latter can be calculated by assuming the same dilution volume as for the inert gas. DLCO is whole lung CO transfer; a useful derived measurement is KCO (=DLCO/VA), CO transfer per litre of accessible lung volume.

b. Pulmonary blood flow Largely a research technique, but worth remembering that the airway gives a useful window onto the pulmonary circulation. If instead of CO a very soluble marker gas (e.g. acetylene, freon-22, nitrous oxide) is mixed with an inert gas to allow for dilution, the uptake of the soluble gas during a rebreathing or single-breath manoeuvre allows calculation of pulmonary capillary blood flow. This is sometimes referred to as effective pulmonary blood flow, that part of right heart output that takes part in pulmonary gas exchange. This is not the same as cardiac output, but in normals is within 95% of it. It will not measure blood shunted right to left at cardiac or pulmonary level. Current availability is limited by the need for sophisticated and expensive gas analysers.

Exercise testing

This has two main purposes. One is diagnostic, covered in part above: does the child drop his peak flow, suggesting asthma, or his saturation in the face of an unchanged peak flow, suggesting an interstitial lung disease? The second is the monitoring of the course of disease or the effects of treatment; how does the child's performance compare with that of matched controls? A therapeutic use is to demonstrate to a child that his performance is in fact better than he thought, to give him confidence to attempt more outside the hospital.

There are numerous different protocols, with stepwise increments at various different time intervals and workloads, or steady state tests. Comparisons between different protocols on the same test apparatus, or between different apparatuses (bicycle, treadmill), is very difficult. The concept of maximal oxygen consumption, although often used, is slightly unreal, in that maximal performance is highly effort- and motivation-dependent. It is valid to record the maximal oxygen consumption reached during a given test; not necessarily to assume that it is the true maximum. Likewise anaerobic threshold is not in my view either clinically useful or related to anything in real life. The concept is to detect an inflection point where CO_2 production starts to rise more abruptly as anaerobic metabolism switches on. In practice, the curve of CO_2 production is smooth, and any inflection is artificial; and the idea of a single point where all exercising muscle switches into anaerobic metabolism is absurd. Many different measurements can be made during and after exercise, including spirometry, oxygen consumption, CO_2 production, and pulmonary capillary blood flow and volume. The choice will depend on the clinical question to be addressed.

Environmental conditions should be standardised as far as possible, and certainly for bicycle and treadmill tests. The room should be air-conditioned and temperature-controlled.

a. Walking The simplest test is a timed walk, with measurement of a distance achieved and final oxygen saturation. A long corridor and a portable oximeter are all that is required. The child is encouraged to keep going at a constant pace as far as possible. This test is simple and reproducible, and may be all that a really sick child, e.g. awaiting lung transplant, may be able to achieve. As with many tests, the motivation of the child is important. To overcome motivation problems, a 3-minute timed step test with measurement of oxygen saturation and rating of perceived exhaustion has been proposed. The equipment is simple and portable, and can even be taken to the child's home.

b. Free running Mainly used to diagnose exercise-induced asthma. The simplest test is literally to make the child run up and down to exhaustion. The test can be refined by using a tape-recording to pace the child, usually getting him to a circuit at ever-increasing speeds. This is a test that even the very young can perform.

c. Treadmill Best for exercise-induced asthma tests, and can also readily be used for measuring O_2 consumption and CO_2 production during exercise. For the former, a 6-minute run, with the child reaching at least 85% maximum heart rate, is ideal. For the latter, the Bruce protocol (3-minute increments, with the increase in incline and treadmill speeds) or a variant is most often used.

WHEN TO CONSIDER EXERCISE TESTING	WHEN NOT TO DO AN EXERCISE TEST
▲ Diagnosis of exercise-induced asthma ▲ Assessment of disability (if any) ▲ Follow progress of disease or effects of treatment.	▲ Hypoxia at rest (they may desaturate dangerously on exercise) ▲ Physical disability making it impractical ▲ Severe airway obstruction.

d. Bicycle Least good for diagnosing exercise-induced asthma, but best if detailed physiological measurements such as pulmonary blood flow are to be made. It is best to use an electronically braked machine. These keep workload constant over a wide range of pedal speeds. The limiting factor in terms of age applicability is often whether the child can reach the pedals.

Measurement of lung compliance

Compliance may be measured using static, quasi-static or dynamic methods, and each measures something different. Compliance may refer to that of the lung, the chest wall, or the integrated respiratory system. This section first describes the different compliance manoeuvres and then the different pressure measurements that can be made. Static compliance is measured by determining pressure (see below) at different lung volumes, measured independently, on a series of different exhalations. The pressure is at steady state, and therefore the effects of inertia and obstruction are minimised. The quasi-static method can be used in the conscious, co-operative child. A slow exhalation is performed into a mouthpiece from TLC. The breath is interrupted instantaneously by a shutter at varying points. The instantaneous relaxation pressure is measured, the shutter lifted and the breath continued. Dynamic compliance is measured during tidal breathing; inertia and obstructive forces are important in the results. This measurement is perhaps the least good guide to lung stiffness. Pressures relative to atmospheric can be measured at the mouth (assumed to equal alveolar pressure) or in the oesophagus with a balloon catheter as a measure of pleural pressure. If the pressure gradient used in the calculations is mouth to atmospheric, then total respiratory system compliance is measured; synchronous pleural and mouth pressure measurements allow separation of lung and chest wall compliance. Mouth pressure will not be the same as alveolar unless airflow has ceased and there is no auto-PEEP due to airway obstruction. This highlights the problems of interpreting 'dynamic' compliance. Commercial systems are used 'on-line' in the intensive care unit in ventilated children. They need to be carefully validated and checked by the unit which proposes to use them. Oesophageal pressure monitoring and the measurement of expired volume may be very difficult; in no other field is it so easy to produce a lot of numbers with little meaning.

When to measure lung compliance

Rarely done, but may be useful in intensive care to optimise ventilation. There is evidence from adult studies in acute lung injury that compliance measurements may be useful in guiding ventilation.

Assessment of respiratory muscle function

a. Using spirometry In the child with suspected neuromuscular disease, the best way of studying respiratory muscle function if feasible is to perform spirometry with the child lying supine and then standing. In normals, the postural drop in vital capacity is less than 25%.

b. Pressure measurements Maximum inspiratory and expiratory mouth pressures can be measured as a global index of respiratory muscle strength. Portable apparatus is available commercially, consisting of a pressure transducer and a mouthpiece with a tiny leak. The leak is important; if the child is asked to blow against a completely closed shutter, glottal closure is likely and the values will be underestimated. Inspiratory pressures are measured from between RV and FRC, with the child sucking as hard as possible; expiratory pressures by blowing from TLC. Although there are excellent theoretical reasons for trying to standardise the lung volumes at which measurements are made, in paediatric practice this is virtually impossible, particularly at the bedside.

A more invasive measurement is that of transdiaphragmatic pressure. The pressure generated by the diaphragm can be measured directly, if invasively, by placing pernasal oesophageal and gastric balloon catheters, connected to pressure transducers. The simplest and most reproducible manoeuvre is to get the child to perform several sniffs, which cause oesophageal pressure to fall and gastric (intra-abdominal) pressure to rise. Transdiaphragmatic pressure is calculated as the difference between these two pressures. This technique will be tolerated by only a minority. Mouth pressure during a sniff may replace these more invasive measurements.

c. Other methods Electrophysiological testing is the most direct method. The phrenic nerves are stimulated in the neck using surface electrodes, and the diaphragm EMG recorded, also using surface electrodes. An absent EMG does not distinguish between disease of nerve, muscle, or neuromuscular transmission, but is very helpful in trying to determine if an elevated hemidiaphragm is due to paralysis or some other cause such as atelectasis. Magnetic coil stimulation of the phrenic nerves in the neck or expiratory muscles (abdomen) is also used, often combined with oesophageal and gastric pressure measurements. Imaging techniques may also be useful. Screening the diaphragms may show paradoxical motion, but have the drawback of irradiation. Ultrasound can also be used to detect abnormal movement. In both cases, misdiagnoses by the inexperienced are common. This is particularly true if the child is very tachypnoeic.

WHEN TO ASSESS RESPIRATORY MUSCLE FUNCTION

▲ Any neuromuscular disorder

▲ Failure of extubation after cardiac or thoracic surgery despite good blood gases

▲ Orthopnoea disproportionate to exercise dyspnoea

▲ High diaphragm(s) on CXR.

ASSESSMENT OF GAS EXCHANGE

Invasive methods

a. Arterial sampling Direct arterial puncture is not much used because it is painful, and thus oxygenation, which is the main variable to be measured, is altered by the act of measurement. Oxygenation is best assessed non-invasively by pulse oximetry, and acid–base status (including pCO_2) by capillary or venous sampling. In intensive care units, where the children will almost invariably have indwelling lines, arterial sampling is routine.

b. Capillary sampling This is usually from an extremity or an earlobe; the latter is almost certainly underused. Peripheral capillary sampling gives reasonably accurate information about acid–base status. To perform earlobe sampling, the lobe is first rubbed with a rubifacient cream for ten minutes, and then incised with a stilette. Blood is collected into a capillary tube; pO_2 is very close to simultaneously measured arterial values. This method has traditionally been used in exercise testing, but there is no reason why it should not also be used on the ward.

c. Venous sampling For many purposes, a venous pCO_2 is adequate; obviously arterial pCO_2 cannot be higher. If doubt remains after a venous sample, then capillary or arterial blood must be obtained. Closer agreement can be achieved by warming the limb for peripheral sampling, or using a central venous sample if a line is available. Since most laboratories no longer measure chloride and bicarbonate, it is worth considering putting a sample through a blood gas analyser when doing a venepuncture. This is particularly relevant in the vomiting child, or the child with CF in whom pseudo-Bartter's syndrome is a possibility.

Non-invasive methods

a. Oximetry The oximeter uses light absorption at two different wavelengths to detect *pulsatile* flow. The commonly-used instruments are attached to a digit, but reflectance oximetry is also possible, for example placing the probe on the supra-orbital artery. The combination of a pulse oximeter with a printer to obtain a continuous recording during sleep is a powerful way of assessing oxygen requirements.

The single most important point to appreciate before using an oximeter is that it is possible to be 100% saturated but nearly dead. If the child is breathing oxygen-enriched mixtures, then oximetry will give no information on the adequacy of ventilation.

If the child is breathing 100% oxygen, and sufficient time has elapsed for alveolar nitrogen to be washed out, by definition:

$$Barometric\ pressure\ (Pb) = saturated\ water\ vapour\ pressure\ (SWVP) + PAO_2 + PACO_2;$$

i.e.,

$$100 = 6.3 + PO_2 + PCO_2\ (pressures\ in\ kPa)$$

hence:

$$PO_2 + PCO_2 = 93.7$$

Because of the sigmoid shape of the oxygen dissociation curve, if PO_2 is more than 15.0, the patient is fully saturated, but pCO_2 may be as high as 78.7 kPa! There is no doubt that pulse oximetry is a major safety advance, but its use and limitations must be understood. If there is any question of a ventilatory problem, it is insufficient to rely only on oximetry, and some way of monitoring

CO_2 should be employed (capnography or transcutaneous CO_2, below). It should also be noted that pulse oximeters are fallible. A recorded saturation of 0.93 means that the true saturation lies between 0.91 and 0.95. There are occasional wildly inaccurate rogue results. As with all machines, if the given answer does not accord with clinical expectation, find out why. There is a delay time of many seconds between change in signal and change in display. Inaccurate results will be obtained if the probe is not placed with meticulous care. Jaundice, anaemia and skin pigmentation do not affect the signal; nail varnish causes false low reading, and bright overhead lighting may falsely elevate the result. Cardiac arrhythmia, shivering, and peripheral vasoconstriction may result in failure to detect the signal.

b. Transcutaneous gases The signal from transcutaneous pO_2 electrodes depends on tissue perfusion, pO_2, and skin thickness. They are most accurate in neonates. Meticulous attention to detail is necessary, including the temperature to which the skin is heated, and the rotation of skin sites. The electrode should be calibrated *in vitro*, but preferably also *in vivo* against an arterial blood sample. Although combined O_2/CO_2 electrodes can be purchased, the evidence is that separate electrodes may be more accurate. Transcutaneous CO_2 electrodes are subject to the same limitations with regard to calibration as O_2 electrodes. However, since CO_2 diffuses through the dermis much more readily than O_2, skin thickness is less important.

c. Capnography This technique finds its place mainly in the operating theatre and intensive care unit. Measurement of expired CO_2 gives useful information about ventilation, and in some circumstances, also about cardiac output. The capnograph should be recorded on-line and inspected regularly.

IMAGING

Chest radiograph including airway imaging

The inspection of the CXR in clinical practice consists first of a technical assessment, then a general overview, followed by a close, targeted look with specific clinical questions in mind. The name and labelling must be correct; the latter is particularly important in children with mirror image arrangement. The quality of the film exposure, the adequacy of inspiration, and whether the child has moved should be assessed.

If the technical side is satisfactory, next all parts of the radiograph should be scrutinised, including the bones and the soft tissues. There are some areas in particular which may be a blind spot. These include the aortic arch anatomy, the bronchial arrangement, the subcarinal region and areas of lung obscured by soft tissue shadows.

Heart size is often commented upon, but small changes are unlikely to be important. Heart size will vary with phase of respiration and cardiac cycle, neither of which can be controlled in routine practice. An obviously huge or small heart will be detected, but subtle abnormalities will not.

The side of the aortic arch may not immediately be obvious, but should be determined, often best by following the tracheal lucency down to the carina; a right-sided arch may be a normal variant, but is a pointer to a vascular ring in a wheezy child.

The bronchial anatomy should be delineated. It is important not to confuse mirror image arrangement with a congenitally small ('hypoplastic') right lung with mediastinal displacement secondary to compensatory distension of the left lung. The presence of isomerism should be noted. A morphological right lung has three lobes, not two, and a short main bronchus with a high take-off of the upper lobe bronchus. Right isomerism (two morphologically right lungs) is associated with asplenia in around 80% of cases, left isomerism with polysplenia in the same proportion. Both are associated with abdominal visceral malrotation and congenital heart disease. Left isomerism may be confused with usual bronchial arrangement with absent right upper lobe bronchus.

A suitable exposed CXR will show an obvious line running very nearly vertically through the mediastinum, from the diaphragm to the carina, the azygo-oesophageal stripe. A mass of subcarinal lymph nodes will obliterate the line below the carina. This may be the only clue to such adenopathy on the plain film.

A further blind area is lung tissue obscured by soft tissues. The classical trap for the unwary is collapse of the left lower lobe. Less well-known traps include the recesses of the lower lobes behind the diaphragms, which may be the site of metastatic deposits or other pathology.

Common pitfalls to avoid: a normal chest radiograph does not exclude an endo-bronchial foreign body; and inspiratory and expiratory films are impossible to obtain in young, uncooperative children. Similarly, extensive segmental mucus plugging may not be detectable on the CXR, if enough air finds its way distal to the obstruction to prevent lung collapse. The diagnosis of bronchiectasis may be suspected on the CXR, and obvious severe cases may be diagnosed, but bronchiectasis cannot be excluded by the plain film alone. If there is clinical suspicion, a CT scan should be performed. Similarly, a normal CXR does not exclude interstitial lung disease. Generally, CT has taught us that the CXR is a very crude form of imaging.

Another pitfall is the 'expiratory' film. Particularly in small children, it is impossible to gate the exposure for the phase of respiration. However, the child who appears not to have taken a deep breath in may in fact have stiff lungs and be unable to do so. It may be virtually impossible to distinguish the increased shadowing of a normal expiratory film from that of interstitial lung disease with low lung volumes.

Rarer traps for the unwary include the apical shadowing caused by Dreadlocks or plaits. Any odd shadow should be carefully traced, to see if it in fact disappears off the edge of the film. Controversial areas include when to perform a CXR in acute asthma, and follow-up films in acute pneumonia. In a known asthmatic who is otherwise well but has an attack which is responding rapidly to oral and nebulised treatment, no film is necessary. A CXR may be performed in very severe exacerbations, or in children who desaturate markedly after nebulised beta-2 agonist, in whom focal consolidation is often seen.

Airway imaging methods include linear tomography and special films such as the Cincinnati view. With the advent of bronchoscopy (below) these investigations are little used. It may be that with virtual reality techniques, airway imaging will make a come-back. The adenoidal pad can be defined with a lateral neck X-ray, although there is only a weak correlation between XR appearances and

WHEN TO PERFORM A CXR

▲ Any child at first attendance at a paediatric respiratory clinic, unless the problem is very trivial or a recent film is to hand.

▲ Follow-up films as dictated by clinical circumstances; if an experienced paediatrician is satisfied that a child has made a complete recovery a follow-up film may not be necessary, but if there is any doubt after apparent recovery from pneumonia it is wise to do a further film to ensure complete clearing.

▲ All acute respiratory admissions, other than an asthma attack in a known asthmatic. If an asthmatic needs an intravenous infusion, or more than a trivial amount of oxygen, then a CXR should at least be considered to exclude pneumothorax or infection.

▲ Marked desaturation after nebulised beta-2 agonist is suggestive of a focal consolidation — consider a CXR.

WHEN NOT TO PERFORM A CXR

▲ Within six weeks of an *uncomplicated* pneumonia — clinical change precedes radiological resolution, and the child will get unnecessary radiation exposure.

funcional disturbance of breathing during sleep. Lateral neck views should not be done in the acutely stridulous child for fear of causing complete obstruction, and anyway they waste time better spent on securing a safe airway. Sinus views including CT may be needed in suspected upper airway disease. Note that in CF virtually all sinus radiographs are abnormal, and changes bear little relationship to symptoms, so routine radiographs are not useful.

Ultrasound

This is the imaging technique of choice for pleural disease. Although CT will show fluid or tumour, and the attenuation number can give an indication as to whether the fluid is clear, purulent or bloodstained, the presence of loculation is best shown by ultrasound. The instruments have the further advantage of being portable.

When performing a diagnostic aspiration or placing a chest drain into an effusion, ultrasound guidance is recommended for all but the largest collections. This

WHEN TO CONSIDER AN ULTRASOUND SCAN

▲ Pleural disease, particularly pleural effusion during attempted aspiration

▲ Mediastinal mass, possibly normal thymus

▲ Suspected diaphragm palsy.

is particularly important if a pleural biopsy is to be performed. Elective blind needling of the chest is rarely desirable.

Ultrasound is not useful for pulmonary pathology, because air in the lung attenuates the signal, and useful images are rarely obtained. An upper mediastinal mass may usefully be imaged with ultrasound if there is doubt as to whether it is a normal thymus. A skilled ultrasonographer may be able to image the diaphragm in cases of suspected paralysis or weakness.

Nuclear medicine techniques

Techniques relevant to clinical respiratory medicine include ventilation perfusion scans and technetium milk scans. Isotope studies for lung deposition and DTPA clearance studies are of research interest. Krypton ventilation scans may be used in children with airway disease (usually CF) who are too young to do conventional pulmonary function tests. Abnormalities may be found which are not detectable either by clinical examination or by CXR. The radiation dose is very low, and information about regional ventilation can be obtained. Perfusion scans require an injection, and probably add little information in primary airway diseases. The low radiation doses make ventilation scans much more attractive to follow the progression of bronchiectasis than CT, but CT remains the *diagnostic* modality of choice.

Perfusion scans using technetium-labelled albumen are valuable in suspected vascular disease, particularly congenital lung disease with a systemic supply to part of the lung and pulmonary arteriovenous malformation. Absent perfusion to a whole lung usually betokens absent main pulmonary artery or veins. Normally, virtually none of the microspheres reach the systemic circulation, being filtered by the lung capillary bed. Quantitative counts over the brain and kidneys should thus be close to zero. If there is a right to left shunt, e.g. due to an arteriovenous malformation, elevation of these values can be used to quantify shunt. A further use of ventilation perfusion scans may be in pulmonary embolism, which is underdiagnosed in paediatric practice. Because it is a rare diagnosis, a confirmatory pulmonary angiogram is usually indicated before starting treatment.

Computed tomography

Modern rapid scanners acquire each image within milliseconds, thus obviating the need for respiratory gating, and thus general anaesthesia in children, and allowing dynamic images to be acquired, e.g. by injecting contrast and scanning repeatedly at the same level. The main lesson that CT has taught us in adult and paediatric respiratory disease is that the CXR is very insensitive, and many abnormalities are missed. Protocols and algorithms for scanning vary greatly; spiral or high resolution, thin section CT, the preferred technique for showing fine detail in the lungs, usually involves scanning cuts of 1–3 mm thickness at 1 cm intervals. Spiral CT scanning with contrast injection is particularly useful for demonstrating filling defects in the large pulmonary arteries.

Thin section CT has completely replaced bronchography in the diagnosis of bronchiectasis. The CXR is notoriously insensitive to all but gross bronchiectasis; CT is indicated if there is a clinical history of chronic daily sputum production or recurrent radiologically-documented infections, particularly if they are always in the same place, looking for an unsuspected area of bronchiectasis or a congenital malformation.

CT also has a place in the diagnosis of interstitial lung disease. In adult patients, the CXR may be normal in up to 10% of cases of documented interstitial lung disease, and is a poor guide to aetiology. Interstitial lung disease is much rarer in children, and no accurate corresponding figure can be given, but if it is suspected, then a thin section CT should be performed, even if the CXR is normal. Unlike in adults, the CT patterns of particular diseases in children are so disparate that confident diagnosis is only possible in a few rare conditions, and a lung biopsy will need to be performed in almost all cases. CT has the disadvantage of relatively high radiation exposure, and thus should not be used for serial studies without a clear-cut reason.

Magnetic resonance imaging

Infants and small children require a full general anaesthetic, and even older children may find the examination quite claustrophobic. It is used for mediastinal imaging, including delineating vascular anatomy.

Angiography

This is usually performed by the radiologist or paediatric cardiologist; the detailed methods will not be discussed here. As well as a diagnostic technique, it may be therapeutic, allowing the occlusion of abnormal vessels. These include aortic collaterals to lung malformations prior to surgery, or even to obviate the need for surgery; and occlusion of hypertrophied bronchial collaterals which have caused haemoptysis in the child with CF. This last is a particularly skilled procedure; the spinal arteries also take origin nearby, and if they are occluded the child may be rendered paraplegic. Angiography carries the risk of a general anaesthetic, and the risk of high doses of contrast, which carry the risk of renal failure. These risks must be balanced against the information to be obtained. For all but the very smallest, sickest infants, the risks are small in experienced hands.

WHEN TO PERFORM ANGIOGRAPHY

▲ Congenital lung disease — definition of anatomy before surgery, and occlusion of abnormal vessels
▲ Pulmonary artery sling to exclude a crossover supply to the right upper lobe
▲ Massive haemoptysis, usually in the context of CF
▲ Suspected pulmonary embolism.

WHEN NOT TO PERFORM ANGIOGRAPHY

▲ Small, sick infants if enough information can be obtained by echocardiography.

GENERAL BLOOD TESTS

Full blood count

In most cases, a full blood count will be performed if a venepuncture is deemed necessary for other purposes. Some clues relevant to respiratory disease in the full blood count will be discussed briefly. Iron deficiency anaemia is almost invariably dietary or gastrointestinal in origin; consider idiopathic pulmonary haemosiderosis and perform a CXR in the child with unusual anaemia. Lymphopenia may be the first clue to severe combined immunodeficiency. Eosinophilia suggests atopy or an allergic state of some sort; if very high in association with CXR shadows, consider the various pulmonary eosinophilic syndromes. Thrombocytopenia, alone or with leukopenia, may be due to hypersplenism in CF.

Immunoglobulins and other tests of immune function

The indications for detailed immune function tests are discussed elsewhere. A common situation is to see a child who has been treated for 'recurrent chest infections' in the community, with no radiological confirmation, and who most likely has asthma. Clues to the presence of an immunodeficiency are summarised in the acronym 'SPUR'; **S**evere, **P**ersistent, **U**nusual organisms, **R**ecurrent infections. Furthermore, a child who is chronically productive of sputum should be considered for an immunological work-up. Although chronic moist cough may be related to postnasal drip, or possible asthma, other more sinister possibilities should be remembered.

A basic immune screen includes white cell count, immunoglobulins, immunoglobulin subclasses, specific antibodies (pneumococcal and haemophilus), and complement profile. If specific antibody levels are low, they should be repeated after appropriate immunisation. Further investigation is performed if either an abnormality is turned up or the child's subsequent clinical course mandates investigation. The pattern of infection gives a clue to the likely type of immunodeficiency.

Serological studies

These have two main purposes. The first is the diagnosis of acute infection, for which paired samples at least ten days apart showing a four-fold rise in titre will be needed. Exceptionally, a very high IgM response on the first sample may be very strongly suggestive of acute infection. The other use of serology is to document evidence of past exposure, and the ability of the host to mount an antibody response to that organism.

ALLERGY TESTING

Probably few subjects engender such polarised views as allergy and its significance. Extremists point out that the scientific basis and clinical utility of conventional allergy tests are few, and the false positive and false negative rate high; others believe them to be of immense diagnostic value. Properly used and understood, allergy tests do have clinical value. A detailed history and targeted use of allergy tests is preferable to a blunderbuss approach.

Skin prick tests

Skin prick tests are used to define whether the subject is atopic; this use is uncontroversial, but in clinical practice may not be valuable. Antihistamines should be discontinued for 3 weeks before testing. Skin tests tell you what happens if you prick allergen into the skin; the connection with what happens if you inhale allergen, or eat it, is more tenuous. A negative skin prick test or RAST is useful for ruling out IgE-mediated allergy; the predictive value of a positive test is less. In children under age 3, skin tests are frequently negative even in the atopic allergic child; if they are positive, they are likely to be significant.

There may be differences between standard allergen preparations, and it is as well to stick with one particular brand. Conventionally, the volar aspect of the forearm is used; in infants, the back may be preferable. A huge range of aero and food allergens can be used. The results are read after 15 and 30 minutes; a positive is defined as a wheal diameter more than 3 mm greater than the negative control. Infants under age 2 produce much smaller wheals, and false negative results become more common.

Other skin tests

Intradermal testing to antigens that the child would have been expected to have encountered previously, e.g. mumps, candida, can be used to demonstrate whether he can mount a T-cell response. Anergy to tuberculin after BCG cannot be taken as evidence of T-cell dysfunction. Skin tests to MMR in an egg-allergic child are not helpful. Such a child can safely be immunised with MMR, however exquisitely sensitive he may be to egg, without recourse to skin testing.

CONTRAINDICATIONS TO SKIN TESTING

▲ History of anaphylaxis to the antigen; severe anaphylaxis can be provoked even by skin prick testing in the susceptible

▲ Eczema — the results will be rendered uninterpretable by non-specific responses

▲ Determining whether to give MMR in an egg-allergic child.

RAST tests

Specific IgE tests are open to the same strictures with regard to sensitivity and specificity as skin prick tests. They can substitute for skin tests in children with eczema and especially anaphylaxis. They are less useful in children under 2. If immunotherapy to insect stings is to be undertaken in an older child (and this is rarely necessary), then a RAST test should be used to confirm the history of which insect actually caused the problem. Total IgE should be measured if RAST tests are being performed, because a very high IgE can cause false positive RASTs.

Other tests

Most challenge testing (either ingestion or airborne) should be undertaken after careful thought and in hospital only. *Prior to the challenge, the dose of adrenaline for anaphylaxis treatment for that child should be calculated, written down in the notes, and actually drawn up ready in a syringe.* Food challenges usually commence with small amounts, working up provided no adverse events are encountered. Aeroallergen challenges should only be done in experienced units, and monitoring continued for many hours to pick up late phase as well as early reactions. Double blind food challenges are the province of experienced units. They require enormous commitment by all concerned, and are only indicated in exceptional circumstances. More usually, open exclusions are tried.

INVESTIGATIONS OF RESPIRATORY SECRETIONS

Sputum examination

Spontaneously expectorated Sputum can usually only be obtained in children aged 7 years or more; younger ones swallow their secretions. A good physiotherapist should be asked to try to ensure a really good sample is obtained. Sputum may be sent for routine bacteriological culture; mycobacterial culture; and cytology (usually for an eosinophil count). Special media are needed if unusual organisms are possible, for example *Burkholderia* genomovars in CF. Close liaison with the laboratory is essential.

Induced sputum

Nebulised hypertonic (5–7% saline) may be given to facilitate sputum production. It is usually wise to pretreat with an inhaled beta-2 agonist. This technique has been used in the immunocompromised child, as well as a research technique. The child's lung function must be carefully monitored to detect any bronchospasm, and the test discontinued if FEV_1 drops by more than 20%. It is unwise to induce sputum if the child has marked airway obstruction.

Upper airway cultures

In the context of CF, and in particular the young child, throat swabs, cough swabs and nasopharyngeal aspirates are used to try to define whether there is lower airway chronic infection. The literature is conflicting, but few would feel able to ignore a positive upper airway culture. If upper airway cultures are negative for *Staph aureus*, *Haemophilus influenzae* and *Pseudomonas aeruginosa*, then bronchoalveolar lavage (BAL) cultures are also likely to be negative. In a symptomatic child, with persistently negative upper airway cultures, most would proceed to a BAL.

Nasopharyngeal aspirates are useful in the diagnosis of viral lower respiratory tract infection, for example respiratory syncytial virus. Pernasal swabs are useful diagnostically only in the early stages of whooping cough.

Indirect methods

Gastric washings may be used to diagnose tuberculosis. There is controversy as to whether this technique is superior to BAL when modern molecular diagnostic techniques are used. FOB has the advantage of allowing direct inspection of the airway, and biopsy of any endobronchial lesions.

SLEEP STUDIES/DETAILED PHYSIOLOGICAL MONITORING

The commonest cause of obstructive sleep apnoea (OSA) in children is adenotonsillar hypertrophy, the vast bulk of which can be managed clinically without recourse to sophisticated physiological measurements. A simple screening test for OSA is overnight pulse oximetry with continuous recording of results. More subtle sleep abnormalities will be missed by oximetry alone. Overnight saturation is a useful test for monitoring O_2 requirement in BPD. It is dangerous to wean off O_2 on the basis of a 'one-off' saturation during the day.

There are many systems available for detailed physiological monitoring or 'full' polysomnography. The instruments incorporated may include oximetry, transcutaneous pO_2 and pCO_2, end-tidal CO_2, nasal airflow, and thoracic and abdominal wall motion, as well as sleep staging. Some systems also allow simultaneous pH monitoring, and others also videotape the sleeping child. The choice of system as always depends on the question being asked. In all cases, it is important to calibrate the equipment carefully, and examine the raw data, so as not to base clinical decisions on artefacts. Apnoeas can be divided into 'obstructive', 'central' and 'mixed'. Obstruction is suggested by continued respiratory effort with cessation of airflow, and an alteration in phase angle between abdominal and thoracic movements. If OSA is detected, then a full anatomical evaluation of the upper airway is mandated. Central apnoea may be due to neuromuscular disease. Periodic evaluation for sleep-disordered breathing is indicated in children with kyphoscoliosis and myopathy and muscular dystrophies.

Detailed overnight monitoring including pH studies is indicated in acute life-threatening events or near-miss cot death.

WHEN TO CONSIDER A SLEEP STUDY/DETAILED PHYSIOLOGICAL MONITORING

▲ Suspected OSA or other sleep-disordered breathing

▲ Near-miss cot death, acute life-threatening events

▲ Pulmonary hypertension with normal CXR

▲ Planning reduction of oxygen therapy

▲ Starting oxygen in airflow obstruction, e.g. CF to exclude hypercapnia

▲ High-risk group for OSA (Downs syndrome, Sickle disease)

▲ Follow-up after surgery for OSA

▲ Severe chest wall disease, e.g. kyphoscoliosis especially with high thoracic curve; early onset of curve; associated muscle weakness or paralysis; and FVC < 40% predicted

▲ Myopathy affecting the respiratory muscles, muscular dystrophies

▲ Checking adequacy of ventilation in those on non-invasive respiratory support.

TESTING FOR CYSTIC FIBROSIS (CF)

Introduction

The diagnosis of CF has gone through many phases. In 1938, when CF was differentiated from other causes of diarrhoea, it was first a pathological diagnosis, and then a clinical one. In the 1950s, the abnormality of sweat electrolytes was appreciated, and the diagnosis became a chemical one, based purely on the sweat test. In the late 1980s, when nasal potential differences, and subsequently genotype analysis, were applied to puzzling cases, it became clear that there were a number of children with borderline or even normal sweat electrolytes who turned out to have CF. Currently the diagnosis of CF is on clinical grounds in some children, since there is at the moment no definite 'rule out' test. This means that the extent to which a diagnosis of CF is pursued, and the tests used, depend on the degree of clinical suspicion, and the clinical context.

Sweat tests

The gold standard for the diagnosis of CF remains the measurement of sweat electrolytes, usually sodium and chloride. Sweat tests should only be performed by someone who is carrying out many tests per week. Meticulous attention to detail in performing the test and interpreting the results is essential. Duplicate estimations, collecting at least 100 mg sweat from each arm, with concordant results, are required. The North American CF Foundation defines sweat chloride > 60 mmol/l as abnormal, 40–60 as borderline and < 40 as normal. However, cases of CF with chloride < 40 are well described. There are a few well-documented cases where the initial sweat test was normal in a child subsequently proven to have CF.

In doubtful cases, the fludrocortisone suppression sweat test may be helpful. The child is given 3 mg/m² fludrocortisone on two successive evenings, and a sweat test is performed on the third day. Patients with CF will fail to suppress into the normal range. There are no normal data for infants, in whom this test is best avoided.

The pitfalls of sweat testing must be remembered. The most important is the experience of the tester. The commonest cause of a wrong diagnosis is an incorrectly-performed test by someone who is not practised in the art. Next comes interpreting the results without regard to the clinical setting, and eczema, which may lead to false positive results. All other problems are minor by comparison. There are a few non-CF causes of elevated sweat electrolytes (e.g. hypothyroidism, fucoscidosis, HIV, mucopolysaccharidoses, malnutrition, type 1 glycogen storage disease, panhypopituitarism, nephrogenic diabetes insipidus, untreated adrenal insufficiency, ectodermal dysplasia), which are not usually a serious diagnostic likelihood.

Nasal potentials

These measurements are performed with varying degrees of sophistication, and should be confined to special centres and highly trained personnel. In brief, electrical potential is measured between an exploring and a reference electrode. The exploring electrode is a double lumen silicone tube which is passed along the floor of the nose. One lumen is filled with an equal mixture of Ringer's lactate and electrocardiographic electrode cream, and connected to a high-impedance voltmeter via a silver/silver chloride electrode. The other lumen can be used to perfuse different solutions, to refine the measurements. The reference consists of a second silver/silver chloride electrode placed on an area of abraded skin on the forearm. The normal nasal potential is 0 to −30 mV, with less than −34 mV being strongly suggestive of CF. The response of the potential difference to amiloride and low chloride/isoprenaline solution may help resolve doubtful cases.

Genotypes

The CF gene was first identified on the long arm of chromosome 7 in 1989. There are considerable racial differences in gene frequency, and type. In white races, delta F508 is present in about 70% CF chromosomes. Most genetics laboratories will routinely test for eight to twelve other mutations, detecting up to 90% of mutations. There are over 900 described in total, so although the finding of two CF genes confirms the diagnosis, a negative gene analysis cannot exclude CF.

Genotype analysis has its main role in antenatal diagnosis. Even if the abnormal gene cannot be identified, linkage studies can usually be used to characterise the pregnancy. For couples who have had a previous child with CF, and who do not want antenatal diagnosis, the best way to determine the status of the new baby is by genetic analysis of cord blood taken immediately after birth. Since the mother is the only person absolutely guaranteed to be present, she should be given an EDTA bottle and a note for the midwife. If this opportunity is missed, a later heel-prick sample can be used.

Other investigations

In most cases, the range of tests listed above will confirm the diagnosis. In puzzling cases, pointers may be provided by pancreatic function tests (discussed elsewhere) and immunoreactive trypsin (IRT). IRT is elevated in many babies with CF, but later in life its specificity for diagnosis is lost. IRT, sometimes combined with determination of common CF mutations, has been recommended for newborn screening. If the child is referred with diarrhoea, measurement of faecal elastase is sensitive and specific for pancreatic insufficiency, and can be used even if the child is taking pancreatic enzyme supplements. In some cases, usually those who are pancreatic sufficient, the diagnosis remains indefinite. In that event, the child should be treated as if he has CF, with aggressive physiotherapy, antibiotics, bronchodilators and inhaled steroids as required.

TESTING FOR PRIMARY CILIARY DYSKINESIA

Saccharine test

This screening test for PCD can only be carried out in older, cooperative children. A 1 mm particle of saccharin is placed on the inferior nasal turbinate of an unblocked nostril, 1 cm from its anterior end. The child must rest with the head tilted slightly forward, particularly if there is marked postnasal discharge, to prevent the saccharine dropping back. The child must not sniff or sneeze. The child is asked to say when a funny taste is noted, and what the taste is (bitter, sweet or sour). If a sweet taste is appreciated within 30 minutes, the test is normal. If no taste is reported, there are several possible explanations. The child may be unable to taste saccharin (rare, and excluded by giving him saccharin into the mouth); the test may be a false positive, or the child may have PCD. If the test is positive, the child should proceed to a nasal brushing. PCD should not be diagnosed on a saccharine test alone.

Nasal and exhaled NO

Although there is considerable interest in the clinical use of NO, the only established role is as a screening test for PCD. Nasal NO < 250 ppb is highly suggestive of PCD, although there is some overlap with CF; a high nasal or exhaled NO virtually excludes PCD. Whatever the levels of NO and also diffuse, if the clinical picture is strongly suggestive of PCD, a brush biopsy is indicated. In addition to the role in diagnosis of PCD, there is a huge research interest in exhaled breath, breath condensate and other techniques for monitoring airway inflammation. However, these are not clinical tools and will not be discussed further in this chapter.

WHEN TO CONSIDER TESTING FOR CYSTIC FIBROSIS

▲ Lower respiratory tract disease — recurrent infection, sputum production, the asthmatic who does not respond to treatment or is 'not quite typical', any child with bronchiectasis, any severe or complicated pneumonia, particularly staphylococcal; 'bronchiolitis' which is unusually severe; any child with *Staph aureus* or mucoid *Pseudomonas aeruginosa* in the sputum, or any pseudomonad unless there is a good reason for nosocomial acquisition.

▲ Upper respiratory tract disease — nasal polyps (ALWAYS), severe sinus disease.

▲ Gastrointestinal disease — diarrhoea, failure to thrive (REMEMBER — 15% thrive), rectal prolapse (ALL CASES without an obvious anatomical abnormality, no matter how well — one in six will have CF), severe gastro–oesophageal reflux, coeliac disease which does not respond to treatment, acute pancreatitis, hepatosplenomegaly, biliary tract disease.

▲ Neonatal disease — bowel atresias, obstruction or meconium ileus equivalent (REMEMBER — this last is seen in pancreatic sufficient CF and a few normal infants with no evidence of CF); prolonged jaundice; haemorrhagic disease in the newborn; circulatory collapse; positive family history.

▲ Other disease — electrolyte disturbance, particularly hyponatraemia, hypokalaemia, chloride deficiency, renal failure; circulatory collapse, and atypical fainting; infertility (or vas deferens not found during herniorrhaphy).

▲ When the mother is convinced her child is not right, and has been reassured by numerous professionals that all is well.

▲ When the child is referred with a diagnosis of CF and the picture is atypical — mistaken sweat test diagnoses are common.

Ciliary function and structure studies

Functional and structural studies should be carried out. Nasal cilia can be sampled by brushing the inferior turbinate with a cytology brush, and separating off the cells by shaking the brush into appropriate medium. The discomfort of the procedure is minimal. The ciliated epithelial cells are spun down and inspected under phase contrast microscopy on a heated stage, and the beat frequency measured. At least ten readings should be taken, and ideally the examination should be videotaped. The commonest cause of abnormal motility is secondary to a bacterial or viral infection; if in doubt, the brushings should be repeated after a one-month course of antibiotics and topical steroids. If there is any doubt as to the diagnosis, then ciliary studies should be repeated several months later.

The cilia are sent for electron microscopy if they are immotile or discoordinate, or if the clinical history is suggestive of PCD. Preferably at least 100 cilia should be examined. Note that the cilia may be structurally normal, but functionally abnormal. Another interesting condition is ciliary disorientation; the individual cilia are structurally normal, but are lined up in a disoriented fashion. This is also commonly seen secondary to infection.

Another potential source of cilia is the bronchial tree. If the child is scheduled for a bronchoscopy, then bushings can conveniently be taken from a segmental carina. Studies have shown that beat frequency is very similar from nasal and bronchial ciliated epithelium. If there is extensive bronchial inflammation, it may be difficult to harvest viable cells.

WHEN TO TEST FOR PCD

▲ Lower respiratory tract disease — bronchiectasis, severe pneumonia, sputum production, the asthmatic who is atypical.

▲ Upper respiratory tract disease — recurrent and refractory serous otitis media, particularly if the ear continues to discharge; nasal polyps; severe sinus disease; persistent rhinitis.

▲ Neonatal lung disease — pneumonia or respiratory distress with no obvious reason, particularly with neonatal rhinitis.

▲ Other indications (particularly if there is an associated suspicious feature) — any disorder of laterality (mirror image, etc.), even if in association with congenital heart disease; severe oesophageal disease (atresia, reflux); biliary atresia; infertility; hydrocephalus; positive family history.

TUBERCULOSIS

Skin testing

There are a number of ways of performing Tuberculin sensitivity testing including the Tine test, the Heaf test and intradermal injections of increasing concentrations of old Tuberculin (Mantoux series). For routine practice, the Heaf test is much the simplest. The Tine test has largely fallen into disrepute because of false negative results. Intradermal testing is time-consuming and not easy to perform in noncooperative children. Most of the British guidelines are based on Heaf testing.

The Heaf test is carried out with a disposable magnetic six-pronged head. The cost is greater than the old flame-sterilised head, but the risk of transmission of infection is not present. The prongs should allow 1 mm penetration (babies and infants) or 2 mm (2 years and over). The skin is cleansed with alcohol and the tuberculin solution (100,000 TU in 1 ml) smeared over an area of about 2 cm^2. The head of the Heaf gun is placed on the tuberculin and fired by pressing firmly down onto the skin. The reaction can be read between 3 and 10 days later, as follows: Grade 0, < 4 discrete papules; Grade 1, at least 4 discrete papules; Grade 2, coalescent popular reaction forming an indurated ring; Grade 3, an area of induration up to 10 mm diameter; Grade 5, induration > 10 mm diameter, or vesiculation of a Grade 3 reaction.

Intradermal testing is probably a slightly more reliable way of detecting skin sensitivity. A dose of 0.1 ml of PPD solution is injected into the volar aspect of the forearm. This should raise a bleb up to 10 mm diameter if done properly. The test is read 48–72 hours later, and only the area of induration is relevant and should be measured in mm, in the diameter perpendicular to the long axis of the forearm. Always start with 1 tuberculin unit (1 in 10,000 Mantoux) for fear of causing a major reaction in the very sensitive. Induration of more than 10 mm is positive.

There are a number of pitfalls to appreciate. There is little correlation between immunity to TB and tuberculin reactivity. Thus even after a satisfactory BCG there may be no skin test reactivity. There may be a delay of up to 8 weeks before seroconversion, or indeed in the immunocompromised, there may be persistent anergy to tuberculin. Thus although tuberculin testing is a valuable guide, in the high risk group (less than 2 years old) treatment may need to be instituted even though the Heaf test is negative.

Other tests

In a child with a contact history, typical radiographic findings and a strongly positive Mantoux, triple therapy may be commenced without further investigation. A culture-proven diagnosis should be sought if drug resistance is suspected and particularly if steroids are to be prescribed. If atypical mycobacteria are suspected, tissue biopsy is essential to distinguish commensal growth from invasive disease.

The tests used will depend on the presentation, with sputum positivity being rare in childhood TB. More invasive tests may include peripheral lymph node biopsy; pleural biopsy; bronchoscopy with lavage and bronchial brushing; and even mediastinoscopy.

Recent advances in molecular biology can facilitate the diagnosis of problem cases of TB. PCR can be used to detect *M. tuberculosis* DNA or RNA within 24–48 hours, faster even than Bactec cultures. PCR of a small region of the rifampicin resistance gene allows determination of rifampicin sensitivity within the same time frame. If the organism is rifampicin sensitive, multi-drug-resistant TB is for practical purposes excluded.

WHEN TO TEST FOR TUBERCULOSIS

▲ Contacts of known cases, particularly if an adult in the same house has TB.

▲ A Heaf test should be considered in virtually all other circumstances, namely *any* respiratory disease unless the diagnosis is totally obvious.

BRONCHOSCOPY

Bronchoscopy should only be performed by experienced operators, and in children is usually carried out under general anaesthetic, performed in accordance with standard protocols. The anaesthetic technique in particular is determined by the question being investigated, and should be discussed in advance between bronchoscopist and anaesthetist.

In most cases it is wise to obtain a full blood count, urea and electrolytes and clotting profile prior to the procedure; clotting studies are mandatory before transbronchial biopsy. In sick children, CO_2 (see above) and blood pressure should also be monitored. If there is an indwelling arterial line, then do a blood gas before and after the procedure. Fibreoptic instruments are solid, and block a considerable proportion of the airway, causing hypercapnia, particularly if the examination is prolonged. A further potential adverse effect is the inadvertent application of end-expiratory pressure, with a fall in venous return and the potential for a rise in intracranial pressure. The haemodynamic effects of a fibreoptic bronchoscopy may last for up to an hour. A permanent record of the examination should be preserved on videotape.

Neonatal fibreoptic bronchoscopy

Instruments available There are two 2.2 mm endoscopes; one is steerable, but contains no suction channel; the other is non-steerable, but has a tiny channel. For all but the smallest preterm babies, a 2.7 mm endoscope with a 1.2 mm channel can be used.

How to do the examination These instruments can be used to examine even the smallest preterm babies. The simplest method is to pass the endoscope down the endotracheal tube of a ventilated baby via a suitable connector. The larynx and proximal structures are not examined. If the baby is extubated, use either a laryngeal mask or pass the bronchoscope through an anaesthetic mask held over the mouth and nose, in both cases allowing ventilation of the baby during the examination. The procedure is best done in cooperation with a senior paediatric anaesthetist.

Diagnostic indications These include stridor, unless it is absolutely characteristic of laryngomalacia; the child who fails to extubate without obvious cause; to exclude concomitant upper airway obstruction in a child with bronchopulmonary dysplasia; localised hyperinflation or atelectasis.

Therapeutic indications The main one is difficulty in intubation (e.g. due to craniofacial abnormalities), especially if a tube change is necessary. The bronchoscope is passed through a new endotracheal tube prior to instrumenting the child. The larynx is visualised, and the tube slid over the bronchoscope into the trachea under direct vision. The position of the tube at the carina can be checked.

If airway secretions are to be sampled, either for diagnostic or research purposes, blind airway lavage is preferable. This is most conveniently done by wedging a fine feeding tube blind down the endotracheal tube, gently injecting 1 ml/kg of normal saline, and hand aspirating.

Fibreoptic bronchoscopy in the infant and older child

Instruments available For infants of more than a few months of age, the instrument of choice is the 2.7 or 3.6 mm external diameter endoscope, with a 1.2 mm suction/biopsy channel. The biopsies obtained are necessarily very small, and at present there are no protected specimen brushes small enough to go down the channel. For older children, particularly if a biopsy is to be performed, it may be preferable to use a 4.9 mm endoscope.

How to do the examination My preference is to perform bronchoscopy under general anaesthesia, either intubated, or via a laryngeal or face mask. If a face mask is used, the bronchoscope is slid through the nose into the pharynx, scrutinising all structures on the way. Next, the vocal cords are inspected. The subglottic structures are best inspected through the vocal cords, before attempting to pass the endoscope into the trachea. Unsuspected severe subglottic stenosis can be seen and appreciated without the risk of precipitating a disaster by traumatising a much-narrowed airway. Once the endoscope has passed the larynx, a suction trap is attached to the bronchoscope. Next, the trachea and all the segmental bronchi are inspected in turn, paying attention to structure and mobility.

Finally, any diagnostic procedures are performed, including bronchoalveolar lavage and bronchial biopsy. At least four, and probably as many as eight biopsies should be taken. Endobronchial biopsy is virtually free of risk, but bilateral biopsies should *never* be performed. Transbronchial biopsy is only indicated in the assessment of lung transplants; the biopsies are too small for diagnostic purposes in most ILD. Oxygen and monitoring are continued for at least 2 hours afterwards. Nothing is permitted by mouth for 3 hours, because of the risk of aspiration.

These instruments can be used in ventilated children, using a suitable adaptor. At least a size 4.5 tube is needed for a 3.6 mm endoscope, and a size 6 for a 4.9 mm instrument. The same monitoring as described above is required.

Diagnostic indications These are expanding all the time. They include suspected airway disease, e.g. malacia, tumour, congenital malformation; recurrent localised infection; interstitial pneumonia, particularly in the immunocompromised; surveillance bronchoscopy after bone marrow transplantation, to exclude occult CMV infection; localised atelectasis or hyperinflation; severe community-acquired pneumonia, or nosocomial infection; and lobar collapse.

Recently the technique of bronchography has been used to demonstrate airway malacia. A small amount of water-soluble contrast is instilled into the airway via the bronchoscope, and the instrument is then withdrawn. Fluoroscopy allows visualisation of airway dynamics without the bronchoscope causing inadvertent continuous positive airway pressure.

Therapeutic indications As with the neonate, difficult intubation is aided by endoscopy. Endobronchial toilet can be performed through a fibreoptic instrument, although the suction channel easily becomes blocked and often a rigid instrument is preferable. Drugs such as surfactant for acute lung injury in the older child can be instilled under direct vision using this technique. Foreign body removal should never be attempted with a fibrescope; if one is found unexpectedly, the examination should be terminated and a rigid bronchoscopy performed.

What is the place of the examination? Fibreoptic bronchoscopy should for the foreseeable future be available within all large paediatric respiratory centres. The same strictures as to indications apply to fibreoptic bronchoscopy in older children as in neonates. Thus the yield of bronchoalveolar lavage in the immunocompromised will be higher if all cases of pneumonitis are endoscoped prior to starting treatment, but it may be better for the patient and more cost-effective for the manager if empirical treatment is started and bronchoscopy reserved for the non-responders.

Rigid bronchoscopy

Instruments available Rigid bronchoscopes are available for even the smallest neonates. The proposal to pass rigid telescopes down an endotracheal tube has little to commend it.

How to do the examination Very few paediatricians will wish to learn this technique, which requires full general anaesthesia. The airway is secure and the child can be ventilated during the procedure. In my practice it is the province of the thoracic surgeons.

Diagnostic indications The main one is exclusion of an endobronchial foreign body. If there is any doubt as to whether the child could have a foreign body, do a rigid bronchoscopy. No other investigation can exclude this diagnosis as well as treat the condition if found. A negative examination does not mean that it should not have been done, any more than removal of a normal appendix is a clinical crime. An H-type fistula or laryngeal cleft is best appreciated using a rigid bronchoscope. For all other indications a fibreoptic examination is preferable. Airway dynamics cannot be assessed easily with the rigid instrument because of the unavoidable end-expiratory pressure applied during the procedure.

Therapeutic indications Removal of foreign body is by far the most important procedure. This should ideally only be attempted by a really experienced thoracic surgeon. Another indication is the balloon dilatation or lasering of acquired tracheobronchial strictures, usually secondary to prolonged intubation of a preterm neonate. There are occasional reports of endobronchial stenting, but this must be considered experimental. Large-volume therapeutic bronchoalveolar lavage for pulmonary alveolar proteinosis requires rigid bronchoscopy. Small children may need to be placed on extracorporeal circulatory support for this technique.

WHEN TO DO A BRONCHOSCOPY	WHEN NOT TO DO A BRONCHOSCOPY
▲ When it will give information which is necessary for the management of the child and which cannot be obtained any other way ▲ Suspected endobronchial foreign body.	▲ When condition (1) above is not met ▲ Beware if the patient is hypoxaemic or has severe pulmonary hypertension.

BIOPSY TECHNIQUES

Bronchoscopic biopsy

This has been discussed in detail above. Airway biopsy is useful in the diagnosis of TB and rarer granulomatous diseases. TBB carries a significant risk of pneumothorax, requires a general anaesthetic, and yields non-diagnostic biopsies so often that it should rarely find a place in paediatric practice outside the monitoring of lung transplant recipients for rejection and obliterative bronchiolitis.

Pleural biopsy

Closed pleural biopsy can be performed provided that there is a reasonably large pleural effusion present. It is particularly useful in suspected cases of tuberculosis and pleural tumour. However, the Abrams needle is large, and the procedure may be painful, so a general anaesthetic is preferable. This also enables the effusion to be drained, and a fibreoptic bronchoscopy performed, under the same anaesthetic.

A diagnostic thoracocentesis is performed under ultrasound control first, to confirm the presence of an effusion and to obtain samples uncontaminated as far as possible with blood. These samples should be sent for culture (looking for aerobes, anaerobes, mycobacteria and fungi) and cytology, for which as large a volume as possible, and certainly at least 50 ml, should be sent. Next, the Abrams needle is inserted, and its intrapleural location confirmed by aspirating more fluid. The needle is fully opened, the pleura engaged and a small sample removed by sharply closing the needle. Biopsies should be taken for mycobacterial culture and histological examination.

Open lung biopsy

Indications for this procedure include undiagnosed interstitial lung disease (below), and pulmonary shadowing in an immunocompromised host who is deteriorating on empirical treatment, and remains undiagnosed after BAL. As with all thoracic surgical procedures in children, open lung biopsy (OLB) should only be performed in units with experience in the care of children, and with access to experienced laboratory and histopathology services. A CT scan prior to biopsy is mandatory, to confirm the presence of disease and to guide the surgeon as to where best to biopsy. With regard to the biopsy itself, thoracoscopic techniques are increasingly replacing minithoracotomy, particularly in the older child. The biopsies should be taken from several sites, guided by the CT, and should include areas that are mildly as well as severely affected. The samples should be sent for culture for the whole range of possible pathogens, as well as sent for histology and electron microscopy. For choice, some of the biopsy, particularly from cases of interstitial lung disease, should be kept frozen in liquid nitrogen in case future immunological studies are suggested.

An alternative biopsy technique is CT-guided, percutaneous biopsy using a 'Tru-cut' needle. This requires a general anaesthetic, and risks bleeding and a pneumothorax. The samples are smaller and non-diagnostic results commoner than with OLB. The evidence is that percutaneous biopsy should be discarded.

OTHER IMPORTANT TESTS IN OVERLAPPING FIELDS

Echocardiography

Transthoracic echocardiography is non-invasive, gives a lot of useful information and thus is widely used in respiratory paediatrics. Transoesophageal echocardiography requires an anaesthetic or heavy sedation, carries a risk, and should only be used if the transthoracic approach fails. A good echocardiogram should be part of the work-up of unexplained recurrent lobar or segmental collapse, recurrent pulmonary shadowing, recurrent atypical wheeze or unexplained tachypnoea or dyspnoea, congenital lung disease, pulmonary embolism, suspected intrapulmonary shunting due to arteriovenous malformation, and in the suspected complications of an indwelling line.

Enlarged cardiac chambers due to left-to-right shunting (for example the left atrium) may cause recurrent lobar collapse with no other manifestation of the abnormal cardiac anatomy. High pulmonary blood flow due to intracardiac shunts may present as recurrent pulmonary shadowing, breathlessness, or atypical wheezing unresponsive to treatment. An echocardiogram is mandatory in all infants with congenital lung disease. Although angiography is the optimal method of delineating the pulmonary vasculature (see above), in the small sick infant it may be deemed wise not to risk this procedure in all cases, but to define pulmonary arterial and venous anatomy using echocardiography, and reserve angiograms for those in whom the anatomy is in doubt. In addition, congenital lung and heart disease may co-exist, and the latter is best defined by echocardiography. Children with bronchial isomerism should have an echocardiogram, in addition to an abdominal ultrasound to assess the spleen.

Pulmonary embolism is unusual in paediatrics, but, as in adults, is underdiagnosed. Sources of embolism which may be found by echocardiography include septic emboli due to infective endocarditis, thrombus around an indwelling line, thrombus formed in the great vessels secondary to a low cardiac output state and right atrial thrombus secondary to cardiac failure or blunt thoracic trauma. The blue infant with a structurally normal heart may have a right-to-left shunt through a pulmonary arteriovenous malformation. Many will have an obvious radiographic abnormality, and the shunt can be confirmed using contrast echocardiography.

Indwelling venous lines are increasingly part of paediatric practice, both in intensive care and in the community (e.g. Hickman lines, Portacaths). Septic complications impact on the lungs and include embolism and abscess formation.

Echocardiographic inspection of the lines should always be performed if embolic complications are suspected.

In addition to the diagnostic uses of echocardiography, estimation of pulmonary artery pressure from physiological tricuspid or pulmonary regurgitation using the Bernoulli equation may give useful prognostic information.

Barium studies

A barium swallow is most useful for the diagnosis of a vascular ring. If reflux is seen, then it is usually significant, but false negatives and positives are possible. Hiatus hernia or malrotation may occasionally present as recurrent vomiting and respiratory infections, and be diagnosed best on barium studies. Suspected varices may be confirmed by barium swallow.

A cine barium swallow is useful in children with neurological impairment and recurrent infections (below); a skilled speech therapist is invaluable if interpretation of the results is to be optimal.

Immune function

The child with genuine recurrent respiratory infections of unknown cause should be referred for more detailed testing. The point at which referral to an immunologist is made will depend on the facilities available locally. The nature and timing of the infections will to some extent determine what detailed immune function tests are subsequently performed. These may include immunoglobulins and subsets, IgA, vacine antibodies, T-cell subsets, neutrophil function tests, and measurement of mannose-binding lectin.

pH monitoring

Gastro-oesophageal reflux can cause respiratory disease, complicate it, or be a coincident irrelevance. Diagnosis is difficult, and false negatives are common. In many instances, if the history is suggestive, then a therapeutic trial may be indicated.

Oesophageal pH monitoring (see also Ch. 9) can define acid but not alkaline reflux. It is invasive, requiring insertion of the probe through the nose, and some means of preventing its being torn out by the child. The position should be about 2 cm above a line joining the cupolae of the diaphragms in the postero-anterior CXR. The length of probe can be calculated from equations, or measured crudely, but in either case the correct position should be confirmed by a CXR. If the pH probe is negative, a milk scan may be performed (above). The finding of many strongly positive fat-laden macrophages on BAL are suggestive of reflux, but not diagnostic; there are many false positive and negative results.

Neurological

Interactions between pulmonologist and neurologist are usually two-way. Referrals from neurology are usually with recurrent respiratory infections in the neurologically-impaired child; the differential diagnosis is usually reflux, pulmonary contamination from swallowing dysfunction, or a coincident condition.

Respiratory referrals to neurologists come under a variety of headings, which include:

▲ The child with apnoeas or blue spells, which might be fits
▲ The child with respiratory muscle dysfunction, for exclusion of a generalised myopathy or neuropathy
▲ The child referred with tachypnoea, who turns out to have a metabolic acidosis of obscure aetiology.

Tests of malabsorption

These are particularly relevant in the case of suspected CF, particularly if atypical. For typical cases, a 2- or 3-day faecal fat will be all that is required to confirm the need for pancreatic enzyme replacement and monitor therapy. For atypical cases, more sophisticated tests of pancreatic function may detect helpful subclinical abnormalities which point to a diagnosis of CF. The child known to have CF who is malabsorbing on pancreatic replacement therapy requires a detailed gastroenterological evaluation to exclude other causes including coeliac disease, Crohn's disease, and the complications of neonatal surgery.

Clinical problems

These are guides only to start off thought. In all cases, the basic tenets of airway, breathing and cardiac output (ABC) are assumed to have been verified. The diagnosis may be obvious in many scenarios, and steps may conveniently be omitted. These schemata are offered as a helpful guide, and are not meant to be prescriptive.

THE BREATHLESS CHILD

Broad categories are given, to widen the diagnostic net beyond the lungs. This algorithm assumes that neither wheeze nor stridor (discussed below) is present. The problem of deterioration in the immunocompromised host is discussed later.

▲ **Question 1** — *Is the child acidotic?* Consider diabetic ketoacidosis, acute renal failure, metabolic diseases.
▲ **Question 2** — *Could there be an acute pulmonary infection?* CXR will show a focal or multifocal abnormality. Viral pneumonitis may not cause CXR abnormalities, at least initially.
▲ **Question 3** — *Could this be 'silent' acute asthma?* It would be very unusual for severe breathlessness with a completely silent chest to be the first presentation of asthma. However, wheeze (and for that matter stridor) require air to be moved by respiratory efforts in significant volumes.
▲ **Question 4** — *Could this be the onset of acute pulmonary oedema (cardiogenic or acute lung injury)?* Acute myocarditis and left ventricular failure, or ARDS after an extra-pulmonary insult.
▲ **Question 5** — *Is pulmonary embolism a possibility?* (see below, Pulmonary hypertension of non-cardiac origin, for a full discussion of embolic disease)

▲ **Question 6** — *Can interstitial lung disease present acutely?* Presentation is usually more subacute, but an acute Hamman–Rich-like syndrome is described in children. Investigations for interstitial lung disease are given later in the chapter.

AIRWAY OBSTRUCTION

This may be predominantly inspiratory, or expiratory. There may be difficulty in both phases of respiration, but the classification may nonetheless be useful in clinical practice.

Difficulty breathing in (stridor)

Acute stridor The main priority is to ensure that the child does not die from an inadequate airway. The differential diagnosis is:

a) Viral or spasmodic croup
b) Acute epiglottitis (rare since HiB immunisation)
c) Foreign body
d) Bacterial tracheitis
e) Diphtheria in an unimmunised child.

No investigations should be done. If the child is on the verge of critical obstruction, then he should be intubated with full facilities available for an emergency tracheostomy. A lateral neck X-ray is useless and dangerous. Suspicion of a foreign body mandates bronchoscopy. Elective bronchoscopy should be considered in cases of recurrent croup; where there are atypical features; and with early onset cases. Children with recurrent spasmodic croup may subsequently develop asthma.

Chronic stridor The differential diagnosis varies with age. In infants, laryngomalacia, congenital laryngeal webs and cysts, and vascular ring should be considered. In older children, foreign body, vocal cord dysfunction, and vascular ring should be considered. In all cases, the definitive investigation for chronic stridor is fibreoptic bronchoscopy. Although radiological investigations may give clues as to aetiology (e.g. a right-sided aortic arch on a CXR with a vascular ring), none are likely to be definitively diagnostic, and merely serve to delay the decisive investigation.

Difficulty breathing out

▲ **Determine the site of obstruction**. The easiest test is the flow volume curve, which should give a clue to large airway problems. The goal of delineating small as opposed to medium airway obstruction has been sought by physiologists, but has not been attained.
▲ **Large airway obstruction** — fibreoptic bronchoscopy.
▲ **Medium/small airway obstruction** — define the cause, which includes asthma, CF, suppurative lung disease (see below); define the reversibility — a formal bronchodilator and even a steroid trial may be indicated.

THE CHILD WITH THE PROBLEM CHRONIC COUGH

▲ **Is there a serious underlying cause?** — History, physical examination, spirometry (if age appropriate) and a CXR are the basic tools for making this most important decision. CF should always be actively considered. Coughing for a few days solely with viral colds is unlikely to be significant.

▲ **Is it asthma?** Cough variant asthma undoubtedly exists, but is greatly over-diagnosed.

   a) Attempt to document variable airflow obstruction with home peak flow monitoring, acute bronchodilator responsiveness or an exercise test. No single test will diagnose asthma, but if all tests are normal, asthma is unlikely.

   b) A therapeutic trial may be indicated particularly in children who are too young to perform lung function. I recommend an inhaled steroid, 400 mcg Budesonide twice daily for two months. If the child responds, stop the treatment. Asthma is diagnosed only if (i) symptoms recur, and (ii) they respond to reintroduction of inhaled steroids. If there is no response to this therapeutic trial, then the diagnosis is highly unlikely to be asthma.

▲ **Is it 'psychological' (older child)?** An important clue is symptomatology that disappears when the child is asleep, and is therapy-resistant when awake. Hidden gains may be obvious. Diagnosis should be a positive one, not just because the doctor is stuck for what to do.

▲ **What is the role of gastro-oesophageal reflux?** The lung and the oesophagus can interact in different ways.

   i) Respiratory symptoms and GOR are both present, but GOR is irrelevant to the respiratory problem

   ii) Respiratory disease is exacerbating or causing GOR; GOR may secondarily exacerbate lung problems

   iii) GOR may be the primary cause of the respiratory presentation, but airway disease may secondarily exacerbate the GOR.

Clues to the importance of GOR may come from the history. In general, if symptoms get better on a holiday to a hot climate the GOR is unlikely to be important. If in doubt, a therapeutic trial is legitimate.

▲ **Is it 'chronic non-specific cough'?** A 'catch-all' diagnosis; treatment is diffi-cult/impossible but prognosis is good. Parents can be reassured, and expensive and useless treatments avoided.

THE CHRONICALLY CYANOSED CHILD

Cyanosis is notoriously difficult to detect clinically. The advent of pulse oximetry has made this less of a problem, but it is not impossible for desaturation to progress markedly before it is detected clinically.

▲ **Is there evidence of chest disease?** Usually symptoms of cough and breath-lessness are present and investigated long before cyanosis occurs. Occasionally in the asthmatic, deterioration is so slow that cyanosis may be present without the family having perceived any other problem. Undoubtedly some but not all instances of so-called 'sudden asthma death' have this as a mechanism.

▲ **Is there evidence of heart disease?** Presentation is usually with a heart murmur or breathlessness. A child whose murmur has not been investigated may present with cyanosis due to the development of Eisenmenger's syndrome.

▲ **Is there evidence of liver disease?** Lung complications of liver disease include primary pulmonary hypertension (see below) and multiple microscopic pulmonary arteriovenous malformations (PAVMs).

▲ **Cyanosed and unwell, no obvious cause** — consider respiratory failure during sleep, either severe obstructive sleep apnoea; central hypoventilation, for example due to posterior fossa abnormality; neuromuscular disease (diaphragm may be the only muscle affected, at least early on); and chest wall disease (scoliosis may be obvious, but the inference drawn from its presence may not be). Primary pulmonary vascular diseases (see pulmonary hypertension of non-cardiac origin, below) should also be considered.

▲ **Cyanosed but well and not breathless, CXR normal** — consider congenital or acquired haemoglobinopathy, e.g. methaemoglobinaemia, and perform a haemoglobin electrophoresis. Multiple microscopic PAVMs enter the differential diagnosis.

▲ **Cyanosed but well and not breathless, CXR shows single or multiple focal defects** — contrast echocardiogram, since macroscopic PAVM is likely.

NON-INFECTIVE CAUSES OF PULMONARY SHADOWING ON THE CXR

The differential diagnosis is wide. Many of these conditions are rare, and infection remains the most common cause of CXR changes in paediatric practice; but before investigating a child for recurrent infection, diseases associated with focal or diffuse abnormalities should be considered.

Diseases usually characterised by focal abnormalities

1. Congenital lung disease, e.g. cystic adenomatoid malformation, bronchogenic cyst (see below)
2. Primary lung, mediastinal or chest wall tumours — CT scan, tumour markers (VMA, β-HCG, α-FP); however, most require biopsy for diagnosis.
3. Pulmonary eosinophilic syndromes — characteristically multiple flitting shadows, associated with blood eosinophilia.
4. Allergic bronchopulmonary aspergillosis — usually in the context of CF (see below), occasionally in asthmatics. Perform total IgE, *Aspergillus* RAST and IgG precipitins, *Aspergillus* skin test, and culture sputum (if any).
5. Atelectasis, which may be secondary to endobronchial disease (e.g. foreign body, mucus impaction), bronchial wall disease (e.g. focal bronchomalacia), or external bronchial compression (e.g. by abnormal mediastinal vessel, tumour or cardiac enlargement). Often needs a bronchoscopy for diagnosis and therapeutic bronchial toilet.
6. Lymphadenopathy from any cause (e.g. lymphoma, tuberculosis, sarcoidosis). Define with a CT scan, which may need contrast administration.

7. Pulmonary embolism (see below), including multiple haematogenous septic emboli; may be single or multiple.
8. Hydatid disease; may be single or multiple. Always consider if a compatible exposure history.
9. Respiratory muscle disease — sitting and supine VC (best); measurements of respiratory muscle strength by mouth pressure.
10. Cardiac disease leading to aneurysm or enlargement of great vessels or cardiac chambers — echocardiography.
11. Large pulmonary arteries due to non-cardiac causes — CT scan with contrast.

Diseases usually characterised by diffuse abnormalities

1. Gastro-oesophageal reflux/aspiration — see Recurrent multifocal (true) infection below.
2. Pulmonary oedema — consider echocardiography to exclude cardiac disease, and remember renal failure and acute lung injury as alternatives. See section below on Acute pulmonary deterioration for the immunocompromised host.
3. Acute lung injury (adult respiratory distress syndrome) — usually a history of antecedent insult.
4. Pulmonary haemorrhage — see sections below for apparently normal host and immunocompromised host.
5. Drug or radiation pneumonitis — should be clear from the history.
6. Interstitial lung disease — see below.
7. Pulmonary veno-occlusive disease — see Pulmonary hypertension of non-cardiac origin, below.
8. Pulmonary burns or smoke inhalation — history obvious; bronchoscopy may be helpful to define the abnormalities.

Disease which may result in focal or diffuse abnormalities

1. Collagen/autoimmune disease (e.g. Wegener's, rheumatoid) — autoimmune workup: ANCA, antinuclear factor, etc.
2. Extrapulmonary malignancy (include lymphoma, discrete secondary deposits, lymphangitis carcinomatosa) — abdominal ultrasound and CT.
3. Blunt chest trauma — history usually obvious, but the changes may be delayed and the history forgotten.
4. Sickle cell disease — full blood count and haemoglobin electrophoresis mandatory in appropriate ethnic groups.
5. Sarcoidosis — angiotensin converting enzyme, CT scan of chest, abdominal ultrasound.
6. Bronchiectasis — see section below.
7. Pulmonary arteriovenous fistula — see The chronically cyanosed child, above.

RECURRENT INFECTION IN THE NORMAL HOST

The commonest cause of 'multiple chest infections' is a fruity cough after a viral cold; the next commonest is asthma. For this protocol to be activated, radiological confirmation of infection is essential.

Recurrent infection in the same sites

Although a systemic immunodeficiency can present this way, and thus the investigations under step 1 below, most likely there is a local anatomical cause.

▲ **Question 1** — *is local airway anatomy normal?* Perform a fibreoptic bronchoscopy.

▲ **Question 2** — *is there a localised parenchymal abnormality (e.g. a congenital cystic malformation?)* Perform a CT scan.

Recurrent multifocal (true) infection

▲ **Step 1** — *Define the organisms, whether the pattern and timing suggests a particular disease, and whether significant extrapulmonary infections are a feature.* Recurrent infection in the lung may signal a local immunodeficiency, or the first presentation of a systemic immunodeficiency. The subsequent investigations should not be haphazard, but guided by the above.

▲ **Step 2** — *Is it cystic fibrosis?* At least a sweat test should be performed; see also equivocal diagnosis of CF, below.

▲ **Step 3** — *Is humoral immunity intact?* Immunoglobulins, subclasses and antibody levels to *Pneumococcus* and *Haemophilus influenzae* should be measured. The specific antibody levels should be repeated after appropriate immunisation if low.

▲ **Step 4** — *Is there recurrent aspiration?* This may be from below (GOR, pH probe); above (incoordinate swallowing, videofluoroscopy; laryngeal cleft, rigid bronchoscopy); or from the side (H-type fistula, tube oesophagram).

▲ **Step 5** — *Is it PCD?* Consider a nasal nitric oxide, or nasal brush biopsy.

▲ **Step 6** — *What about other immune defects?* Consider the involvement of a specialist paediatric immunologist.

ACUTE PULMONARY DETERIORATION IN THE IMMUNOCOMPROMISED HOST

The differential diagnosis is wide, comprising:

a) A wide spectrum of infections, e.g. *Pneumocystis carinii, cytomegalovirus*
b) Pulmonary haemorrhage
c) Pulmonary oedema (fluid overload, cardiomyopathy)
d) Acute lung injury (ARDS)
e) Recurrence of the original disease
f) Pulmonary drug or radiation toxicity
g) Graft versus host disease (post bone marrow transplant — usually other features present, e.g. typical skin rash).

Remember that in neutropenic patients pulmonary shadowing may be disproportionately minimal compared with the degree of illness. In any case, the CXR appearances are likely to be very non-specific. A systematic approach to investigation comprises:

▲ **Step 1** — *Full blood picture and clotting profile*; if pulmonary haemorrhage is likely, then a rebreathing measurement of CO transfer should be considered if the child is old enough to perform the measurements; it will be elevated for up to 72 hours after a bleed.

▲ **Step 2** — *Is cardiac dysfunction or fluid overload likely?* An echocardiogram to assess left ventricular function and left atrial dimensions may be helpful.

▲ **Step 3** — *Fibreoptic bronchoscopy.* The timing will vary with the clinical picture. Many units will give empirical therapy with antibiotics and anti-fungals, and so the diagnostic yield of bronchoscopy will be lower. Lavage should be submitted for the full range of microbiological and cytological investigations. Most would not perform transbronchial biopsy (TBB) for fear of bleeding.

▲ **Step 4** — *If the patient is deteriorating and the BAL is negative.* In this situation, a repeat BAL is highly unlikely to be useful, and the patient should have an open lung biopsy.

INTERSTITIAL LUNG DISEASE

▲ **Step 1** — *Is an interstitial lung disease present?* A high resolution CT scan con-firms this, and guides the site of future biopsy. Occasionally the appearances may be diagnostic (e.g. pulmonary haemosiderosis) but this is unusual.

▲ **Step 2** — *Non-invasive investigations.* A minority can be diagnosed on blood tests (e.g. Wegener's granulomatosis on ANCA, allergic alveolitis on finding IgG anti-bodies to appropriate allergens, sarcoidosis on angiotensin converting enzyme).

▲ **Step 3** — *Fibreoptic bronchoscopy.* The yield is so poor that for most children a separate anaesthetic for this procedure is unjustified. The diseases which can be diagnosed on BAL include Langerhans cell histiocytosis, pulmonary haemosiderosis, and surfactant protein B deficiency. TBB is only useful in rare cases with highly specific features, for example alveolar microlithiasis.

▲ **Step 4** — *Lung biopsy.* Most cases of interstitial lung disease require a biopsy for diagnosis. My own choice is open lung biopsy, rather than TBB or trans-thoracic needle biopsy (see above).

CONGENITAL LUNG DISEASE

This is becoming an increasingly important part of paediatric pulmonology, as antenatal diagnosis of these lesions is made. The choice of investigations is wide, and should be considered under several headings.

▲ **Is significant bronchial tree disease present?** Consider penetrated CXR (bronchial situs), fibreoptic bronchoscopy (wall calibre and compliance), tube oesophagram (H-type fistula), CT or MRI (parenchymal abnormality).

▲ **Is significant vascular disease present?** Consider echocardiography, pul-monary and aortic angiography, CT with contrast, MRI, V:Q scan.

▲ **Is significant lymphatic disease present?** Open lung biopsy, for the rare congenital lymphatic disorders.

▲ **Are other organ systems abnormal?** The heart, great vessels, chest wall, abdomen, and neuromuscular system may all harbour relevant disease. Remember multisystem diseases such as tuberous sclerosis in appropriate cases.

The most important principle before contemplating surgery is to describe completely the abnormality and the state of the tissue around it. Knowledge of (for example) vascular anatomy is essential to prevent surgical disaster in apparently simple and isolated cysts.

PULMONARY HYPERTENSION OF NON-CARDIAC ORIGIN

Most children with pulmonary hypertension have cardiac disease, which can be diagnosed on transthoracic echocardiography, or obvious end-stage lung disease, such as cystic fibrosis. If neither is present, then consider the following:

▲ **obstructive sleep apnoea** — screening overnight pulse oximetry as a minimum
▲ **occult interstitial lung disease** — CT scan (10–20% may have a normal CXR)
▲ **primary pulmonary vascular disease** — primary pulmonary hypertension; pulmonary thrombo- or other embolic disease; pulmonary veno-occlusive disease; (rare) invasive capillary haemangiomatosis. The investigation of such patients is best left to specialist units.

> **Step 1** — *Is pulmonary hypertension present?* Right heart catheterisation with reversibility of elevation of pulmonary vascular resistance to nitric oxide, intravenous adenosine or prostacyclin, or other agent as appropriate. If pulmonary capillary wedge pressure is high, with normal left heart function, then pulmonary venous disease is likely (e.g. pulmonary veno-occlusive disease, pulmonary venous stenosis).
>
> **Step 2** — *Is embolic disease present?* Pulmonary angiography may be performed, and is the gold standard, but carries a risk in severe pulmonary hypertension. The alternative is a spiral CT scan. Embolism may be difficult to distinguish from in situ thrombosis. If embolism is likely, follow algorithm (a) immediately below. For pulmonary hypertension due to vascular disease not related to embolism, see (b) below.

Investigation of embolic disease

a) *Is thromboembolism likely* — common causes are intravascular foreign body (e.g. Broviac line) and vascular stasis.
b) *Thromboembolism with no obvious cause* — investigate for congenital or acquired coagulopathy.
c) *Non-thromboembolic pulmonary hypertension* — consider tumour emboli (especially Wilm's); schistosomiasis if there is a history of tropical travel; talc emboli in an adolescent who abuses drugs intravenously; and fat emboli after major trauma.

Investigation of non-embolic pulmonary hypertension

Look for evidence of associated diseases, including liver disease, connective tissue disease and HIV infection. Consider open lung biopsy to confirm the diagnosis.

PLEURAL EFFUSION

This section describes the approach to the infant and child, excluding the complications of trauma, including iatrogenic. Probably the commonest cause encountered in paediatric practice is effusion complicating pneumonia, in which case some steps below can be bypassed. Congenital pleural effusions are not discussed.

▲ **Step 1** — *Confirm that a significant effusion is present.* Pleural ultrasound is far superior to CT scan for imaging pleural space disease. A CT scan is indicated if an underlying tumour is suspected.

▲ **Step 2** — *Eliminate obvious causes from the differential diagnosis.* Particularly if the effusions are bilateral, consider hypoalbuminaemia and heart failure as a cause. TB should not be forgotten, and if in doubt a Mantoux and gastric washings performed.

▲ **Step 3** — *Drain and analyse the fluid, including where appropriate a closed pleural biopsy.* This step is most often performed in large unilateral effusion. In my hands, pleural space procedures are painful. With the child under a short general anaesthetic, and under ultrasound control, I would carry out the following:
  a) a diagnostic aspiration (protein content; microscopy and culture, including for tuberculosis; PCR may also be indicated; bacterial antigens if available; cytology. I have not routinely measured pleural fluid pH, glucose, or LDH)
  b) a closed pleural biopsy, part of which should be cultured for TB
  c) drain the fluid to dryness, often leaving a chest drain in place
  d) inspect the airways and perform a BAL with the fibreoptic bronchoscope

▲ **Step 4** — *Investigation of a transudate.* Heart failure and hypoalbuminaemia should be excluded if not already considered.

▲ **Step 5** — *Investigation of an exudate.* The commonest causes should have been elucidated by the above. Options now include:
  i)   an open (or thoracoscopic) pleural biopsy, with lung biopsy as appropriate
  ii) a trial of treatment, usually anti-tuberculous chemotherapy.

BRONCHIECTASIS

▲ **Step 1** — *Confirm that bronchiectasis is present, and the extent of the problem.* The CXR may be normal or near normal unless bronchiectasis is severe. A CT scan should be performed; this investigation may show that the bronchiectasis is localised and amenable to surgery (although surgery for bronchiectasis is rarely performed).

▲ **Step 2** — *Define function, including presence or absence of airway reactivity and hypoxia.* This requires:
  a) Spirometry at least, and consider lung volumes
  b) Bronchodilator and oral steroid trial should be considered
  c) Overnight saturation study (pulse oximeter with memory)

▲ **Step 3** — *Define the underlying cause.* See Recurrent multifocal (true) infection, above.

▲ **Step 4** — *Define whether complications are present.* Consider echocardiography to assess pulmonary hypertension; a pH study to assess reflux (see interactions between airway and oesophagus under Child with problem chronic cough, above).

EQUIVOCAL DIAGNOSIS OF CYSTIC FIBROSIS

Usually the problem is in a child with suggestive features of the disease, an equivocal sweat test, and possibly a single CF mutation detected.

▲ **Step 1** — *Repeat the sweat test in an experienced centre*; 98% of patients with CF can be diagnosed on a properly performed sweat test. Pitfalls:
  a) eczema (not enough sweat)
  b) inexperienced operator
  c) rare disease such as fucoscidosis
  d) sweat chloride of 40 in a neonate is in the 'normal' range, but is at least 6 SDs away from the mean, and likely abnormal
  e) Occasional indubitable negative sweat tests in children who later turn out to have CF.

▲ **Step 2** — *In the older child, perform a fludrocortisone suppression test.* There are no normal data for infants.

▲ **Step 3** — *Perform an extended genotype.* Usually least helpful when most needed.

▲ **Step 4** — *Make measurements of ion transport.* Nasal potential differences, and the responses to amiloride and low chloride/isoprenaline solutions may be very helpful, but are available in a few centres only. Definitely for experts.

▲ **Step 5** — *Look for supportive evidence of subacute organ dysfunction.* Tests include a thoracic CT scan to detect occult bronchiectasis; BAL to try to culture organisms suggestive of CF, such as *Staph. aureus* or *Ps. aeruginosa*; semen analysis in male adolescents for azoospermia; and sophisticated pancreatic function tests.

▲ **Step 6** — If the matter is still undecided, continue to follow-up the child, and treat any complications aggressively (e.g. lung infection with antibiotics and physiotherapy). It may be useful to re-investigate after a year.

FURTHER READING

Gozal, D. (2000) Pulmonary manifestations of neuromuscular disease with special reference to Duchenne muscular dystrophy and spinal muscular atrophy. *Paediatric Pulmonology* 29: 141–150.

Zach, M., Carlsen, K-H., Warner, J.O., Sennhauser, F. (1997) *New Diagnostic Techniques in Paediatric Respiratory Medicine.* European Respiratory Monograph 1997.

11

Cardiology

E Baker and J Skinner

1. Physiology/anatomy

Congenital heart disease is commonly divided into cyanotic and non-cyanotic types. A better classification is into defects with left to right shunts (Table 11.1), cyanotic defects with bi-directional shunts (Table 11.2) and defects that do not have a shunt (Table 11.3).

Some cardiac malformations are complex and cannot be described using these simple labels. To simplify the description of these hearts, sequential segmental analysis has been developed (Ho et al. 1995). The heart is divided into four segments, the great veins, the atria, the ventricles, and the arterial trunks.

Table 11.1 Acyanotic defects with left to right shunts	
	Relative incidence
Ventricular septal defect	28%
Persistent ductus arteriosus	10%
Atrial septal defect	7%

Table 11.2 Cyanotic defects with bi-directional shunts	
	Relative incidence
Transposition of the great arteries	6%
Tetralogy of Fallot	5%
Double outlet right ventricle	1%
Truncus arteriosus	1%
Pulmonary atresia	2%
Mitral atresia	1%
Tricuspid atresia	1%
Total anomalous pulmonary venous drainage	1%

Table 11.3   Acyanotic defects which usually have no shunt

	Relative incidence
Aortic stenosis	5%
Pulmonary stenosis	5%
Coarctation of the aorta	*5%*

Table 11.4 Sequential segmental analysis of the heart

Segment	Examples
Atrial situs	Solitus
	Inversus
	Left isomerism
	Right isomerism
Venous connections of the atria	Total or partial anomalous pulmonary venous connection
	Anomalous systemic venous connection
Atrioventricular connection	Concordant
	Discordant
	Absent left connection (mitral atresia)
	Absent right connection (tricuspid atresia)
	Double inlet left ventricle
Ventriculo-arterial connection	Concordant
	Discordant (transposition)
	Double outlet right ventricle
Associated anomalies	Ventricular septal defect
	Atrial septal defect
	Pulmonary or aortic stenosis
	Coarctation of the aorta

Abnormalities are described in each of these segments and in the connections between them (Table 11.4). A concordant connection is one that would be expected from the morphology (e.g. the right atrium connected to the right ventricle), while a discordant connection is the reverse of the expected (e.g. left ventricle connected to pulmonary trunk).

Acquired heart diseases in children include the cardiomyopathies, which may be dilated, with reduced contractility of the left ventricle, or hypertrophic, in which there is reduced compliance of the left ventricle. Viral myocarditis presents as an acute dilated cardiomyopathy with the onset of heart failure in a previously well child. Arrhythmias may cause clinical problems because of bradycardia or tachycardia. In either case, an insidious or abrupt fall in the cardiac output precipitates heart failure or syncope.

List of tests

CARDIAC STRUCTURE AND FUNCTION

Echocardiogram
   Trans-oesophageal cardiogram
   Fetal echocardiography
MRI
Radionuclide angiography
Cardiac catheterisation
Myocardial biopsy

CARDIAC RHYTHM

Electrocardiogram
Ambulatory electrocardiography
Exercise electrocardiography
Tilt testing
Electrophysiological study

OTHER TESTS

Chest X-ray
Haemoglobin/haematocrit
Hyperoxia test
Barium swallow
Pulmonary perfusion scan

ABBREVIATIONS USED IN THIS CHAPTER

IVC — inferior vena cava
LCA — left coronary artery
LVOT — left ventricular outflow
   tract

RCA — right coronary artery
RVOT — right ventricular outflow
   tract

---

2. Tests

CARDIAC STRUCTURE AND FUNCTION

Echocardiogram

Echocardiography is used in all age groups, but imaging is often less easy in older children and adults as the echocardiographic window may be more limited. Structural imaging is very precise in young children, and even in complex conditions is sufficient to plan surgical management. Doppler measurements are used for measuring the severity of stenoses in valves and arteries, and are particularly important in the follow-up of aortic valve stenosis. Doppler is also used for estimating the pulmonary artery pressure in congenital heart defects, such as ventricular septal defect or patent ductus arteriosus. It can also often be used for detecting pulmonary hypertension in respiratory disease, usually by estimating the right ventricular pressure from the Doppler trace of any tricuspid incompetence.

Measurements of left ventricular size (usually using M-mode) are important for assessing incompetent aortic and mitral valves. The shortening fraction is a measurement of the percentage change in the size of the left ventricle during contraction, and therefore the systolic function. It is not very reproducible, but is widely used (normal value 35–45% in infants, 28–38% in older children). It is also possible to estimate the left ventricular ejection fraction (normal value 55–75%), but this is not an accurate or reproducible measurement when made echocardiographically. There are many other echocardiographic derived functional indices. None are widely used clinically.

Echocardiography is also important for the identification of intracardiac masses and vegetations and pericardial effusions.

Trans-oesophageal echocardiogram
An imaging probe is passed on an endoscope through the oesophagus and into the stomach to obtain a good window on the heart from behind. This is useful in older patients when the window from the front is poor. It is also used in younger patients to image the pulmonary veins and the mitral valve. It is particularly useful in the monitoring of cardiac function during surgery and in positioning catheters and other devices during interventional procedures.

Fetal echocardiography
Up to a third of infants with congenital heart disease can be detected before birth and those with serious disorders delivered at a cardiac centre. From 18 weeks of gestation most major structural heart defects can be diagnosed accurately. In-utero treatment for arrhythmias is routine, but prenatal treatment for structural defects has yet to be shown to be effective (see Allan et al. 1994).

Magnetic resonance scan
Magnetic resonance imaging (MRI) is used for studying abnormalities of the great arteries and the major veins. Very accurate functional measurements can be made (Elliot 1991).

Radionuclide angiography
Radionuclide imaging is invaluable for measuring ventricular function and superior to echocardiography in this respect. It can also be used to measure left to right shunts and myocardial perfusion (see Baker 1994).

Cardiac catheterisation
The indications for a diagnostic cardiac catheterisation in children are few. It is important for estimation of pulmonary vascular resistance. Selective angiography is used to study cardiac anatomy that cannot be imaged by other techniques, principally coronary artery anatomy and complex pulmonary artery anomalies (Ho et al. 1995).

Myocardial biopsy
Transcatheter endomyocardial biopsy has been used in children with suspected myocarditis and in the assessment of transplant rejection.

CARDIAC RHYTHM

Electrocardiogram

Standard electrocardiograms have limited value in structural abnormalities of the heart and are mainly used to investigate the cardiac rhythm. They are often used as screening tests for structural heart disease, if echocardiography is not available. Atrial or ventricular hypertrophy, or abnormalities of QRS axis, may indicate structural problems, but are rarely specific (Park and Gunteroth 1987).

Ambulatory electrocardiography

Twenty-four hour ECG recordings are used to detect transitory rhythm disturbances, correlating them with symptoms, and monitoring treatment. If arrhythmias are not detected on 24-hour recordings, patients can be given ECG event recorders over a longer period, which they activate when symptoms occur. Event recorders are much more likely to detect arrhythmias than 24-hour recordings.

Exercise electrocardiography

Some arrhythmias are induced by exercise. Older children can be exercised on a treadmill while their ECG is recorded. This is also of value in the assessment of exercise tolerance and in deciding about exercise restriction.

Tilt testing

This is used as a test for vaso-vagal syncope. The test takes place in a semi-darkened quiet room. The ECG and blood pressure are monitored. The child lies on a tiltable table and is raised from supine to a 60 degree head-up tilt and kept at that angle for an extended period. A positive tilt test is indicated by syncope or pre-syncope with severe bradycardia, hypotension or both. Drugs may be given intravenously during the test to improve the sensitivity of the test. The test is neither highly specific nor sensitive – it is important to know that a positive tilt test does not exclude other significant pathology, such as long QT syndrome.

Electrophysiological study

An invasive test of the electrical pathways in the heart used to detect causes of paroxysmal arrhythmias or to induce arrhythmias to demonstrate their origin. Transcatheter ablation of abnormal pathways is often possible.

OTHER TESTS

Chest X-ray

A good chest X-ray can show cardiomegaly and increased or decreased pulmonary blood flow. It will show visceral situs and cardiac position. It is valuable as a screening test for cardiac disease, but it is not of great value in the diagnosis of specific structural abnormalities.

Haemoglobin/haematocrit

Arterial desaturation in cyanotic heart disease causes polycythaemia. Measurement of this gives an indication of the severity of the chronic hypoxia.

Except in the neonatal period, this is a more important measure than an instantaneous measurement of arterial oxygen saturation.

Hyperoxia test
The hyperoxia, or nitrogen washout, test is a sensitive way of detecting a right to left shunt. Cyanotic heart disease, severe respiratory disease and persistent pulmonary hypertension can all cause right to left shunts in neonates. A hyperoxia test is occasionally of value if it is uncertain whether a structural heart anomaly is present.

Barium swallow
A barium swallow is a useful screening test for a vascular ring in a child with stridor. MRI, if available, is a better alternative.

Pulmonary perfusion scan
Pulmonary perfusion can be very abnormal in children with complex congenital heart disease. Radionuclide pulmonary perfusion may be used, but the scan can only be interpreted correctly if the anatomy of the pulmonary arteries is known.

3. Clinical problems

Heart disease in children presents with:

- Asymptomatic murmur
- Clinical heart failure, with dyspnoea, failure to thrive or exercise intolerance
- Central cyanosis or cyanotic attacks
- Palpitations or syncope

Heart disease may be suspected because of other malformations or syndromes. In children it rarely presents with anginal type chest pain.

Asymptomatic murmur
Any child who is clinically judged to have a structural heart anomaly, however minor, should have an echocardiogram.

Clinical examination including palpation of the peripheral pulses and measurement of the blood pressure should demonstrate that most asymptomatic murmurs are innocent. In the majority of children clinical examination should be sufficient to diagnose an innocent murmur. Clinically innocent murmurs do not need investigation or follow-up. If a murmur is not thought to be innocent a GP should refer to a paediatrician.

A paediatrician who is not sure a murmur is innocent should refer on to a paediatric cardiologist or arrange an echocardiogram by someone skilled in paediatric echocardiography. A chest X-ray and ECG are usually obtained if echocardiography is not readily available. While a normal chest X-ray and ECG support the diagnosis of an innocent murmur, they do not rule out structural heart disease. Chest X-ray features that suggest structural heart disease are enlargement of the heart (on a good quality posterior–anterior film), abnormal cardiac position such as dextrocardia, abnormal abdominal situs and abnormal pulmonary vascular markings. Minor variations in the shape of the heart are not usually of great significance. Some patterns are noteworthy. An apparently enlarged right atrium, a narrow mediastium (characteristic of transposition) or the combination of reduced size pulmonary arteries and right ventricular enlargement (tetralogy of Fallot) all point to structural heart disease.

If the standard 12-lead ECG is abnormal, an echocardiogram is essential. Ventricular or atrial hypertrophy or an abnormality of QRS axis are all significant (Figs. 11.1, 11.2, 11.3, 11.4). A normal QRS axis (approximately 0–90 degrees) is indicated by both lead 1 and aVF having predominantly upright QRS waves. This rule does not hold true in young infants, where a degree of right axis deviation is to be expected.

A so-called partial or incomplete right bundle branch block pattern is often a normal variant, but can point towards an atrial septal defect. Left ventricular voltages are often tall in normal children and the diagnosis of left ventricular hypertrophy should only be made if the voltages are very tall or there is T-wave inversion (Fig. 11.5).

At the tertiary centre clinical assessment and echocardiogram is often all that is necessary, even if surgery is required. Other investigations depend upon the structural diagnosis.

Heart failure

Initial investigations are chest X-ray and ECG. The chest X-ray will usually show an enlarged heart. If there is a left-to-right shunt there will be increased pul-

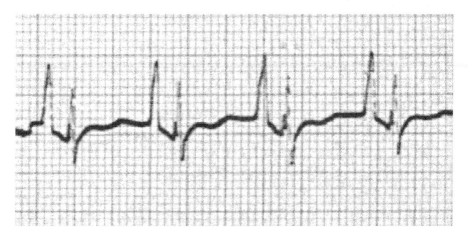

Fig. 11.1 **Right atrial hypertrophy: giant p waves (greater than 3 mm) in lead 2.**

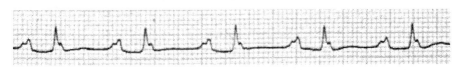

Fig. 11.2 **Left atrial hypertrophy: bifid p waves (wider than 0.1 seconds)**

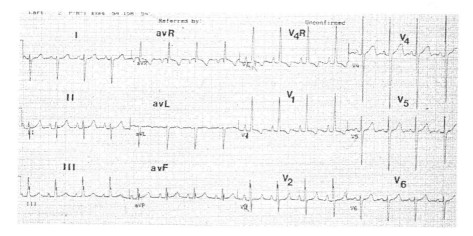

Fig. 11.3 **Right ventricular hypertrophy. Note the tall R wave in lead V1 and the deep S wave in lead V6. The deep S wave in lead I indicates that there is right axis deviation.**

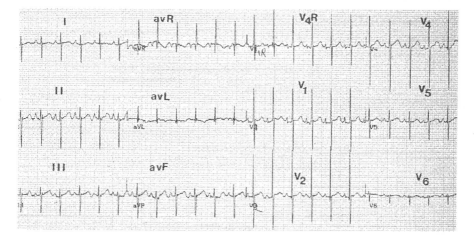

Fig. 11.4 **Abnormal axis: this ECG has a very abnormal QRS axis. Except in the neonatal period you expect the QRS to be predominantly positive in both lead I and aVF (i.e. the QRS axis is between 0 and 90 degrees). In this case both are negative, so the axis is opposite to normal, sometimes called a North-West axis.**

monary arterial markings. If the heart failure is due to a cardiomyopathy or myocarditis there will be pulmonary venous engorgement or even pulmonary oedema. An ECG may identify the presence of an arrhythmia, which may be amenable to immediate treatment. Tachyarrhythmias may be narrow complex or, less commonly, wide complex. Administration of adenosine intravenously is an important diagnostic tool for tachyarrhythmias (Fig. 11.6). Rarely an ECG in a child

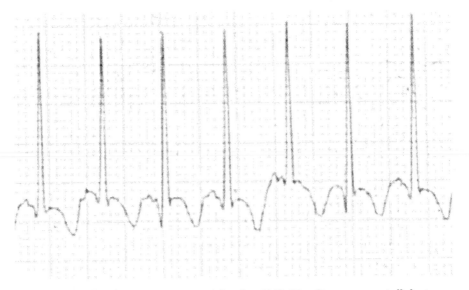

Fig. 11.5 **Left ventricular hypertrophy: lead V6. The R waves are tall, but more importantly the T-waves are inverted.**

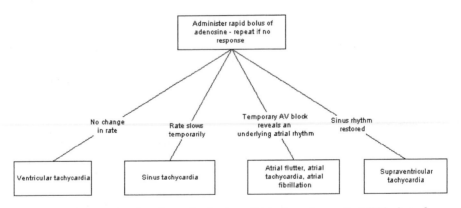

Fig. 11.6 **Diagnosis of tachyarrhythmias with adenosine: a fast IV bolus of 50 to 250 microgram/kg of adenosine is given to cause transient block at the atrioventricular node. It can be repeated after 2 minutes, if necessary. The ECG is monitored and recorded during the bolus administration. From the response the cause of the arrhythmia can be determined.**

with heart failure may show ischaemic changes if cardiac dysfunction is caused by a coronary anomaly either congenital or secondary to Kawasaki's disease. In cases of new-onset heart failure, urgent assessment at a specialist unit is usually essential.

Central cyanosis
Cyanotic heart disease needs urgent specialist assessment. A chest X-ray, ECG, echocardiogram, arterial oxygen saturation and haematocrit are the initial investigations. A hyperoxia test is used where, usually in a neonate, it is unclear

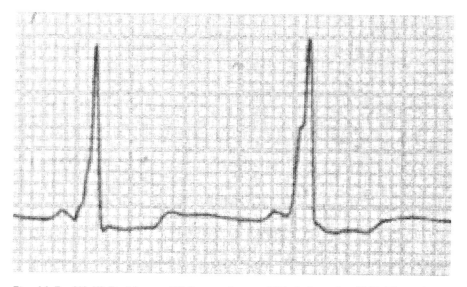

Fig. 11.7 **Wolff–Parkinson–White syndrome. This is from lead V4. There is a short PR interval and a delta wave — a slurred upstroke to the QRS complex revealing the presence of an accessory pathway; the commonest cause of supraventricular tachycardia in children.**

whether the hypoxia is respiratory in origin or caused by a right to left shunt. It is not a test for structural heart disease, since right to left shunts can occur in structurally normal hearts. A hyperoxia test is not needed if there is other evidence of structural heart disease.

Palpitations

A paediatrician should do a 12-lead ECG. Abnormalities of the P wave, the PR interval, pre-excitation — delta waves (see Fig. 11.7), or prolongation of the QT interval (see Fig. 11.8) should be sought. If the ECG is abnormal or the history is strongly suggestive of an arrhythmia a 24-hour ECG should be done.

A specialist unit will do an echocardiogram, further ambulatory ECG recording and, possibly, an exercise test and electrophysiological study.

Syncope

An ECG might show evidence of structural heart disease or an arrhythmia. Abnormalities of the T waves may be present in cardiomyopathies and long QT syndrome. Syncope thought to be cardiac in origin (more likely when associated with or following exercise) should be referred directly to a specialist centre. An echocardiogram and ECG would be the initial investigations. Tilt testing, ambulatory ECG and exercise testing are possible further investigations. The choice would depend on whether the cause was a structural abnormality or an arrhythmia.

Chest pain

The history will usually not indicate a cardiac origin and no tests are necessary in most cases. If cardiac chest pain is suspected a paediatrician should do an

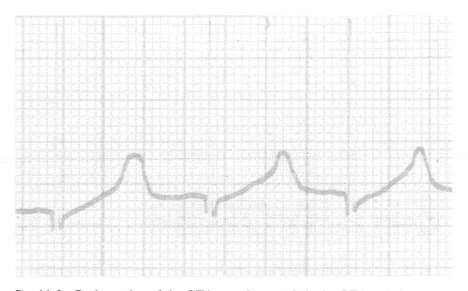

Fig. 11.8 **Prolongation of the QT interval: not only is the QT interval very long, occupying more than half of the R–R interval, but the morphology of the ST segment and T wave is very abnormal. QT interval is 500 msec, R–R interval is 760 msec. The heart rate corrected QT interval (QT/$\sqrt{R\text{–}R}$) is 570 msec (normal is < 450 msec in infants, < 440 msec in children and < 425 msec in adults).**

ECG, looking for evidence of structural heart disease, arrhythmia, cardiomyopathy or, rarely in children, ischaemia, and arrange specialist echocardiography.

A specialist centre might do an exercise ECG and radionuclide myocardial perfusion study.

3. Practical details of tests

Echocardiogram

A child must lie reasonably still for an echocardiogram. Sedation is often required in young children, particularly in the 1–3 years age group. The value of the examination depends critically on the skill and expertise of the operator. Experience with and knowledge of congenital heart disease is vital.

Positioning the probe for specific views

There are, by convention, a number of 'standard views' obtained from a variety of sites on the chest and upper abdomen. These will be covered in turn, highlighting variations that can be obtained where appropriate. The positioning of the ultrasound probe is limited to echocardiographic 'windows' where there is little or no air (lungs) between the probe and the heart; ultrasound does not travel well through air. These windows are subcostal, apical, parasternal and suprasternal.

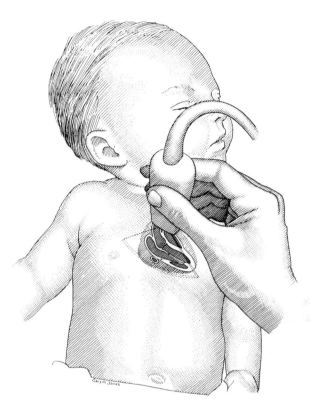

Fig. 11.9   **The position of the transducer and orientation of the scanning plane to provide a parasternal long-axis image of the heart.**

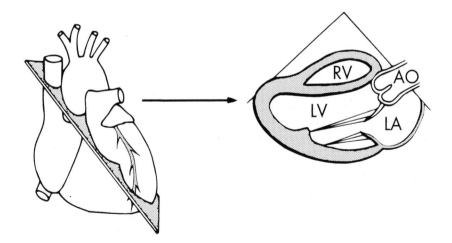

Fig. 11.10   **Parasternal long-axis view. Reproduced with permission from Park (1995).**

There are three axes which are conventionally used in describing cross-sectional images. These cut the heart in **long-axis, short-axis** and **four-chamber** planes. These three planes are at *right angles* to each other and, generally speaking, it is possible to view most of the structures of the heart through images obtained in these planes.

The apex of the heart is usually in the left chest, although in the neonate the bulk of the heart is often more midline. It is important to define not just the position but also the orientation of the heart, as this has implications for other structures both within and without the heart. The orientation can be defined in terms of the direction of the apex and the position of the great vessels. Only once the position and orientation are known can the transducer be manipulated to obtain the standard echocardiographic views.

Long-axis plane

The scanning plane transects the heart along its longitudinal axis (Figs 11.9–11.10) from the base and root of the aorta towards the apex (akin to slicing a green pepper longitudinally, leaving the stalk protruding from the slice). This provides an image of the left heart structures from the left atrium to the aorta with the interventricular septum and a small part of the right ventricle anteriorly.

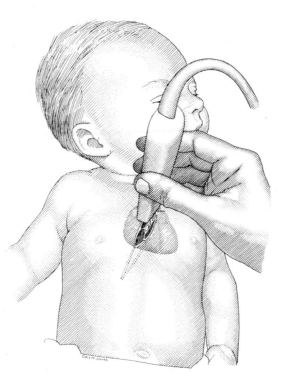

Fig. 11.11 The position of the transducer and orientation of the scanning plane to provide a parasternal short-axis image of the heart at the aortic valve level.

Short-axis plane

The short axis is at 90° to the long axis and cuts the heart transversely (rather like slicing rings from the green pepper). Short-axis views are obtained from the parasternal position by rotating through 90° from a long axis (Fig. 11.11). Tilting of the probe allows different structures to be visualised (Fig. 11.12). The standard 'midlevel' cut provides an image of the right heart as it wraps round the left ventricle and outflow tract. The right atrium, tricuspid valve, right ventricle, RVOT and main pulmonary artery can be seen around the central aortic valve and coronary arteries. By tilting up towards the sternal notch a higher cut demonstrates the right ventricular outflow, pulmonary arteries and, if present, the arterial duct. Tilting down towards the apex brings the left ventricle into view in a cross-section with the mitral valve structures gaping like a 'fish mouth' as the leaflets open and close. Further manipulation of the probe in this position

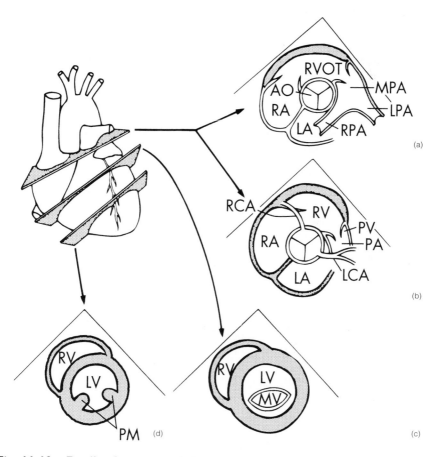

Fig. 11.12   Family of parasternal short-axis views sweeping from the base of the heart: (a) shows the bifurcation of the pulmonary arteries, RPA and LPA; (b) shows the right and left coronary artery origins (RCA and LCA); (c) cuts through the mitral valve, and (d) cuts through the two papillary muscles near the apex of the left ventricle. Reproduced with permission from Park (1995).

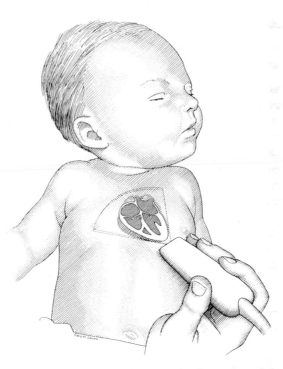

Fig. 11.13 **The position of the transducer and orientation of the scanning plane to provide an apical four-chamber view of the heart.**

allows better views of RVOT, pulmonary arteries, duct and descending aorta. Short-axis images are often obtained from the parasternal position, but can also be obtained subcostally.

Four-chamber plane

This third plane is at 90° to the other two and provides further images along the long axis of the heart, cutting through the four chambers of the heart. Four-chamber views are possible from the apex and subcostal positions (Figs 11.13– 11.16) but not from the parasternum. The probe is placed at the apex in a near coronal plane (at 90° to the orientation that allows a 'longitudinal axis' view and parallel to the bed the infant is lying on). Tilting up towards the front of the chest brings the left ventricular outflow tract (LVOT) into view, providing the so-called 'five-chamber' view (the fifth 'chamber' being the aorta). Tilting back may bring the coronary sinus into view behind the left atrium.

The subcostal position allows these views to be developed and is a good position for examining the interatrial septum and much of the interventricular septum as they lie at 90° to the ultrasound waves and thus are maximally echogenic. By tilting the probe anteriorly and posteriorly much of the atrial and ventricular septa can be seen. With posterior tilt the floor of the atria and the entry of the pulmonary veins into the left atrium can be seen, as can the coronary sinus running in the atrioventricular groove behind the left atrium and opening into the right atrium.

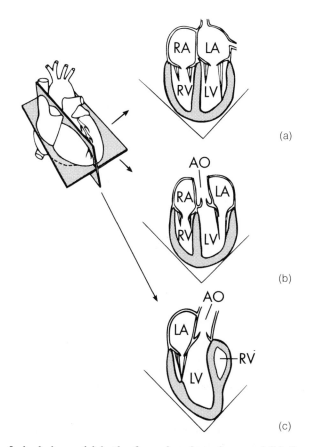

Fig. 11.14   Apical views. (a) is the four chamber view, and (b) the apical five chamber view including the aorta, from an anterior tilt. (c) is ninety degrees to (a) and (b) and is an apical long-axis view. Reproduced with permission from Park (1995).

Rotating the probe anticlockwise in the subcostal position brings the RVOT into view anteriorly, with the right atrium posteriorly and aorta centrally. This is then a subcostal short-axis view and is analogous to the 'right anterior oblique' view in cardiac catheterisation. Tilting the probe in this orientation allows other short-axis views to be obtained from the base to the apex of the heart.

Great vessels
The origin of both pulmonary arteries can usually be seen in the standard short-axis views.

The LVOT and some of the descending aorta can be seen in some of the views described above, but the ascending aorta, arch and descending aorta can only be seen in their entirety from the suprasternal window. It is often useful to extend the infant's neck by placing a small roll under the shoulders so that the scanning

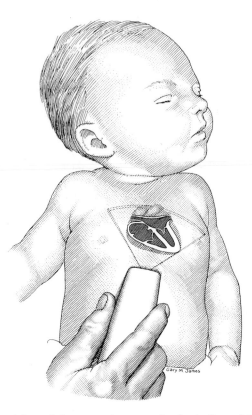

Fig. 11.15 **The position of the transducer and orientation of the scanning plane to provide a subcostal four-chamber image of the heart.**

head can be placed in the suprasternal notch (Fig. 11.17). The probe is angled so that the scan plane follows the line of the aorta. This is titled and rotated slightly from a sagittal cut (towards the left shoulder) since the ascending arch passes to the right of the midline and the descending aorta lies to the left of the midline. By tilting the probe in this plane the aortic valve, ascending aorta, arch and descending aorta can be seen along with the distal end of the arterial duct. The right pulmonary artery is seen in cross-section as it passes underneath the ascending aorta.

A transverse cut in the suprasternal position, angled slightly posteriorly, demonstrates the innominate vein as it comes across anteriorly from the left subclavian vein to join the superior vena cava.

The inferior vena cava, in its course through the liver, can be seen well from the subcostal position by scanning in a sagittal orientation, vertically through the liver. Angulation allows the vessel to be followed into the right atrium. The IVC is a right-sided structure and by tilting the probe slightly to the left, the descending aorta can be brought into view in a more posterior position. The mesenteric and coeliac axis arteries can often be seen in this view as they arise anteriorly from the descending aorta.

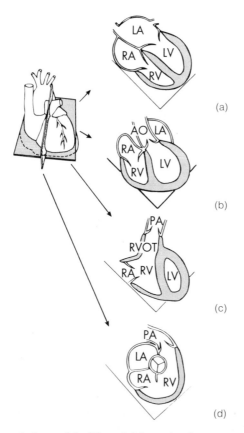

Fig. 11.16 **Subcostal views. (a), (b) and (c) are in the transverse or four-chamber plane. (a) shows the four chambers. (b) is obtained with a slight anterior tilt to show the aortic outlet ('five chamber view') and (c) is further anterior showing the right ventricular outlet. To obtain the view in (d), the transducer is rotated anticlockwise through ninety degrees and shows a subcostal short axis view. Reproduced with permission from Park (1995).**

The pulmonary veins can usually be seen entering into the back of the left atrium. However, it is often not possible to identify all four veins in a single image, and a number of cuts from different positions may be necessary.

Trans-oesophageal echocardiogram
General anaesthesia is used in children.

Magnetic resonance scan
Sedation is generally required in young children. Some centres use general anaesthesia. The presence of pacemakers and some metal implants preclude the use of MRI. MR scanners can be very noisy. Boredom and, occasionally, claustrophobia cause problems in some older children.

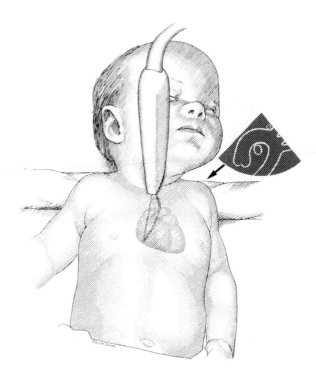

Fig. 11.17 **The position of the transducer and orientation of the scanning plane required to obtain views of the aortic arch with a conventional left-sided aorta. Note that a roll has been placed behind the shoulders to extend the neck.**

Radionuclide angiography

Intravenous access is needed. Sedation is generally required in young children.

Cardiac catheterisation

Cardiac catheterisation is usually performed under general anaesthesia, but can be performed under sedation. Most commonly access is from percutaneous puncture of the femoral artery and vein. Occasionally access is from a brachial, axillary or jugular approach. Overnight admission afterwards is usual, although some catheters are done as daycase procedures.

Electrophysiological study

Access is similar to cardiac catheterisation. It is usually performed under general anaesthesia in children.

Hyperoxia test

An infant is given greater than 80% oxygen to breathe for more than 10 minutes. If the arterial PO_2 rises to more than 20 kPa (150 mmHg) a right to left shunt is unlikely; if it rises to more than 27 kPa (200 mmHg) a right to left shunt is not present.

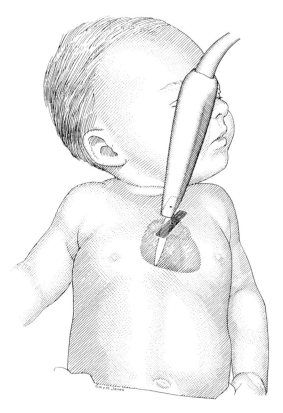

Fig.11.18 **Movement of the foot of the probe is required to bring the ductal view, roughly half-way between a parasternal short-axis view at the aortic valve level and an suprasternal view of the aortic arch.**

3. Checklist

Heart failure, cyanotic heart disease:

- ECG to exclude arrhythmia, chest X-ray, arterial oxygen saturation
- Refer to specialist centre

Arterial hypoxia, but no other evidence of heart disease:

- If no respiratory signs consider hyperoxia test to exclude right to left shunt

Other evidence of structural heart disease:

- Arrange for specialist paediatric echocardiography, consider referral to specialist centre depending on diagnosis

Probable innocent murmur:

- Discharge on clinical grounds if confident
- Consider chest X-ray, 12-lead ECG
- Echocardiogram if still unsure

Palpitations:

- 12-lead ECG
- Consider ambulatory ECG, exercise ECG or event monitor

Syncope:

- If history suggests cardiac cause, 12-lead ECG, chest X-ray, echocardiogram
- Consider ambulatory ECG and event monitor
- Consider exercise ECG
- Consider tilt testing

Chest pain:

- Consider non-cardiac causes
- If history suggests cardiac cause, 12-lead ECG, chest X-ray, echocardiogram
- Consider exercise ECG

ACKNOWLEDGEMENTS

Some of the text and figures on echocardiography are taken with permission from Chapter 1.4 in *Echocardiography for the Neonatologist* (ref), including contributions from Dr John Madar and Dr Stewart Hunter.

REFERENCES

Allan, L.D., Sharland, G.K., Milburn, A. et al. (1994) The prospective diagnosis of 1006 consecutive cases of congenital heart disease in the fetus. *Journal of the American College of Cardiologists* 23: 1452–1458

Baker, E.J. (1994) Congenital heart disease. In: Murray, I.P.C., Ell, P.J. *Nuclear Medicine in Clinical Diagnosis and Treatment*, pp 1229–1236. London: Churchill Livingstone.

Elliot, L.P. (1991) *Cardiac Imaging in Infants, Children and Adults*. Philadelphia: Lippincott.

Ho, S.Y., Baker, E.J., Rigby, M.L., Anderson, R.H. (1995) *Color Atlas of Congenital Heart Disease*. London: Mosby Wolfe.

Park, M.K., Guntheroth, W.G. (1987) *How to Read Pediatric ECGs*. Chicago: Year Book Medical Publishers

Skinner, J., Alverson, D.C., Hunter, S. (2000) *Echocardiography for the Neonatologist*. London: Churchill Livingstone.

12

Neurology

F Kirkham and V Ganesan

Introduction

The importance of making a diagnosis in a child presenting with neurological symptoms or signs lies not only in the potential for treatment but also in giving the family information in order to help them plan for the future. Neurological symptoms and signs are always worrying for the patient and family. As there is very little guidance on the appropriate use of investigations there is a temptation to perform all possible tests to make sure that nothing is missed. This may lead to unnecessary expense, and more importantly, discomfort to the child and distress to the family. There are also a number of important conditions which can be recognised clinically, but for which there is no diagnostic test. In reality, there is no substitute for a competent clinical history and examination.

This chapter attempts to provide a guide to the appropriate investigation of common neurological conditions. The emphasis is on the recognition of the constellation of signs, symptoms and positive investigation results in such conditions, whether congenital or acquired. Acute presentations, where decisions on appropriate treatment may prevent death or handicap, are particularly stressed. Mention is made of important conditions which are often overlooked, rather than attempting to be comprehensive. There is often a case for excluding important treatable conditions urgently and then either following the child for some time or asking the opinion of a paediatric neurologist, a geneticist or a developmental paediatrician.

I Physiology / anatomy / biochemistry

DEVELOPMENT OF THE CENTRAL NERVOUS SYSTEM

Development of the central nervous system (CNS) is a complex process which extends beyond intrauterine life to the early childhood years. It is dependent on a myriad of genetic and environmental factors at each stage. Both the nature and timing of insults to the developing nervous system influence the nature of the resultant malformation, and thus disorders can be considered as affecting neural tube closure, diverticulation, or neuronal migration, or involving destruction of formed structures. Prenatal insults may cause significant postnatal morbidity; this represents the thin end of the wedge, as up to 25% of all conceptuses are thought to have a developmental disorder of the CNS. These disorders contribute to the high rate of early fetal loss.

Broadly speaking, the causes of maldevelopment of the CNS can be thought of as being due to either genetic factors, factors affecting the intrauterine environment, or a combination of the two. Defective genetic material in the form of chromosomal anomalies, deletions or mutations leads to incorrect instructions being issued for CNS development; in the presence of normal genetic material, factors interfering with the interpretation of the genetic information can also have the same end result. Finally, the normal development of the nervous system may be disrupted by an insult and the resultant repair, or lack of repair, may lead to CNS maldevelopment.

The intrauterine environment can be contaminated by a number of factors which harm the developing nervous system. These include drugs (e.g. sodium valproate/phenytoin) or other substances such as alcohol ingested by the mother. Adequate intrauterine nutrition is also crucial for brain development. The effect of prenatal infections such as toxoplasmosis or rubella depends on the relative timing of the insult; infection early in gestation tends to produce more severe malformations, often not limited to the nervous system. Developmental anomalies in other organs or systems frequently coexist with neurological malformations. These may or may not be part of a recognised syndrome.

In 60% of infants with maldevelopment of the CNS the cause remains obscure. Although single gene defects and chromosomal anomalies are recognised aetiological factors, they account for only about 13% of all cases. Polygenic factors, in which there is an interaction between genes and environment, account for 20%, and environmental teratogens are identified in a further 3.5%. Accurate aetiological diagnosis in brain malformations rarely influences therapy for the individual affected; however, recognition of cause is helpful both in helping parents understand the mechanism of their child's handicap and in providing them with an estimate of the risk of recurrence in future pregnancies. The advent of prenatal diagnostic techniques, e.g. amniocentesis/chorionic villous sampling, has further increased the drive to understand the aetiology of neurological maldevelopment.

ANATOMY OF THE CSF PATHWAYS

CSF is an ultrafiltrate of plasma produced within the choroid plexus in the lateral and third ventricles at a rate of 0.5 ml/kg/h. Resorption of CSF from the subarachnoid space is via the arachnoid granulations. Blockage of the CSF within the ventricular system may cause obstructive hydrocephalus and acutely raised intracranial pressure. Blockage may occur at the foramen of Monro, in the third ventricle, at the aqueduct of Sylvius between the third and fourth ventricles, in the fourth ventricle or at the foraminae of Luschka and Magendie. Blockage may be secondary to a genetic anomaly (usually X-linked in association with flexed and adducted thumbs), malformation, tumour, bleeding or inflammation, e.g. secondary to meningitis. If CSF does not re-enter the blood at the arachnoid granulations freely, then communicating hydrocephalus results, which may also cause raised intracranial pressure, although often less acutely.

INTRACRANIAL PRESSURE

The pressure inside the head depends on the volume of three intracranial components: brain, blood and CSF (the Munro–Kellie doctrine). The fontanelle closes between six and eighteen months, and thereafter the skull is a rigid box, which cannot increase in size to accommodate any increase in volume. Baseline intracranial pressure (ICP) is up to 5 mmHg in infants, 10 mmHg in older children, and 20 mmHg in adults; this may increase for short periods, e.g. during coughing or sneezing. If the volume of one of the components increases, there may be some compensatory reduction of one of the other components. For example, blood volume may be slightly reduced, or CSF may be absorbed more quickly, or shunted into the subarachnoid space around the spinal cord, where it is also reabsorbed. Whether or not this compensation is able to take place depends partly on the size of any volume change and also on its rapidity. Once the compensatory reserve has been exhausted, the ICP may rise exponentially with small increases in the intracranial volume, putting the patient at risk of herniation of the temporal lobes through the tentorium, or the cerebellar tonsils through the foramen magnum. Cerebral perfusion pressure (CPP) equals mean arterial pressure minus ICP. ICP monitoring in the ITU situation enables optimalisation of CPP; the usual goal is to maintain ICP below 20 mmHg and to maintain CPP above 60–70 mmHg.

CEREBRAL BLOOD FLOW AND METABOLISM

Cerebral blood flow (CBF) varies between about 45 and 65 ml $100 \text{ g}^{-1} \text{ min}^{-1}$, although it may be higher than this value in mid-childhood and lower in neonates and infants. CBF is regulated over a wide range of perfusion pressures, approximately 50–150 mmHg in healthy adults, but probably narrower and with lower upper and lower limits in children. Below the lower limit and above the upper limit of autoregulation, CBF varies directly with perfusion pressure. The lower limit of autoregulation is lower when ICP is increasing than when blood pressure is decreasing. If CPP falls below the autoregulatory range, there is a significant risk of global ischaemia, although before this occurs there is usually a compensatory increase in oxygen extraction. The autoregulatory range may be altered by factors such as carbon dioxide (CO_2) tension, by drugs and in pathological circumstances such as coma, seizures or ischaemia.

CBF varies directly with arterial carbon dioxide tension ($paCO_2$) over a range of $paCO_2$s of approximately 2.5–8 kPa. Below 2.5 kPa and above 8 kPa, there is little change in CBF. The response of the cerebral circulation to $paCO_2$ is preserved under most circumstances but may be abolished at low perfusion pressure, by drugs such as indomethacin, and occasionally by very severe traumatic or ischaemic insults. CBF varies little with arterial oxygen tension (paO_2) over a very wide range of paO_2 but increases exponentially below a paO_2 of approximately 4 kPa.

CBF is closely coupled to the metabolic demand of the tissue and regional CBF increases during motor and cognitive tasks and sensory, e.g. visual, stimulation. Non-functioning or poorly functioning areas of tissue may have a low metabolic demand, therefore a low CBF. During seizures, the metabolic demand for oxygen and glucose increases manyfold, and under most circumstances CBF increases in parallel. CBF may be mapped using positron emission tomography (PET), single photon emission computer tomography (SPECT) and MR perfusion imaging. In patients with focal epilepsy, the epileptogenic focus often has a relatively low CBF between seizures (inter-ictally) and a relatively high CBF ictally, compared with the surrounding tissue. Changes in regional haemodynamics secondary to appropriate stimulation form the basis of functional magnetic resonance imaging (fMRI) studies.

2 Available tests and techniques

The tests available in paediatric neurology, together with their indications, requirements and limitations, are set out in Table 12.1. Individual tests are described later in the chapter.

ABBREVIATIONS USED IN THIS CHAPTER

ASOT — antistreptolysin O titres
AT — ataxia telangectasia
BSAEP — brain-stem evoked potentials
CBF — cerebral blood flow
CFAM — cerebral function analysing monitor
CMAP — compound muscle action potential
CPP — cerebral perfusion pressure
EMG — electromyography
ERG — electroretinogram
FA — Friedreich's ataxia
fMRI — functional MRI
HMSN — hereditary motor and sensory neuropathy
ICP — intracranial pressure
IDM — infant of diabetic mother

LBW — low birth weight
MELAS — mitochondrial encephalopathy with lactic acidosis
MUP — motor unit potential
NAI — non-accidental injury
PCR — polymerase chain reaction
PET — positron emission tomography
SOL — space-occupying lesion
SPECT — single photon emission computed tomography
SSEP — somatosensory evoked potentials
SSPE — subacute sclerosing panencephalitis
TBM — tuberculous meningitis
VEP — visual evoked potentials

CRANIAL ULTRASOUND SCAN

In young infants with an open fontanelle, cranial ultrasound using a B mode or sector scanner is a non-invasive means of visualising intracranial structures. The advantages of this technique are that it is easily performed at the bedside,

Table 12.1 Neurological tests and techniques

Type of test	Test	Main indications	Limitations	Requirements/notes
Imaging	Plain skull X-ray	Skull fracture Craniosynostosis	CT more appropriate for intracranial calcification	
	Plain X-ray spine	Suspicion of spina bifida occulta e.g. hairy/pigmented patch over spine	Normal study does not exclude spinal dysraphism; bifid L5/S1 common, not necessarily pathological	
	Ultrasound head	Neonatal • Haemorrhage • Ischaemia • Infarction • Hydrocephalus Infant • Hydrocephalus	May miss subdural effusions and malformations; operator dependent, therefore CT or MR often required for confirmation or exclusion of pathology	Open fontanelle
	Transcranial Doppler ultrasound • Diagnostic • Continuous monitoring	• Cerebrovascular disease (screening e.g. in sickle cell anaemia) • Vasospasm e.g. subarachnoid haemorrhage, meningitis • Change in velocity with physiological changes e.g. blood pressure, pCO_2, seizures	Some patients do not have acoustic window Cannot measure CBF as diameter of vessel not known	

Table 12.1 (continued)

Type of test	Test	Main indications	Limitations	Requirements/notes
	Computed tomography (CT scan)	Haemorrhage Tumour Abscess Ischaemia (focal stroke or global) Oedema Non-accidental injury Infarction (after 24 hours) Calcification Malformation Demyelination	Limited resolution; poor visualisation of posterior fossa structures. Radiation dose, therefore try to avoid frequent repeats or undertaking in susceptible patients e.g. those with Ataxia telangiectasia	Sedation/general anaesthesia for young or uncooperative children, although diagnostic scan may be obtained in many as time required often very short
	Contrast CT	Inflammation e.g. meningitis, tumour	Avoid in ischaemia if possible	
	Bone windows	Skull fracture		
	CT angiography	Cerebrovascular disease		Diagnosis or exclusion in ?NAI
	Magnetic resonance (MR scan) MR imaging	Spinal imaging e.g. tumour, trauma Posterior fossa tumour, inflammation, ischaemia Tumour Malformations Neuronal migration defects Ischaemia (focal or global) Haemorrhage Inflammation Demyelination Characteristic genetic disease e.g. Pelizaues Merzbacher, Hallervordan–Spatz	Poor delineation of areas of calcification. Must examine carefully for haemorrhage	Sedation/general anaesthesia for young or uncooperative children as scan usually takes around 1 hour

Table 12.1 (continued)

Type of test	Test	Main indications	Limitations	Requirements/notes
	MR angiography (circle of Willis and/or neck vessels)	Cerebral arterial circulation		
	MR venography	Cerebral venous sinuses		
	MR spectroscopy	Characteristic genetic disease e.g. Canavan's, guanidinoacetate methyltransferase deficiency		
	MRI with FLAIR sequence	Inflammation e.g. *Herpes simplex*		
	MRI with coronal cuts through temporal lobes and hippocampi, T2 mapping of hippocampi, MP-range	Hippocampal sclerosis, dysembryoplastic neuro-ectodermal tumour, cortical dysplasia in patients with intractable complex partial seizures		
	3D data sets			
	Diffusion MRI	Acute ischaemia		
	Perfusion MRI	Focal reduction in CBF		
	Functional MRI (fMRI)	Mapping of changes in functional topography of the brain e.g. after stroke		
	Cerebral angiography	Haemorrhagic stroke — arteriovenous malformation, aneurysm	1% risk of associated neurological event	Main use is to detect small vessel disease or plan surgical management
		Ischaemic stroke — occlusion (with or without moyamoya), stenosis, dissection of large vessels, small vessel vasculitis		
	Single photon emission computed tomography (SPECT)	Focal areas of reduced perfusion e.g. associated with cortical dysplasia in patients with intractable epilepsy or distal to large-vessel disease	Requires isotope	

Table 12.1 (continued)

Type of test	Test	Main indications	Limitations	Requirements/notes
	Ictal SPECT	Focal area of increased perfusion at the site of seizure onset in patients with intractable focal complex partial seizures	Injection should be made during seizure if possible or immediately afterwards, although scan may be done a few hours later	
	Position emission tomography (PET)	Focal areas of reduced perfusion e.g. associated with cortical dysplasia in patients with intractable epilepsy	Requires isotope with short half-life, therefore isotope must be generated on-site and scan must be done immediately	
	Barium swallow	Hiatus hernia	Does not exclude reflux oesophagitis	
	Video fluoroscopy	Sucking and swallowing inco-ordination		Needs to be carried out in conjunction with speech therapist
	Video-urodynamics	Neuropathic bladder e.g. in association with spina bifida or cerebral palsy	Risk of urinary infection	Cover with 2/7 course of oral antibiotics
Neurophysiology	Electroencephalography (EEG)	Epilepsy Degenerative disease Coma Encephalitis	Normal EEG does not exclude epilepsy	Sleep record may be useful in specific situations
	Electroretinogram (ERG)	Batten's Retinitis pigmentosa Visual impairment		May be diagnostic before clinical retinitis pigmentosa apparent e.g. in Laurence Moon–Biedl or Senior syndrome

Table 12.1 (continued)

Type of test	Test	Main indications	Limitations	Requirements/notes
	Visual evoked potentials (VEP)	Optic neuritis Visual impairment Degenerative disease	May recover after acute insult, therefore of limited use prognostically	
	Brain-stem evoked potentials (BSAER)	Degenerative disease Hearing impairment Prognosis for coma	Not if wave I absent	Requires expert interpretation
	Somatosensory evoked potentials (SSEP)	Prognosis for coma Monitoring in spinal cord surgery		Requires expert interpretation
	Electromyography (EMG)	Myopathy Myasthenia (single fibre study/ repetitive stimulation), Botulism (repetitive stimulation) Myotonic dystrophy Denervation (anterior horn cell disease)	Uncomfortable, therefore difficult to repeat; repetitive stimulation may require general anaesthesia Often normal in neonate	Requires expert performance and interpretation in the context of the clinical symptoms and signs Examine mother of neonate for example Spinal muscular atrophy, Polio
	Nerve conduction	Neuropathy e.g. Guillain–Barré syndrome (GBS)	Uncomfortable, therefore difficult to repeat	More useful for diagnosis of Guillain–Barré than CSF protein
Lumbar puncture	Opening pressure	Meningitis, benign intracranial hypertension, communicating hydrocephalus, post-haemorrhagic hydrocephalus in neonate	Contraindicated in early stages of acute coma; must cover with third generations cephalosporin if febrile and anti-TB treatment if hydrocephalus	Clinical assessment to assess safety of procedure + CT scan to exclude space-occupying lesion, obstructive hydrocephalus or severe cerebral oedema
	Glucose	Distinction between bacterial or tuberculous (low glucose) and viral meningitis (normal glucose)		Must do simultaneous true blood glucose — CSF glucose should be greater than 2/3 of blood glucose

Table 12.1 (continued)

Type of test	Test	Main indications	Limitations	Requirements/notes
	Protein	Tuberculous meningitis Tumour Inflammation	Protein usually normal early in Guillain–Barré syndrome therefore nerve conduction is investigation of choice	Neonate — normal <1.2 g/L Age 6/12 — normal <0.25 g/L Age >1 year — normal <0.4 g/L
	White cell count and differential	Meningitis (bacterial, viral, tuberculous, Lyme and other)		Lymphocytes $>$ polymorphs may imply TB meningitis or partially treated bacterial meningitis rather than viral meningitis or encephalitis
	Red blood cells	Non-accidental injury Subarachnoid haemorrhage Meningitis Encephalitis		After a traumatic tap, the blood should be less in the third bottle
	Ziehl–Neelsen staining Lowenstein–Jensen culture	Tuberculous meningitis	Searching for acid-fast bacilli may take hours; culture may take several months	Anti-TB treatment required if high index of suspicion
	Indian ink stain	Cryptococcus meningitis		Consider in immunodeficient patients or those infected with HIV
	Bacterial/viral PCR	Meningitis/encephalitis e.g. TB, *Herpes simplex*, enteroviruses	Very sensitive to environmental contamination, frequent false positives	
	Meales antibody	Subacute sclerosing panencephalitis		
	Cytospin	Tumour Neuroblastoma Leukaemia		

Table 12.1 (continued)

Type of test	Test	Main indications	Limitations	Requirements/notes
	Oligoclonal bands	Demyelination Inflammatory disease		Send simultaneous blood sample
	Lactate	Encephalopathy, muscle weakness, pigment retinopathy, external ophthalmoplegia, hearing impairment		High levels suggest mitochondrial disease
	Glycine	Neonatal convulsions		High — Non-ketotic hyperglycinaemia
Blood tests	Chromosomes including fragile X	Learning difficulties Dysmorphic syndromes	Fragile X testing relatively expensive and detection rate <1% if undertaken in all children with learning difficulties	Fragile X indicated if poor eye contact, friendly personality, echolalic, large protuberant ears, long face, wide forehead, hyperextensible joints, tall slim physique, eunuchoid habitus or family history of learning difficulties
	DNA analysis	High level of suspicion for disorder where specific defect is recognised	Expensive, requires careful liaison with laboratory	e.g. Angelman's, Prader–Willi, Friedreich's ataxia, ataxia telangiectasia
	Alpha-feto protein	Ataxia		Raised in ataxia telangiectasia
	DNA fragility in irradiated lymphocytes	Ataxia		Used in diagnosis of ataxia telangiectasia

Table 12.1 (continued)

Type of test	Test	Main indications	Limitations	Requirements/notes
	Full blood count and film	Ataxia Progressive disease e.g. cognitive deterioration with epilepsy, extrapyramidal disorders		*Vacuolated lymphocytes* e.g. juvenile neuronal ceroid lipofuscinosis. *Acanthocytes* e.g. abetalipoproteinaemia, Hallervordan–Spatz, neuroacanthocytosis
	Creatinine	Epilepsy Developmental delay		Low in guanidinoacetate methyltransferase deficiency, a treatable inborn error of creatine metabolism
	Blood gas	Acute/chronic encephalopathy		Acidosis in organic acidaemias
	Creatine kinase	Muscular dystrophy, Myopathy Inflammatory muscle disease		High in muscular dystrophy; may be normal in dermatomyositis; AST may be more useful
	Acetylcholine receptor antibodies	Ptosis, ophthalmoplegia, bulbar weakness,		High in myasthenia gravis
	Lactate	Encephalopathy, muscle weakness, pigment retinopathy, external ophthalmoplegia, hearing impairment	Normal blood lactate does not exclude mitochondrial disease	High in mitochondrial disease
	Ammonia	Encephalopathy Hypoglycaemia		Urea cycle defects Organic acidaemia
	Amino acids			Disorders of amino acid metabolism

Table 12.1 (continued)

Type of test	Test	Main indications	Limitations	Requirements/notes
	Very long fatty chain acids	Hypotonia, Dysmorphic features, Chondrodysplasia punctata, Leucodystrophy		Peroxisomal disorder (e.g. Zellwegger syndrome, adrenoleukodystrophy)
	Biotinidase	Seizures, visual impairment, stridor, alopecia		Low in Biotinidase deficiency Treat with biotin until result received
	Acid phosphatase			High in infantile Gaucher's
	White cell enzymes	Progressive disease (p 342)	Expensive often worth screening first — e.g. with blood film	Must inform laboratory of clinical history and examination
Urine Tests	Amino acids	Encephalopathy Movement disorder Spastic paraparesis Microcephaly (check mother for PKU)		Aminoaciduria Fanconi-type tubulopathy e.g. in mitochondrial disease, Lowe's oculocerebrornal syndrome
	Organic acids	Encephalopathy Hypoglycaemia	Exclusion of disorders may require high performance liquid chromatography	Organic acidaemia
	Mucopolysaccharides	Learning difficulties (± coarse facies)		Hunter's, Hurler's, Sanfilippo
	Metachromatic granules	Ataxia Leucodystrophy	Urine needs to be fresh	Metachromatic leucodystrophy
	Urinary N acetyl aspartate	Macrocephaly and leucodystrophy		Canavan's disease
	Sulfite	Neonatal seizures		Sulfite oxidase deficiency, molybdenum cofactor deficiency

Table 12.1 (continued)

Type of test	Test	Main indications	Limitations	Requirements/notes
	Sialic acid	Progressive disease (p 342)		Salla disease
Biopsy	Muscle	Myopathy Muscular dystrophy Inflammatory muscle disease Mitochondrial disease	Needle muscle biopsy may be difficult in toddlers or if muscle mass is very reduced; open biopsy usually required for enzymology	Close liaison between operator/surgeon and laboratory to ensure that specimen is transferred to laboratory quickly and correctly processed
	Nerve	Peripheral neuropathy		Expert histopathological interpretation
	Skin	Mitochondrial disease Degenerative disease		Enzyme measurement in cultured fibroblasts (e.g. in cytochrome oxidase deficiency); electron microscopy for inclusions in Batten's disease, Infantile/juvenile neuroxonal dystrophy Abnormal sweat glands in Lafora body disease
		Progressive myoclonic epilepsy		
	Rectum	Visual impairment Dementia Myoclonic epilepsy Degenerative disease	Invasive, therefore reserved for typical cases with negative skin or conjunctival biopsy	Neuronal ceroid lipofuscinosis (Batten's disease)
	Conjunctiva	Degenerative disorder		Neuronal ceroid lipofuscinosis (Batten's disease), Infantile/juvenile neuroxonal dystrophy
	Sweat glands	Pain insensitivity Degenerative disorder		Lafora's disease

Table 12.1 (continued)

Type of test	Test	Main indications	Limitations	Requirements/notes
	Liver	Intractable epilepsy and abnormal liver enzymes		Alper's disease
Therapeutic trial	Pyridoxine	Seizures in neonates and children up to the age of 2 years	Extreme caution if test dose is given IV as this may lead to electro-cerebral silence in patients with true pyridoxine dependency.	Pyridoxine deficiency or dependency. Oral dose is 200 mg/day for 3–5 days
	Biotin	Seizures in neonates and infants		Biotinidase deficiency
	L-DOPA	Movement disorder with diurnal variation		Dopa responsive dystonia (Segawa syndrome)
	Tensilon test	Ptosis, ophthalmoplegia, bulbar weakness, recurrent apnoeas, generalised weakness		Myasthenia (gravis or congenital)
Autonomic testing		Hypotonia, poor feeding, lack of tears, insensitivity to pain		Riley–Day syndrome

without the need for sedation or exposure to ionising radiation. Serial studies can be performed easily. Coronal, sagittal and parasagittal views can be taken, and enable study of the size of CSF spaces and, to a more limited extent, parenchymal tissue. Ultrasound is of particular value in looking for and monitoring hydrocephalus; other abnormalities such as haemorrhage within or outside the ventricles and, to a more limited extent, anomalies of structure can also be seen. The limitation of cranial ultrasound is that the signal is reflected and refracted better at interfaces than within cerebral parenchymal tissue. Collections in the subdural or subarachnoid space may also be missed. The technique is also extremely operator-dependent. A normal cranial ultrasound should not be interpreted as excluding structural or parenchymal abnormalities.

COMPUTERISED TOMOGRAPHY

Computerised tomography of the brain is widely available and will in most instances be the first-line modality for neuroimaging. The commonest practical difficulty encountered in scanning children is the necessity for sedation in order that the child lies still for a sufficient period of time to enable the investigation to be performed. However, in modern scanners brain imaging can usually be achieved in around 10 minutes.

Communication of clinical information to the radiology department is important, to ensure that the optimal form of imaging is carried out. CT of the brain is usually carried out in the axial plane with slices taken 5–10 mm apart but in specific situations it may be appropriate to take thinner slices for visualisation of specific structures, e.g. orbital cavity/pituitary fossa. Intravenous contrast may be given to further clarify the nature of any abnormalities or in the appropriate clinical situation where no abnormality is visualised on the non-enhanced scan.

In the emergency situation, the CT scan is helpful in the detection of intracranial haemorrhage, infection, hydrocephalus, cerebral oedema or space-occupying lesions. Thus it enables detection of most pathology needing emergency treatment, and is the modality of choice in the acutely ill child.

In many childhood diseases the CT scan will be helpful diagnostically or may serve as a pointer for the direction of further investigations. However, in some situations the precise nature of pathology may not be immediately apparent and it may be necessary to follow the temporal progression of the neuroimaging before diagnostic information is obtained. It is important to bear in mind that white matter lesions or defects of neuronal migration are better visualised on MRI, as are posterior fossa structures. It may therefore be helpful in selected clinical situations to progress to MRI for further clarification of cerebral pathology.

MAGNETIC RESONANCE IMAGING

Magnetic resonance imaging allows detailed imaging of intracranial structures, including cerebral vessels, without exposure to ionising radiation. As with CT, the patient is required to be still for the investigation, and sedation or anaesthesia may be required in young children. The duration of the investigation is longer, particularly for spinal cord imaging.

The signal in magnetic resonance images is derived from the protons in hydrogen. These are most abundant in body water. Tissue contrast is dependent not only on the concentrations of free and bound water in the area under study but also on the sequence used for imaging. The terms T1 and T2 refer to the relaxation times used in a particular sequence. The determination of the most appropriate sequence depends on the nature of the clinical problem under consideration and it is therefore important that the full clinical picture is drawn to the attention of the neuroradiologist.

Images are usually taken in three planes, sagittal, coronal and axial. Intravenous gadolinium may be given as a contrast agent. MRI is useful in detection of structural pathology, in detecting ischaemic changes, in looking for white matter pathology and in detailed visualisation of posterior fossa structures.

Magnetic resonance angiography (MRA) enables visualisation of the cerebrovascular tree down to vessels of 1 mm calibre. This technique can be used for detection of cerebrovascular disease and can therefore be used to screen populations at risk, e.g. children with sickle cell disease. Visualisation of the venous circulation can also be achieved and this is useful for detection of sagittal sinus thrombosis, e.g. in nephrotic syndrome. There are limitations to this technique and there is still a role for contrast angiography, for instance for the diagnosis of vasculitis, which often involves the small vessels, or for imaging of the posterior circulation. Dissection of the carotid or vertebral arteries may be diagnosed using fat-saturated MRI of the neck, but may require conventional arteriography.

There are other techniques of magnetic resonance imaging — FLAIR sequences, MR spectroscopy, MR diffusion and MR perfusion imaging and functional MR imaging, which are at present research techniques but will, within the near future, revolutionise our investigation and understanding of cerebral pathophysiology.

NEUROPHYSIOLOGY

I. EEG

EEG enables assessment both of global cerebral function and of focal abnormalities. The role of the EEG in clinical practice is not therefore limited to the investigation of epilepsy. The technique of obtaining recordings in young children requires a sympathetic and opportunistic approach and the presence of their parents may provide reassurance. It is preferable to obtain an unsedated record if at all possible, although in some situations sleep records may provide useful additional information. Stick-on electrodes are better tolerated by children and may be correctly placed for the International 10–20 electrode placement system within a specially-designed cap. Comments can be made about the background activity, the presence of normal rhythms, the responses to activation procedures and the type, distribution and electroclinical correlates of any abnormal rhythms or discharges.

It is important to realise that the normal EEG matures during childhood and therefore has to be interpreted accordingly. Abnormalities of rhythm can also show age-related patterns, e.g. hypsarrhythmia in young infants. Procedures such as photic stimulation, overbreathing or eye closure may be helpful in eliciting both physiological responses and patterns suggestive of pathology. Drugs, both sedative and anticonvulsant, can affect the EEG and an accurate drug history must be provided. The administration of pyridoxine under EEG control can be diagnostic in pyridoxine-dependent seizures. However, this should be done with extreme caution as it may precipitate cardiorespiratory collapse in patients with pyridoxine dependency.

The EEG remains the cornerstone of investigation in epilepsy. Firstly, it can help to determine whether or not paroxysmal clinical phenomena have an epileptic basis. This may be particularly difficult to determine by clinical judgement alone, especially in the young infant. Simultaneous video and EEG recording during an episode is of particular value in this context. A 24-hour recording may provide evidence for epileptiform discharges, but must be interpreted alongside the carer's documentation of events. In children with epilepsy, the EEG enables definition of the particular electroclinical syndrome affecting the patient, e.g. infantile spasms and hypsarrhythmia. This gives information which is of value in determining aetiology, treatment and prognosis. It should, however, be borne in mind that a normal EEG does not exclude epilepsy; this is particularly true in cases where the semiology is suggestive of complex partial seizures.

Although a recording during an episode is helpful, it is not always practicable, and most recordings take place in the inter-ictal period. The recent occurrence of a seizure is sometimes quoted as a reason for not carrying out a recording on the grounds that the post-ictal slowing will obscure any other abnormalities; in fact this rarely lasts for more than a few hours providing there are no complications resulting from the seizure. The nature of the problem may not be immediately apparent after the initial recording, and it may therefore be helpful to repeat the investigation at an appropriate interval; the progression observed in the sequential recordings may conform to a recognised pattern and thus provide clarification.

In children with epilepsy the EEG may enable localisation of the epileptogenic focus, thus targeting imaging and other investigations into aetiology. In the situation where seizures are resistant or control has deteriorated, studying the evolution of the EEG can be helpful in management; for example, the first EEG may have demonstrated a focal onset although subsequent EEGs appear generalised. Sleep-deprivation may reveal an underlying focal epileptiform discharge in some patients.

Convulsive status epilepticus is usually clinically apparent; the EEG may be helpful in identification of any localisation phenomena. In the obtunded or paralysed, ventilated child the EEG can be the only means of identifying ongoing seizure activity of the effect of drug therapy. Monitoring can also be helpful in preventing overdosage of anaesthetic drugs as levels which produce electrocerebral silence can be associated with unwanted cardiovascular side-effects. Continuous monitoring can be carried out using a device such as the cerebral function analysing monitor (CFAM).

Non-convulsive status epilepticus should be suspected in the context of fluctuating consciousness, motor inco-ordination, cognitive or behavioural deterioration in a child with a history of seizures. The discrepancy between clinical symptoms and the EEG abnormality can be very striking and diagnosis depends on having a high index of clinical suspicion. In other children with cognitive or behavioural regression, either the awake or sleep EEG may be abnormal; possible syndrome diagnoses include Landau–Kleffner and electrical status in slow-wave sleep. The potential benefits of switching off the epileptiform discharges, regardless of whether they are associated with clinical seizures, is the subject of ongoing research.

In acute encephalopathies, the EEG is used both diagnostically, e.g. in *Herpes simplex* encephalitis (localised repetitive discharges), and to give prognostic information, e.g. after cardiac arrest. Regardless of aetiology, the EEG findings are of varying degrees of slow activity. Focal slowing can guide the search for aetiology, such as a space-occupying lesion. The EEG can be used as an adjunct to other methods in the determination of brain-stem death.

The role of the EEG in the investigation of structural, neurometabolic and vascular diseases in the paediatric neurology is vast and cannot be covered here. The clinical neurophysiologist must be given the full clinical picture in order to interpret the EEG also in order to decide whether or not complementary neurophysiological investigations would be helpful. The role of the EEG in non-epileptiform disorders is often underestimated; the EEG can give valuable clues which may guide other more invasive investigations, and in some situations may provide the only 'handle' on aetiology, for example high-voltage slow activity on passive eye closure in Angelman syndrome.

2. Evoked potentials

Measurement of evoked potentials allows the evaluation of the integrity of sensory pathways. It can also assist localisation of pathology, e.g. assessment of brain-stem auditory evoked potentials (BSAEPs), in looking for objective evidence of brain-stem dysfunction.

Visual evoked potentials (VEPs) allow assessment of the visual pathways from the eye to the occipital cortex. In older children or adults the stimulus used is a pattern (checkerboard); in younger children or infants, where co-operation is not possible, the response to a flash stimulus may be recorded. A flash stimulus can also be used to elicit an electroretinogram (ERG), thus enabling simultaneous assessment of retinal function. Patterns of dysfunction may be suggestive of a specific diagnosis, e.g. absent ERG in Batten's disease. Each response can be assessed either from monocular stimulation, necessitating closure of one eye, or by binocular stimulation.

BSAEPs can be recorded over the vertex in response to a click stimulus presented to the ear. The auditory pathway, from cochlea to brainstem, can be assessed. It is useful to note that BSAEPs are not affected by the state of arousal of the patient and can therefore usefully be carried out under sedation, possibly coinciding with sedation for other investigations. This is particularly useful in young children with learning difficulties and possible hearing impairment.

Somatosensory evoked potentials (SSEPs) are recorded from the scalp in response to stimulation of a peripheral nerve. Measurement of SSEPs allows assessment of the integrity of the afferent input into the cortex. SSEPs are particularly useful during spinal surgery (e.g. for scoliosis) in order to ensure that the integrity of the spinal cord is not deranged.

All evoked potentials mature over the early childhood years. It is important to bear this in mind when interpreting results so that false conclusions are not drawn. A combination of BSAEPs and SSEPs, together with EEG, may be used to predict outcome in unconscious patients, but expert interpretation is required.

3. Nerve conduction and electromyography

These investigations enable study of the peripheral nerves and the muscles and enable investigation of pathology involving the anterior horn cells, roots, plexuses, peripheral nerves, neuromuscular junction and muscles. Patterns of abnormality can suggest the nature of the underlying pathophysiology but, as with all investigations, a specific diagnosis can only be reached if the information is interpreted in the light of the clinical picture. It is usually useful to carry out both nerve conduction studies and EMG simultaneously and to regard these as complementary methods of investigating the peripheral nervous system.

Impulses are carried down peripheral nerves at a rate that is determined by the degree of myelination of the largest and fastest conducting fibres. Loss or deficiency of myelin will therefore slow the conduction velocity along a motor or sensory nerve. The size of the evoked action potential is dependent upon the number of anterior horn cells and the number of axons conducting the impulse. Axonal degeneration will, therefore, result in a reduction in the amplitude of this action potential. Conduction block is a term that refers to a local disruption of conduction, either because the nerve is trapped or because there is segmental demyelination.

Conduction in peripheral nerves is assessed by stimulating a peripheral nerve and measuring the resultant action potential in nerve or muscle. The stimulus is a brief electrical pulse, which is delivered through a surface pad electrode. The magnitude of the stimulus determines the number of responding fibres; a supramaximal stimulus is necessary for exciting all the fibres underlying the stimulus. The response is similarly usually recorded by means of surface electrodes. The characteristics of the response measured are the amplitude, form and distal motor latency (stimulus to response time). Motor conduction velocity can be measured by measuring the difference in distal motor latencies between two points a known distance apart. The amplitude of the action potential is a measure of the number of medium/large myelinated nerve fibres adjacent to the recording electrode.

Normal values for motor conduction in the adult are 50–70 m/s in the upper limb and 40–60 m/s in the lower limb; in the term infant these values are approximately halved. Adult values are reached at about 3 years. Nerve conduction velocity can be artificially slowed if the limb being studied is cold.

The compound muscle action potential (CMAP) is recorded in response to the stimulation of motor nerves. The amplitude of the CMAP is dependent on muscle mass and the synchrony of the discharges from the various motor units stimulated.

Electromyography is the study of the spontaneous, voluntary and evoked activity of the motor unit. The usual type of electrode used is called a concentric needle electrode; the recording is obtained by placing this into the area of muscle under study. 'Single fibre' EMG utilises a very fine needle electrode to study a small area in greater detail.

Spontaneous activity at rest can represent the fibrillation potentials seen in denervated muscle. In children with myotonic dystrophy, the spontaneous activity can take on the form of a 'dive bomber' discharge, although infants may not have a typical pattern and it is usually more useful to study the mother.

Voluntary activity of the motor unit is studied in the form, duration, amplitude, stability firing rate and relation to effort of the motor unit potential (MUP). Individual MUPs can be studied during weak effort or with stronger effort the overlapping of a number of MUPs creates an interference pattern, analysis of which can provide useful information about the site of the lesion. Tibialis anterior is the muscle usually sampled.

In myasthenic syndromes the clinical syndrome of fatiguability has an electrical correlate of a decremental response to repetitive stimulation of the motor nerve. This can be a useful step in the diagnosis of congenital myasthenia, but may require general anaesthesia in young children, as it is painful.

EXAMINATION OF THE CEREBROSPINAL FLUID

CSF examination remains crucial in the investigation of neurological diseases. The usual route of sampling is by lumbar puncture and the importance of measuring the opening pressure every time a lumbar puncture is carried out cannot be overemphasised. This is often neglected in paediatric practice and can therefore lead to a further lumbar puncture being carried out solely to determine pressure. Opening pressure is measured by means of a transducer or manometer attached to the spinal needle before any CSF has escaped. Most hospitals have disposable manometers used for the purpose of measuring central venous pressure (CVP) if no specific equipment is available. The normal opening pressure of lumbar CSF should be less than 15 cm of water. If the child is struggling or crying this value may be falsely elevated, therefore the procedure is usually performed under appropriate sedation, e.g. with intravenous Midazolam, and/or local anaesthesia.

The CSF should always be sent for estimation of its cellular content by microscopy. Culture of the CSF should also always be performed. Use of the polymerase chain reaction (PCR) to detect DNA from viruses or bacteria may be useful but it is important to discuss the case with the laboratory so that the appropriate organisms are sought. PCR has not superseded other investigations, in part because the sensitivity of the technique makes environmental contamination, and therefore false positive results, a common problem. Good communication with the laboratory will also ensure that appropriate staining and antibody tests are not neglected such as Ziehl–Neelsen stain for tuberculosis. In addition to the detection of organisms, determination of specific antibody titres in the CSF can also be helpful, e.g. titres of antibodies to measles virus where SSPE (subacute sclerosing panencephalitis) is suspected.

Normal CSF should contain fewer than 5 cells/mm^3. If the tap is traumatic, the white count will increase by 1 for every 700–800 red cells present. The presence of red cells must not always be taken to indicate a traumatic procedure; subarachnoid haemorrhage or HSV infection can cause the presence of blood in the CSF.

Routine biochemical analysis of the CSF consists of the estimation of the protein and glucose content of the fluid. Physiologically, the level of CSF protein is elevated in the neonatal period due to the increased permeability of the blood-brain barrier and can reach levels of 1.2 g/L; it then falls so that at 6 months the upper limit of normal is 0.25 g/L. In older children the upper limit of normal is the adult value of 0.4 g/L. The presence of blood in the CSF can elevate the protein. In addition to the determination of total CSF protein, which consists mostly of albumin, the determination of the presence of oligoclonal bands of immuglobulin may be helpful. These are indicative of specific antibody synthesis within the CNS and can therefore be detected in infectious, inflammatory and immunological conditions. The usual indication for looking for the presence of oligoclonal bands is the suspicion of a demyelinating or inflammatory disorder. It is important to remember that the presence of oligoclonal bands in the CSF can reflect 'spillover' from the blood, and therefore serum should be taken simultaneously for immunoglobulin estimation.

CSF glucose values can only be estimated in the light of blood glucose, which should always be measured simultaneously. CSF glucose should be two-thirds of blood glucose.

Where a mitochondrial cytopathy is suspected, the estimation of CSF lactate is a valuable diagnostic aid. This may be the only abnormal finding and may be elevated even if the plasma lactate is not raised. Given that the presentations of mitochondrial disease are so variable in childhood, the assessment of CSF lactate is useful in the investigation of many neurological syndromes.

Measurement of CSF glycine should form part of the investigation of neonatal seizures. In non-ketotic hyperglycinaemia, the plasma glycine may be normal, whereas the raised CSF glycine is diagnostic. The plasma: CSF glycine ratio may be useful in resolving equivocal cases; the normal ratio is <0.025.

GENETICS

The karyotype is useful in diagnosis of trisomies, deletions and translocations, e.g. Down syndrome. In individuals with developmental delay and characteristic clinical features (see Table 12.1), a search for fragile sites on the X chromosome should be instituted, as fragile X syndrome is one of the commonest causes of mental handicap in males, with an incidence of around 1:5000. Learning difficulties can, however, also affect female carriers.

The genetic basis of many diseases is now recognised, and this information is useful in confirmation of the diagnosis in affected individuals. Genetic tests do not provide a means of screening; rather they are highly specific investigations and the onus remains on the clinician to request the appropriate investigation in a patient with typical clinical symptoms and signs. Examples of conditions in which genetic confirmation of diagnosis is required are Fragile X syndrome, Duchenne muscular dystrophy, Prader–Willi syndrome, Angelman syndrome, Friedreich's ataxia, HMSN type 1, and myotonic dystrophy.

3 Investigation of diseases and symptoms

ACUTE PROBLEMS

Coma

Any reduction in the level of consciousness in a child is an acute emergency, particularly if the aetiology is unknown. History and examination are often diagnostic. It is essential to record vital signs, especially blood pressure, coma score, brain stem signs and any focal features. A CT scan should be performed before the lumbar puncture, particularly if the child is not localising pain, and/or there are signs of incipient cerebral herniation and/or the child is non-febrile. EEG is helpful in the management of status epilepticus as well as being of considerable diagnostic and prognostic help. It is well worth saving freshly frozen specimens of plasma, CSF and urine for later toxic or metabolic analysis.

Causes of coma are listed in the information box.

CAUSES OF COMA

- Accidental head injury
  Extradural haematoma
  Intracerebral haematoma
  Diffuse brain oedema
  Penetration, e.g. gunshot

- Non-accidental injury
  Subdural haemorrhage/
  effusion
  Intracerebral haemorrhage
  Hemispheric ischaemia
  secondary to carotid
  occlusion
  Diffuse brain oedema

- Infections
  Meningitis
  Pneumococcus
  Haemophilus
  Meningococcus
  Tuberculous
  Encephalitis
  Herpes simplex
  Enteroviruses
  Mycoplasma
  Cerebral malaria
  Cerebral abscess

- Shock
  Meningococcal shock
  Toxic shock syndrome
  (*Staphylococcus*)
  Haemorrhagic
  shock/encephalopathy

- Diabetic encephalopathy
  Ketotic
  Diffuse brain oedema

- Drug-induced coma/poisoning

- Status epilepticus

- Hypertensive encephalopathy
  Preceded by visual symptoms
  and seizures

- Hypoxic–ischaemic
  encephalopathy

- Hepatic encephalopathy
  Mild encephalopathy
  accompanied by foetor/flap
  Viral hepatitis

- Space-occupying mass
  Spontaneous intracerebral
  haemorrhage
  Ischaemic stroke — large
  hemispheric or brain-stem
  Tumour

Investigations of coma are detailed in Table 12.2.

Table 12.2 Investigation of coma

Investigation	Indication	Possible abnormality	Further investigation if abnormal	Possible diagnoses	Action
Dextrostix Blood Glucose	All	Low	Blood glucose Liver function tests Blood ammonia Blood lactate Blood and urine amino acids Urine organic acids	Hypoglycaemia a secondary to • Fasting • Severe illness • Reye's syndrome • Organic aciduria • Fatty acid oxidation defect • Haemorrhagic shock & encephalopathy	Intravenous dextrose
Blood sodium	All	Low High	Urinary sodium	Hypo/hypernatraemia ± dehydration	Appropriate fluids
Blood urea	All	High	Blood creatinine Blood film	Dehydration Haemolytic–uraemic syndrome	Dialysis, plasmapheresis
Aspartate transaminase	All	High	Blood ammonia	Reye's syndrome Hypoxic–ischaemic insult	
Blood ammonia	All	High	Blood orotic acid Urine organic acids	Urea cycle defect Organic acidaemia	Sodium benzoate

Table 12.2 (continued)

Investigation	Indication	Possible abnormality	Further investigation if abnormal	Possible diagnoses	Action
Full blood count and film	All	Low Hb	Hb electrophoresis	Anaemia	Transfusion
		High WBC		Infection	Antibiotics
		Low platelets		DIC, infection	
		Sickle cells		Sickle cell disease	
		Burr cells		Haemolytic–uraemic syndrome	Dialysis, plasmapheresis
		Parasites on thick/thin films		Malaria	Antimalarials
		Basophilic stippling		Lead encephalopathy	Chelation
Blood culture	All				
Mycoplasma titres	All		Chest X-ray		Erythromycin
Viral titres, PCR	Analyse if unexplained				
Urine for toxicology screen	Analyse if unexplained		Blood film	Poisoning	Antidote
Blood lead	Analyse if unexplained		Wrist X-ray for lead lines		Chelation
CT scan without contrast		Bleed	Skull X-ray/skeletal survey/clotting screen	NAI	Neurosurgical referral
		• Subdural			Child protection
		• extradural			
		• intracerebral			
		Space-occupying lesion		Tumour	Neurosurgical referral
		Hydrocephalus	CSF examination	Consider tuberculous meningitis, space-occupying lesion	Neurosurgical referral
		• obstructive			
		• communicating			

Table 12.2 (continued)

Investigation	Indication	Possible abnormality	Further investigation if abnormal	Possible diagnoses	Action
		Abscess	Culture aspirate Contrast CT/MRI		Anaerobic cover
		Swelling Focal low density		Cerebral abscess, H. simplex, stroke, ADEM	Mannitol 0.25 g/kg
		Abnormal basal ganglia	Plasma/CSF lactate, blood gas	Leigh's syndrome, hypoxic–ischaemic, striatal necrosis	
Lumbar puncture • Pressure measurement • Microscopy • Bacterial culture • Glucose • Protein • PCR for viruses, TB	If no clinical or radiological evidence of raised ICP (delay and treat if doubt)	High High WCC High RBC		Meningitis/encephalitis Haemorrhage/encephalitis	
Lactate	Abnormal breathing/ eye movements, basal ganglia lucencies		Muscle biopsy	Leigh's syndrome	
EEG	All	Epileptiform discharges Asymmetrical foci of spikes on slow background		Status epilepticus H. simplex encephalitis	IV benzodiazepines, phenytoin, thiopentone IV acyclovir

Stroke

Approximately 50% of children presenting have no previously diagnosed underlying condition. Fifteen percent of children presenting with acute focal neurological signs suggestive of arterial ischaemic stroke have alternative aetiologies, e.g. cerebral venous sinus thrombosis, hemiplegic migraine, metabolic disease, e.g. mitochondrial cytopathy or ornithine carbamoyl transferase deficiency. Risk factors are listed in the box.

RISK FACTORS FOR ISCHAEMIC STROKE IN CHILDHOOD

- Infection (chickenpox, tonsillitis)
- Head or neck trauma (arterial dissection)
- Hyperhomocystinaemia
- Prothrombotic disorders, e.g. Factor V Leiden, antiphospholipid syndrome (more evidence for role in venous thrombosis)
- Hyperlipidaemia (cholesterol or lipoprotein (a))
- Hypoxaemia and reactive polycythaemia in sickle cell disease and cyanotic congenital heart disease
- Immunodeficiency, e.g. HIV

Investigations

1. *Neuroimaging.* Haemorrhage must be excluded by CT or MRI. MRI detects smaller ischaemic lesions in symptomatic and asymptomatic high-risk patients and is particularly useful for separating ischaemic stroke from alternative pathologies. MR angiography (MRA) allows diagnosis of some of the possible underlying cerebrovascular abnormalities, e.g. demonstrating turbulence or occlusion in the distal internal carotid or proximal middle cerebral arteries. MR venography may demonstrate occlusion of the large venous sinuses, e.g. in sagittal sinus thrombosis. Fat-saturated MRI of the neck may demonstrate dissection of the carotid artery. Conventional arteriography may be required to diagnose arteriovenous malformations or aneurysms in patients with haemorrhage, or to delineate the cause of stroke in ischaemic cases if MRA is normal or not diagnostic, e.g. in arterial dissection or vasculitis. Patients with an infarct in the territory of the vertebrobasilar circulation usually require formal arteriography and should have an X-ray of the cervical spine in flexion and extension to look for subluxation and developmental anomalies such as an arcuate ligament or so odontoideum.
2. *ECG and echocardiography,* although relatively few children with stroke have previously unrecognised cardiac abnormalities.
3. *Screening for underlying prothrombotic and metabolic disorders* which might predispose to recurrent stroke: full blood count and ESR; activated protein C resistance; DNA testing for factor V Leiden, thermolabile methylene tetrahydrofolate reductase and prothrombin 20210; plasma total homocystine; anticardiolipin antibodies and lupus anticoagulant; cholesterol; immunodeficiency,

nocturnal hypoxaemia. There is no evidence for an association between deficiencies of protein C, protein S, antithrombin III, heparin cofactor II or plasminogen and arterial stroke in childhood, but the tests may be worth doing in patients with cerebral venous sinus thrombosis.

4. Patients with acute focal signs but without an infarct in a typical vascular distribution should have metabolic investigations, e.g. ammonia (to exclude ornithine carbamoyl transferase deficiency), plasma and CSF lactate (to exclude mitochondrial encephalopathy with lactic acidosis (MELAS).

Acute ataxia

Although ataxia implies a cerebellar lesion, it may be very difficult to distinguish cerebellar ataxia from a peripheral neuropathy, action myoclonus or dystonia in a young child. Horizontal nystagmus and past pointing suggest involvement of the cerebellum whereas areflexia indicates a peripheral neuropathy. Causes and investigations in ataxia are given in the information boxes.

CAUSES OF ACUTE ATAXIA

Posterior fossa space-occupying lesion (may be accompanied by head tilt)
- Tumour, e.g. medulloblastoma
- Extradural or subdural haematoma
- Infarct

Acute cerebellitis, e.g. mycoplasma

Post-infectious cerebellitis, e.g. chickenpox

Guillain–Barré syndrome (see under acute weakness)

Non-convulsive status epilepticus

Drugs and toxins — phenytoin, carbamazepine, lead

INVESTIGATIONS IN ATAXIA

CT scan/MRI

Toxicology screen

Blood film (acanthocytes)

α-fetoprotein

Plasma lactate

Urine amino acids

EEG (to exclude non-convulsive status epilepticus)

Nerve conduction to exclude Guillain-Barré syndrome if reflexes reduced

Acute generalised weakness

Causes and investigations are presented in the information boxes.

CAUSES OF ACUTE GENERALISED WEAKNESS

1. Guillain–Barré syndrome

2. Dermatomyositis

3. Viral myositis

4. Myasthenia gravis

5. Cervical cord lesion, e.g. acute disseminated encephalomyelitis, trauma, tumour

6. Botulism — associated with fixed, dilated pupils

7. Other toxins, e.g. lead, vincristine

8. Poliomyelitis — usually asymmetrical weakness

9. Acute presentation of chronic weakness, e.g. hereditary sensorimotor neuropathy

---

INVESTIGATIONS IN ACUTE GENERALISED WEAKNESS

1. Creatine kinase (CK) to diagnose dermatomyositis, viral myositis

2. Nerve conduction to diagnose Guillain–Barré
   — May be normal in initial phase of illness
   — CSF examination is usually unnecessary as the protein is not raised until a few days after onset in Guillain–Barré
   — Other conditions, e.g. botulism, may have characteristic features

3. Exclusion of myasthenia

4. MRI cervical spine if suspicion of cord lesion, e.g. if bladder involvement

---

NON-ACUTE PROBLEMS

Floppy neonate and infant

Clinical examination of mother and baby often yields diagnostic clues which may guide logical investigation. In many cases, relatively painful or invasive investigations, such as EMG/nerve conduction and muscle biopsy, may be avoided if clinical suspicion of a particular condition is high and the results of the initial blood, urine and imaging tests are pending. Unless the child is deteriorating rapidly or there is a need to know the genetic implications urgently there is often a case for delaying muscle biopsy, even if aetiology is obscure, at least until the second half of the first year when the clinical picture may be clearer and it may be easier to

CAUSES OF FLOPPY NEONATE/INFANT

- Dystrophia myotonica
- Congenital muscular dystrophy
- Myopathies, e.g.
  - Pompe's disease (Glycogen storage disease type II)
  - Nemaline myopathy
  - Myotubular myopathy
- Spinal muscular atrophy type I (Werdnig–Hoffman)
  - Autosomal recessive
  - Anterior horn disease
  - Survival motor neurone gene on chromosome 5q13
- Congenital and neonatal myasthenia gravis
- Peripheral neuropathies
- Spinal cord disease
  - Trauma
  - Congenital malformation
- Central
  - Chromosomal, e.g.
    - Down's
    - Prader–Willi
      - Genomic imprinting with interstitial deletion in paternal 15q1.1–1.3
- Metabolic
  - Peroxisomal
    - Zellweger
    - Neonatal adrenoleukodystrophy
- Structural brain malformation
- Cerebral haemorrhage
- Sepsis

CLINICAL QUESTIONS IN FLOPPY NEONATE/INFANT

1. History — maternal illness, e.g. myasthenia, other family history, pregnancy and birth history, fetal movements
2. Examination of infant — typical facial appearance, posture, degree of truncal, limb and facial weakness, reflexes, tongue fasciculation
3. Examination of parents, especially mother —
   Dystrophia myotonica — ability to bury eyelashes, myotonia exacerbated by cold
   Myasthenia — ptosis and weakness

obtain a diagnostic specimen. The information boxes present causes, clinical questions to be raised, and investigations.

Detailed investigations in floppy baby and acute and chronic weakness appear in Table 12.3.

INVESTIGATIONS IN FLOPPY NEONATE/INFANT

1. Molecular genetic studies for characteristic condition, e.g. Prader–Willi, dystrophia myotonica
2. Creatine kinase
3. Echocardiography, e.g. for Pompe's
4. X-ray knee to look for patellar calcification/stippling in peroxisomal disorders
5. Appropriate biochemistry for metabolic condition, e.g. very long chain fatty acids for peroxisomal disorders or plasma/CSF lactate for mitochondrial disease
6. Electromyography and nerve conduction studies
   Single fibre for myasthenia gravis
7. Neuroimaging of brain to exclude structural brain abnormality, either isolated or in association with muscle disease, e.g. white matter abnormality in Fukuyama congenital muscular dystrophy
8. Muscle biopsy may be essential if diagnosis cannot be secured by an alternative method

Chronic and progressive weakness in the older child

Causes are set out in the information box.

CAUSES OF CHRONIC AND PROGRESSIVE WEAKNESS IN OLDER CHILD

Muscle disease
Dystrophies
   Duchenne and Becker forms
   — X-linked recessive
   — Dystrophin gene on X chromosome
   — Majority of boys with dystrophy have abnormality dystrophin
   — Affected girls — manifesting carriers
   Limb girdle
      Abnormalities of sarcoglycans ($\alpha,\beta,\gamma,\delta$)
            calpain 3
   Fascioscapulohumeral
   Emery–Dreifuss
   Dystrophia myotonica
   Myopathies, e.g. Nemaline
Myasthenia gravis
Anterior horn cell disease
   Kugelberg–Welander form of spinal muscular atrophy

Neuropathies
Hereditary motor and sensory neuropathy type I (HMSN I) (Charcot–Marie–Tooth)
HMSN II

Table 12.3 Investigation of floppy baby (and acute and chronic weakness)

Investigation	Findings	Clinical clues	Possible diagnosis	Confirmatory investigation
DNA studies	• Deletion on chromosome 15 • Triplet repeat	• Poor suck and swallow • Fish-shaped mouth, mum cannot bury eyelashes or release handshake	Prader-Willi syndrome Myotonic dystrophy	
Karyotype	Chromosomal anomaly	Dysmorphic features	e.g. Down's syndrome	
CPK	High		Congenital muscular dystrophy	Muscle biopsy
TSH	High	Tongue protrusion	Congenital hypothyroidism	
Calcium, alkaline phosphatase	Low calcium, high alk.phos.		Rickets	
Urine reducing substances	Present	Cataracts	Galactosaemia	
Urine organic acids	Characteristic patterns		Methylmalonic acidaemia	
Urinary mucopolysaccharides	Characteristic patterns	Hepatosplenomegaly, coarse features		
Plasma biotinidase	Low	Alopecia, rash, seizures	Biotinidase deficiency	
Plasma very long chain fatty acids	High	High forehead, poor vision	Peroxisomal disorder	Plasmalogens Renal ultrasound, patellar X-ray
CSF lactate	High	Acidosis, abnormal eye movements	Mitochondrial disorder	Muscle biopsy
CT scan/MRI	Destructive lesion Malformation • Cerebellar hypoplasia • Vermis aplasia	Eye and respiratory abnormality	Joubert's syndrome	

Table 12.3 (continued)

Investigation	Findings	Clinical clues	Possible diagnosis	Confirmatory investigation
Nerve conduction/EMG	Large amplitude voluntary motor unit potentials	Normal face, bell-shaped chest	Spinal muscular atrophy	SMN deletion
	'Dive-bomber' discharges	Fish-shaped mouth	Myotonic dystrophy	DNA studies for triplet repeats
	Brief, small amplitude polyphasic potentials		Myopathy	
	Slow velocities, prolonged distal latencies		Peripheral neuropathy	
		Irritability, stiffness	Hypomyelinating neuropathy	Sural nerve biopsy — demyelination
EMG with repetitive nerve stimulation	Decremental response	Ptosis, peripheral contractures	Myasthenia	
		Fixed dilated pupils	Botulism	*Clostridium botulinum* in stool
Tensilon test			Myasthenia gravis	Neostigmine trial, single fibre

The information boxes give clinical questions and investigation in chronic and progressive weakness.

CLINICAL QUESTIONS IN CHRONIC AND PROGRESSIVE WEAKNESS.

1. History of weakness, family history, associated features, e.g. learning difficulties, cardiac manifestations
2. Examination — Gower's manoeuvre to demonstrate proximal weakness, distribution of weakness, facial involvement including ptosis, presence or absence of muscular hypertrophy, additional features including scoliosis, cardiac involvement, learning difficulties
3. Examination of family members, e.g. both parents in HMSN I

INVESTIGATION IN CHRONIC AND PROGRESSIVE WEAKNESS

1. Creatine kinase
2. Edrophonium test and acetylcholine receptor antibodies if myasthenia likely
3. Molecular genetic studies:
   Duchenne — dystrophin deletion on X chromosome
   Dystrophia myotonica — CTG expansion on chromosome 19
   HMSN I — duplication of 1.5-Mb region of chromosome
   17 including the peripheral myelin protein 22 gene
4. Electromyography and nerve conduction. May need to include single fibre studies if initial studies are not diagnostic and myasthenia is likely
5. ECG and echocardiogram
6. Muscle biopsy to include appropriate stains, e.g. for dystrophin

---

Macrocephaly

The majority of children with large heads at birth do not require further investigation, although since ultrasound is non-invasive, there should be a low threshold for investigating if there is any doubt over clinical symptoms and signs. An increase in head size during the first year of life should always be investigated with ultrasound, and if this is normal with CT scan, in view of the high probabil-

---

CAUSES OF MACROCEPHALY

Familial
Hydrocephalus
Subdural haemorrhage or effusion
Metabolic-glutaric aciduria type I
Degenerative:
   Alexander's disease
   Canavan's disease (N-acetylaspartic aciduria)

ity of subdural effusions secondary to non-accidental shaking injury. Progressive increase in head size is rare in older children, but hydrocephalus should be excluded in such cases. A large head may suggest the diagnosis of Canavan's or Alexander's leucodystrophy in a child with dementia.

Causes and clinical approach in macrocephaly appear in the information boxes.

CLINICAL APPROACH IN MACROCEPHALY

Measure head and plot serially on centile chart
Measure parents' head circumferences and plot them

Ultrasound if:
- head greater than 3 standard deviations
- head circumference increasing across the centiles
- vomiting
- poor visual attention
- any other uncertainty

CT scan:
- to exclude subdural effusions, e.g. if sudden increase in head circumference in an older infant
- to plan surgical management of hydrocephalus

MR scan:
- if suspect associated metabolic disorder

Toxoplasma titre in idiopathic hydrocephalus
Urine for glutaric acid (large head ± frontal atrophy ± progressive dystonia after intercurrent illnesses)
N-acetyl aspartate (urine) if leucodystrophy demonstrated on MR scan, for diagnosis or exclusion of Canavan's disease

---

Microcephaly

The information box gives the clinical approach in microcephaly.

Headache

The majority of children with headache have either a mild intercurrent illness or migraine and do not need neuroimaging, provided that a thorough clinical history and examination are performed on presentation. If the headaches persist after an interval of a few weeks or if there is any doubt, a CT scan should be carried out. The information box lists the clinical approach.

Epilepsy

(i) Neonatal convulsions

The common causes of neonatal convulsions include hypoxic–ischaemic encephalopathy, particularly if the convulsions start between 12 and 48 hours, hypoglycaemia, hypocalcaemia, and structural malformations of the brain. The

---

CLINICAL APPROACH IN MICROCEPHALY

Measure head and plot on centile chart
Review birth history including CTG traces

a) *Small head size at birth*
- Chromosomes
- TORCH screen in young infants
- Urine for Cytomegalovirus culture
- Maternal phenylalanine
- Ultrasound head to exclude gross destruction or malformation
- CT scan to exclude calcification and structural malformations of the brain (delay if possible)
- MRI scan if CT scan not diagnostic and genetic issue important
- Genetic opinion for syndrome diagnosis and for counselling family about high recurrence risk if investigations normal

b) *Normal head size at birth, progressive decrease*
- Chromosomes including high resolution studies of chromosome 15 (Angelman's)
- Urine amino acids (phenylketonuria)
- Plasma biotinidase (biotinidiase deficiency)
- CT/MRI scan
- Human immunodeficiency virus (HIV) testing after counselling
- Electroretinogram (infantile Batten's)
- In girls, developmental opinion and perhaps genetic testing ?Rett syndrome
- Genetic opinion about syndrome diagnosis

---

labour and delivery notes, including CTG traces, should be carefully reviewed. Although IV pyridoxine may abolish seizures in patients with pyridoxine dependency, this should be done with extreme caution and with full cardiorespiratory monitoring. It is worth giving a trial of oral pyridoxine for at least 3–5 days even if the response to IV pyridoxine is not dramatic. In cryptogenic cases it may also be worth giving biotin until the results of the biotinidase assay are available. The other metabolic causes of neonatal convulsions are not treatable at the present time. Although investigation is less urgent, conditions such as non-ketotic hyperglycinaemia and peroxisomal disorders should be excluded in cryptogenic cases, since the parents need counselling about the extremely poor prognosis and about the risks for future pregnancies. If the cause remains obscure, the prognosis may depend on whether the seizures remain intractable. These children should be followed up carefully so that developmental progress can be reviewed and a more accurate prognosis given, and so that the diagnosis can be re-considered. It is, for example, often worth delaying the MRI scan or repeating it after the first year of life, when malformations may be more obvious (with increasing myelination and improved technology).

Table 12.4 sets out investigation of neonatal convulsions.

CLINICAL APPROACH IN HEADACHE

- Careful history looking for features suggestive of raised ICP, e.g. nocturnal or early morning headache, nausea or vomiting
- Careful examination including blood pressure, visual fields, visual acuity and fundi
- CT scan if history suggestive of raised ICP or any abnormal neurological signs, or occasionally to reassure family
- Lumbar puncture after CT scan (sometimes during same sedation)
  - to exclude meningitis
  - to measure pressure if symptoms and signs suggestive of raised ICP but CT scan normal (pseudotumour cerebri, also known as benign intra-cranial hypertension)
- MR including angiogram and/or venogram to exclude arteriovenous mal-formation (e.g. migrainous headaches) or venous thrombosis (in child at risk e.g. with nephrotic syndrome)
- If imaging not performed, review child in three months for full neurological examination, including visual fields, visual acuity and fundi
- If headaches considered to be psychogenic clinically, try to avoid multiple investigations which may reinforce the child's concerns, but continue to follow in parallel with psychological services and re-examine neurological system periodically

---

(ii) Infantile spasms

The common causes of infantile spasms are tuberous sclerosis, porencephaly, perina-tal asphyxia, and structural malformations of the brain. In cryptogenic infantile spasms an MRI scan is worthwhile, and if this is normal then metabolic tests may be worth performing, although the diagnostic yield if there is no other clue is very poor.

Tests include the following:

- Careful examination of the skin with a Wood's light
- EEG
- Routine biochemistry
- Trial of pyridoxine
- Biotinidase
- MRI scan
- Ammonia
- Urine amino acids and organic acids.

(iii) Febrile convulsions

- No investigations if generalised
- EEG and CT scan if focal.

Table 12.4 Investigation of neonatal convulsions (and intractable epilepsy in older child)

	Investigation	Clinical Clues	Further investigations	Possible diagnoses	Implications
Blood	Glucose	Low birth weight, infant of diabetic mother (IDM)	If not LBW or IDM, MRI scan head	LBW, IDM, hyperinsulinism, septo-optic dysplasia/ hypopituitarism	Glucose infusion
	Sodium				
	Calcium				Supplement
	Magnesium				Supplement
CSF	Microscopy, cells, culture	Prolonged rupture membranes		Infection, haemorrhage	
	Viral titres			Infection	
	Lactate	Metabolic acidosis		Mitochondrial disease	
	Glycine	Prenatal onset of seizures	Plasma glycine for CSF: plasma glycine ratio (normal <0.025)	Non-ketotic hyperglycinaemia	Early death Prenatal diagnosis
EEG	Routine EEG	EEG — burst suppression pattern	Birth asphyxia		
	Pyridoxine 100 mg IV during EEG	Status epilepticus, sibling death in status		Pyridoxine dependency	Oral pyridoxine 100 mg/day
Ultrasound		Prematurity		Intraventricular and periventricular haemorrhage	
		Large head		Hydrocephalus	
Hair	Microscopy — Pili torti	Boy, sparse hair, cherubic face	Low serum copper	Menkes	X-linked
MRI scan				Malformation, e.g. lissencephaly, agenesis corpus callosum Tumour (e.g. primitive neuroectodermal)	
		Birth trauma		Subarachnoid and subdural haemorrhage	

Table 12.4 (continued)

	Investigation	Clinical Clues	Further investigations	Possible diagnoses	Implications
Urine	Amino acids Organic acids Sulfite	Hyperammonaemia Hypoglycaemia		Amino aciduria Organic acidaemia Sulfite oxidase deficiency — Molybdenum co-factor deficiency	
Blood:	Very long chain fatty acids, bile acids	Hypotonia, poor vision, high forehead	Plasmalogens, patellar X-ray, renal ultrasound, fibroblast studies	Peroxisomal disorder	
second-line tests	Amino acids Lactate Ammonia			Amino aciduria Mitochondrial disease	
	Urate		Low plasma urate and urinary urate	Molybdenum co-factor deficiency	
	Biotinidase	Alopecia, dry skin, stridor		Biotinidase deficiency	Oral biotin 10 mg/day Prenatal diagnosis

(iv) Generalised tonic–clonic seizures

- EEG only
- Neuroimaging rarely indicated.

(v) Absence seizures

- EEG with hyperventilation and photic stimulation
- Consider sleep-deprived or 24-hour EEG in developmentally delayed children with possible absences.

(vi) Partial seizures

- History (differentiation of benign from symptomatic partial epilepsies, localisation, lateralisation, family history)
- Examination (neurocutaneous stigmata, and any evidence of hemiparesis or facial weakness
- EEG (but interictal EEG commonly normal in children with symptomatic partial seizures)
- Sleep-deprived EEG/sleep EEG
- Ictal EEG (cassette or telemetry)
- CT scan if symptomatic partial epilepsy but unnecessary if history is typical of benign Rolandic or benign occipital seizures (yield is much higher with MRI)
- MRI if intractable partial epilepsy to include:
  - scans through the hippocampi in the coronal plane looking for evidence of hippocampal sclerosis or atrophy
  - T2 maps for the diagnosis of hippocampal sclerosis
  - Careful analysis of cortical architecture, e.g. with 3D MP-range datasets, particularly in children with a history compatible with epilepsy arising in the extratemporal regions.

(vii) Epilepsies with multiple seizure types (including Lennox–Gastaut syndrome, myoclonic astatic epilepsy, epilepsy with myoclonic absences, etc.)

- EEG for attempted syndrome diagnosis; sleep EEG often helpful
- Opthalmological opinion to exclude associated retinopathy, Cherry red spot
- ERG and blood film for vacuolated lymphocytes if Batten's disease is a possibility
- Chromosomes to exclude ring chromosome 14 or 20 (or Angelman's if typical clinical or EEG features)
- Urine sialic acid to look for sialuria
- MRI scan with a careful look at the cortical architecture, e.g. with 3D datasets
- Blood and CSF lactate to exclude mitochondrial disease
- Mitochondrial mutations
- Consider DNA analysis for Baltic myoclonus (Unverricht–Lundborg disease)
- Consider white cell enzymes for Juvenile Gaucher's if hepatosplenomegaly
- Consider
  - muscle biopsy to look for mitochondrial disease
  - liver biopsy to provide evidence for Alper's disease

— skin biopsy to look for amyloids in the sweat glands in Lafora body disease or spheroids in the skin in juvenile neuroaxonal dystrophy.

Cerebral palsy

Investigation of underlying aetiology should be considered, particularly if there are no obvious perinatal risk factors and/or if there is a genetic issue. Although CT scanning may yield important information about aetiology, MRI is an excellent method of distinguishing between congenital malformations and acquired ischaemia. Birth asphyxia may underlie spastic and dystonic quadriparesis, and prematurity is a major risk factor for diplegia, but any of these patterns of cerebral palsy can arise from other causes and there are a number of important inherited conditions causing ataxic cerebral palsy. Hypotonia is often prominent in infancy in those who later develop dystonic, dyskinetic and ataxic forms of cerebral palsy; whether or not to investigate those with apparently typical cerebral palsy must depend on the likelihood that an important condition might be missed clinically. The threshold for investigating dystonic, dyskinetic and ataxic forms should be much lower. Investigations worth doing despite low yield include therapuetic trial of L-DOPA in the dystonic/diplegic group and α-fetoprotein in the ataxic group. MRI of the cervical spine may be indicated if a child with a dystonia or dystonic quadriparesis deteriorates, as cervical trauma has been described in association with os odontoideum and degenerative disease of the cervical spine. MRI of the head with appropriate vascular imaging (see under Stroke) may also be appropriate in this situation, as vertebrobasilar dissection is a possibility. Prothrombotic abnormalities, e.g. Factor V Leiden, may be risk factors for congenital hemiparesis (see under Acute stroke).

Table 12.5 presents investigations in idiopathic or atypical cerebral palsy.

Movement disorders in a previously well child

The diagnosis of an extrapyramidal disorder is often made simply by observing the posture of the child at rest. Extrapyramidal disorders improve during sleep and examination under anaesthesia may be required to assess whether or not a deformity is fixed. The slow writhing movements of athetosis are a form of dystonia and may be distinguished from the rapid movements of chorea, although the two may occur together. There may be more difficulty in distinguishing some of the other movement disorders.

Table 12.6 presents treatable causes of extrapyramidal movement disorders.

Some other causes of extrapyramidal movement disorders, and investigations, are set out in the boxes.

Progressive movement disorders

Table 12.7 outlines the investigation of acquired or progressive movement disorders.

In Table 12.8, treatable causes of intermittent or progressive ataxia are listed.

The information boxes outline other causes of progressive ataxia, and relevant investigations.

Table 12.5 Investigations to consider in idiopathic or atypical cerebral palsy

Pattern of CP	Investigation	Clinical clues	Possible cause	Confirmatory test	Implications
Spastic quadriparesis	Chromosomes CT or MRI	May be dysmorphic	Chromosome abnormality Structural malformation		
Dystonic/dyskinetic quadriparesis	Chromosomes Trial of L-DOPA	May be dysmorphic Classically fluctuates throughout day	Chromosome abnormality Segawa syndrome	CSF homovanillic acid, DNA testing	Rx L-DOPA
	PH studies Barium swallow	Dystonia in infancy	Reflux oesophagitis		Rx medical/surgical
	α-fetoprotein	Deterioration in static CP ± ataxia ± infections	Ataxia telangiectasia	Chromosome fragility	Autosomal recessive Rx infection/neoplasia
	Plasma/urine uric acid	Self mutilation	Lesch–Nyhan syndrome	Low hypoxanthine guanine phosphoryl transferase	X-linked recessive, antenatal diagnosis
	Urine, glutaric acid (repeat if strong clinical suspicion)	Large head, presents during intercurrent illness	Glutaric aciduria	Low glutaryl coA dehydrogenase (fibroblasts)	Autosomal recessive, antenatal diagnosis Rx diet/drugs
	MRI — hypomyelination Urine sulfite, plasma urate	Rotatory nystagmus	Pallizaeus — Merzbacher Molybdenum cofactor deficiency	DNA testing Enzyme testing on cultured fibroblasts	X-linked recessive Autosomal recessive
Diplegia	MRI—hypomyelination	Rotatory nystagmus	Pelizaeus–Merzbacher	DNA testing	X-linked recessive, antenatal diagnosis possible
	Caeruloplasmin/urinary copper	Older child; late diagnosis of CP	Wilson's disease		Rx Penicillamine
	Chromosomes		Chromosome abnormality		Structural malformation
	Trial of L-DOPA	Classically, diurnal variation but not necessarily No hand involvement	Segawa syndrome	CSF homovanillic acid	

Table 12.5 (continued)

Pattern of CP	Investigation	Clinical clues	Possible cause	Confirmatory test	Implications
	MRI spine	Cutaneous stigmata, bladder involvement	Spinal lesion		
	CT or MRI		Leukodystrophy		
	Skull X-ray		Basilar impression		
	Urinary amino acids		Arginase deficiency		
Ataxia	Chromosomes	Oculomotor apraxia ± dystonia ± infection ± telangiectasia	Chromosome abnormality	Chromosome fragility	Avoid CT scan (risk of neoplasia), Auto recessive
	α-fetoprotein		Ataxia telangiectasia	Immunoglobulins (IgA)	
	Full blood count and film — acanthocytes	Diarrhoea, poor vision	Abetalipoproteinaemia	Full blood count ERG, low total lipids, cholesterol, β-lipoprotein	Rx Vitamin E Autosomal recessive
	EEG	Often previous epilepsy	Minor status		Rx Anticonvulsant
	MRI		Hydrocephalus Tumour Malformation — Cerebellar hypoplasia — Vernis hypoplasia Basilar impression Narrow foramen magnum Pelizaeus-Merzbacher hypomyelination		
	Urine amino acids		Maple syrup urine Hartnup disease		
	Urine succinylacetone		Tyrosinaemia	Fumarylacetoacetate WBC	Rx liver transplant
	Urine metachromatic granules		Metachromatic leukodystrophy	Arylsulphatase A (WBC)	Autosomal recessive

Table 12.5 *(continued)*

Pattern of CP	Investigation	Clinical clues	Possible cause	Confirmatory test	Implications
	Urine sialic acid		Salla disease		Autosomal recessive
	Nerve conduction	Depressed or absent reflexes Pes cavus	Peripheral neuropathy — HMSN I, II	Distinguish by DNA testing and nerve conduction	May be familial
		± pyramidal signs	Spinocerebellar degeneration — Friedreich's	ECG, ECHO	
			— Tyrosinaemia	Abnormal nerve conduction	
				Famarylacetoacetate (WBC)	
			— Metachromatic leukodystrophy	Arylsulphatase A (WBC)	
	White cell enzymes — Hexosaminidase A and B — β galantosidase		Juvenile Sandhoff disease Juvenile GM1 or GM2		

Table 12.6   **Treatable causes of extrapyramidal movement disorders**

Condition	Diagnostic test	Treatment
Wilson's disease	Plasma copper, caeruloplasmin	Penicillamine
Sydenham's chorea	Antistreptococcal titre	Penicillin
Segawa syndrome	Trial of L-DOPA Molecular genetics in 70%	L-DOPA
Systemic lupus erythematosus	Antinuclear antibodies, lupus anticoagulant	Immunosuppression
Moyamoya (see Stroke)	MR angiography	Revascularisation
Arteriovenous malformation	Contrast CT, MRI Conventional arteriography	Surgery, embolisation Radiotherapy
Tumour	Neuroimaging	Radiotherapy
Glutaric aciduria type I	Urinary organic acids	Protein restriction Carnitine
Homocystinuria	Plasma total homocysteine, methionine	Pyridoxine Methionine restriction Betaine
Infections	Mycoplasma, CMV, HIV	Antimicrobials
Drugs and toxins	Urine and blood screening	Withdrawal
Hysteria	Exclusion of alternatives, observation	Rehabilitation
Sandifer syndrome (reflux)	pH studies, barium swallow	Omeprazole, Nissen fundoplication

SOME OTHER CAUSES OF EXTRAPYRAMIDAL MOVEMENT DISORDERS

Hypoxic–ischaemic damage (may be delayed or worsen after initial stability)

Post cardiopulmonary bypass

Trauma (may be delayed)

Ataxia telangiectasia

GM1 and GM2 gangliosidoses

Mitochondrial disease, e.g. Leigh's syndrome

Hallervordan–Spatz disease

Huntington's chorea

INVESTIGATIONS IN EXTRAPYRAMIDAL MOVEMENT DISORDERS

1. Clinical: accurate description of movement disorder and any associated behavioural manifestation (video and further opinions may be helpful); slit lamp examination by ophthalmologist for Kayser–Fleischer rings
2. Neuroimaging (may include MRA to exclude moyamoya)
3. Plasma copper and caeruloplasmin, ASOT, plasma amino acids, urine organic acids, plasma lactate, alpha fetoprotein
4. May need CSF lactate, white cell enzymes, pH studies and barium swallow, DNA testing for Huntington's chorea or ataxia telangiectasia if clinically indicated

Table 12.7 **Investigation of acquired or progressive movement disorders**

	Possible diagnosis	Diagnostic investigation
Dystonia	Wilson's disease	Plasma caeruloplasmin Slit lamp examination for Kayser–Fleischer rings 24-hr urine for copper
	Segawa syndrome	Trial of L-DOPA
	Lesch–Nyhan syndrome	Uric acid
	Glutaric aciduria type I	Urine organic acids
	Mitochondrial cytopathy	Plasma/CSF lactate
Chorea	Sydenham's	ASO titre
	Juvenile Huntington's disease	MRI brain (DNA studies for triplet repeat — requires careful genetic counselling)
	Ataxia-telangiectasia Benign non-progressive familial chorea	AFP, DNA fragility studies
Myoclonus	Myoclonic epilepsy	EEG
	Mitochondrial disease	Plasma/CSF lactate
	Batten's disease	VER/ERG, enzyme/DNA studies
	Lafora body disease	Sweat gland biopsy
	Spinal tumour	Spinal MRI

Table 12.8 Treatable causes of intermittent or progressive ataxia		
Cause	**Diagnosis**	**Treatment**
Posterior fossa tumour	Neuroimaging	Surgery, radiotherapy, chemotherapy
Drugs and toxins	Urine drug screen	Stop drugs
Hartnup disease	Urine amino acids	Nicotinamide
Maple syrup urine disease	Urine amino acids	Thiamine
Biotinidase deficiency	Urine organic acids Plasma biotinidase	Biotin
Hereditary paroxysmal cerebellar ataxia	Gene on 19q	Acetazolamide
Refsum disease	Plasma phytanic acid	Dietary
Pyruvate dehydrogenase complex deficiency	Plasma/CSF lactate Enzyme assay Gene on Xp22	Thiamine may help
Primary Vitamin E deficiency		Vitamin E (+A+K)
Secondary Vitamin E deficiency		
— Abetalipoproteinaemia	Acanthocytosis	
— Hypobetalipoproteinaemia	Plasma triglycerides Plasma lipoproteins	
— Alpha-tocopherol transfer protein	DNA testing	

OTHER CAUSES OF PROGRESSIVE ATAXIA

Hereditary sensory and motor neuropathy

Ataxia telangiectasia (AT)

Ataxia-oculomotor apraxia (also abnormality of AT gene)

Friedreich's ataxia (FA-abnormality of Frataxin gene)

Early onset ataxia with preserved deep tendon reflexes (also abnormality of Frataxin gene)

Metachromatic leukodystrophy, other leukodystrophies

GM1 and GM2 gangliosidoses

INVESTIGATIONS IN PROGRESSIVE ATAXIA

1. Neuroimaging
   - should be urgent if there is reduced visual acuity (secondary to raised intracranial pressure), vomiting or headache
   - should be avoided if the patient is areflexic and clinically has a peripheral neuropathy or telangiectasia

2. Nerve conduction to diagnose peripheral neuropathy and to distinguish hereditary motor and sensory neuropathies from Friedreich's ataxia (FA)

3. Alpha-fetoprotein and immunoglobulins to screen for Ataxia telangiectasia (AT)

4. White blood cell chromosome fragility (AT), gene probes for e.g. AT, FA; urine amino and organic acids, plasma amino acids; plasma and CSF lactate, biotinidase; phytanic acid; triglycerides and lipoproteins; white cell enzymes

---

Learning difficulties

The majority of children with learning difficulties make steady progress through their developmental milestones but at a slower speed than normal. Development slowing, arrest or regression is more likely to be caused by a treatable condition, e.g. epilepsy or hydrocephalus, than by a degenerative disease, although it is important to take a careful history and to perform a full physical examination to exclude the latter. A detailed developmental assessment should be undertaken to determine the cognitive profile, as the causes of specific learning difficulties, e.g. in language, may be different from those causing global delay. In some cases the cognitive profile may be specific for the underlying diagnosis, e.g. relatively well-preserved verbal ability in children with Williams syndrome. Parents may find the associated behavioural difficulties, e.g. hyperactivity or behaviour within the autistic spectrum, more difficult to deal with than the learning difficulties. Some children with learning difficulties have dysmorphic features, which may be diag-

---

ESSENTIAL INVESTIGATIONS INTO LEARNING DIFFICULTIES

1. Chromosomes. If a diagnosis such as Angelman, Prader–Willi or fragile X syndrome is considered likely clinically, it is often appropriate to request more specific genetic investigation

2. Urine amino acids

3. Other metabolic investigations suggested by clinical features, e.g. mucopolysaccharides

4. EEG if epilepsy

5. Neuroimaging may be fruitful if there are additional clinical features, e.g. epilepsy, microcephaly, neurocutaneous stigmata

Table 12.9 Selective investigation of learning difficulties

Presentation	Possible cause	Investigation
Mental retardation	Chromosome abnormalities	Chromosomes
	Fragile X syndrome	Fragile X
	Structural malformation of the brain	CT/MRI scan
	Duchenne muscular dystrophy	CK
	Lesch–Nyhan syndrome	Uric acid
Language delay	Landan–Kleffner	EEG
	Kleinfelter's	Chromosomes
		Possible Fragile X
Language regression	Landan-Kleffner	EEG
	Tumour	CT/MRI scan
	Neurocutaneous syndrome	Careful examination of the skin
Autism	Neurocutaneous condition e.g. tuberous sclerosis	Careful skin examination including Wood's light
	Structural malformation	CT/MRI scan
Autistic regression	Neurocutaneous problem	Careful examination of the skin including Wood's light
	Associated epilepsy	Sleep deprived EEG
Cognitive deterioration	Undiagnosed epilepsy	EEG (including sleep)
	Wilson's disease	Plasma caeruloplasmin 24-hr urine for copper
	Mucopolysaccharidosis	Urine for mucopolysaccharides
	Leukodystrophy	CT or MRI if confirmed, urine for N-acetyl aspartate
	Subacute sclerosing panencephalitis	CSF for measles antibodies
	Creutzfeld–Jakob disease	CSF 14-3-3 protein, brain biopsy

nostic. Those with neurocutaneous stigmata may have other associated problems, such as epilepsy or the risk of malignancy. Epilepsy should be managed carefully, as frequent fits may reduce the child's potential for learning. Other children with learning difficulties may have cerebral palsy (see appropriate section), with implications for aetiology and therapy. Serial measurement of head circumference is important from the diagnostic point of view, as microcephaly recognised at birth is very likely to be recessively inherited (see appropriate section), while acquired microcephaly may be due to birth asphyxia or Rett syndrome.

Table 12.9 and the information box set out investigations in learning difficulties.

4 Practical details of tests

WOOD'S LIGHT

The patient is taken into a small room which can be darkened. The patient is undressed and Wood's light is switched on and is used to highlight any depigmented patches on the skin.

TENSILON TEST

The aim of this procedure is to make a diagnosis of myasthenia gravis by relieving specific symptoms or signs after administration of a short-acting anticholinesterase (edrophonium or Tensilon). It is useful to have identified a specific clinical symptom or sign to use as a marker and to video the procedure, as interpretation can be very difficult, especially in young infants. A negative Tensilon test does not exclude the diagnosis of myasthenia gravis and it is worth considering a trial of a longer-acting anticholinesterase if there is clinical or neurophysiological support for this diagnosis.

The procedure should be carried out in a clinical area with facilities for cardiorespiratory resuscitation readily available. The patient's heart rate should be monitored with a cardiac monitor as excess cholinergic drive may precipitate bradycardia. It is therefore wise to have a vial of atropine available close by. The edrophonium is initially administered in a test dose of 20 mcg/kg; if this is well tolerated by the patient, a further 80 mcg/kg is administered and the chosen clinical marker is closely observed. Ideally the procedure should be carried out with a placebo (normal saline) and with Tensilon and the observer should be unaware of which of these is being administered. It may be difficult to be certain about the result during the procedure and it is therefore worth reviewing the video carefully.

SKIN BIOPSY

After freezing the skin with local anaesthetic spray, a small piece of skin is picked up with a pair of tweezers and is cut off with a scalpel. The specimen is transported in saline, not formalin.

MUSCLE BIOPSY

Muscle biopsy remains one of the two most important investigations in establishing the diagnosis in paediatric neuromuscular conditions (along with specific mutation analysis). It may be performed as an open surgical procedure or via a needle technique under sedation (e.g. with IV Midazolam) and local anaesthetic.

The biopsy is usually taken from the quadriceps (left leg for a right handed person and vice versa) using a Bergström needle (size 5 is usual). The site of entry is midway between knee and groin, a centimetre or so lateral to the midline of the thigh. Local anaesthetic cream is applied and, when effective, removed. With the child under Midazolam sedation, the site is cleaned and further local anaesthetic is infiltrated around the incision site and in the deep tissues. When ready, a 1 cm incision is made in the thigh with the axis of the incision running superiorly-inferiorly. The incision is extended deeply to pierce the muscle sheath.

The Bergström needle is in three parts, an outer casing, an inner cutting cylinder and a solid rod. The outer casing and inner cutting cylinder are assembled together and the needle inserted through the incision with the bevel laterally (to avoid neurovascular structures). It is pushed through the muscle sheath into the muscle. The inner cutting cylinder is withdrawn 1–2 cm to allow muscle to bulge into the aperture, the process being encouraged by squeezing the thigh with the free hand. The inner cutting cylinder is then pushed down and usually reaches its lowest position with a satisfactory 'snip' when muscle is obtained. The cylinder may be rotated to disengage any strands of connective tissue. The needle is withdrawn and pressure applied to the incision and biopsy site.

The muscle sample (which may be only 0.2–0.3 cm in diameter) is transferred to a sterile pot containing gauze soaked in normal saline. It should then be transferred without delay to the pathology laboratory for freezing, sectioning and storage.

The incision is closed with steristrips and a dressing is applied over this. The incision site should be kept dry for 5 days.

Complications of the procedure include bleeding, and failure to obtain muscle in about 1–2% in experienced hands. As the procedure is 'blind', misdirection of the needle by untrained hands can lead to damage to more important structures.

FURTHER READING

Anderson, P.-B., Rando, T.A. (1999) Neuromuscular disorders of childhood. *Current Opinion in Pediatrics* 11: 497–503.

Collier, J.E. (1998) The recognition, diagnosis and management of neurodegenerative disorders. *Current Paediatrics* 7: 163–166.

Crouchman, M. (2000) Principles of management of cerebral palsy. *Current Paediatrics* 10: 167–171.

Index

Note: Page references in **bold** refer to Tables and Figures